AF574356

Neuropsychiatric Symptoms of Neurological Disease

Series editor
José M. Ferro
Serviço de Neurologia Stroke Unit
Hospital de Santa Maria
Lisboa
Portugal

Health care professionals are starting to realize the importance of managing neuropsychiatric complications in neurological disease, they disturb the process of care and are indicators of poor outcome, they also produce significant caregiver burden. This series will describe neuropsychiatric symptoms of major neurological diseases including new drugs (new anti-psychotics, mood stabilizers, antidepressants, cholinergic agents) that are available and other interventions for the management of these complications.This series will be targeted at neurologists, geriatricians, psychiatrists, internists, hospitalists, intensive care MDs, psychologists ad neuropsychologists, research and specialised nurses, clinical researchers and methodologists. Each volume will provide an up to date comprehensive review of the neuropsychiatry of major neurological diseases by active authorities in the field internationally. Emphasis will be placed on the diagnostic and management issues to serve as a tandard reference book for clinicians of several specialities.Volumes will feature:- Critical appraisal of the methodological aspects and limitations of current research including ongoing controversies in the field.- Focus on the pharmacological aspects of management to provide robust information on drug dosages, side effects and interaction.

More information about this series at http://www.springer.com/series/10501

Marco Mula
Editor

Neuropsychiatric Symptoms of Epilepsy

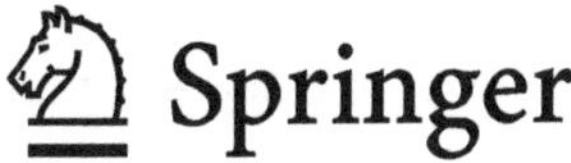

Editor
Marco Mula
Atkinson Morley Regional Neuroscience
Centre, Epilepsy Group
St George's University Hospitals
NHS Foundation Trust
London
UK

ISSN 2196-2898 ISSN 2196-2901 (electronic)
Neuropsychiatric Symptoms of Neurological Disease
ISBN 978-3-319-22158-8 ISBN 978-3-319-22159-5 (eBook)
DOI 10.1007/978-3-319-22159-5

Library of Congress Control Number: 2015953159

Springer Cham Heidelberg New York Dordrecht London

Printed on acid-free paper

Springer International Publishing AG Switzerland is part of Springer Science+Business Media (www.springer.com)

Preface

Epilepsy is a neurological condition that knows no geographic, social, or racial boundaries, occurring in men and women, affecting all ages, though more frequently affecting young people in the first two decades of life and people over the age of 60 years. It has been estimated that worldwide there are at least 50 million people who have epilepsy and more than 80 % of people with epilepsy live in developing countries where the condition remains largely untreated. These people could live normal lives if properly treated, but the majority of them do not receive any effective treatment. Most importantly, epilepsy is now recognized as a disorder of the brain characterized not only by an enduring predisposition to generate epileptic seizures but explicitly also by the neurobiological, cognitive, psychological, and social consequences of this condition, and for this reason, although seizure freedom is of course still the goal where possible, "More than seizures" was the theme for the European Epilepsy Day in 2014. Psychiatric disorders are relatively frequent comorbidities in epilepsy, with a lifetime history identified in one of every three patients, but these problems are, more often than not, ignored, unless they are severe enough to cause major disability. This seems to be due to multiple factors, including the patients' reluctance to volunteer spontaneously information about existing psychiatric symptoms, a paucity (or total lack) of a specific training of the treating neurologist to recognize these psychiatric comorbidities, and a lack of time in very busy clinics to screen for them. Nonetheless, psychiatric problems in epilepsy have a deleterious impact on quality of life, morbidity, and mortality.

Traditionally, among all different neurological subspecialties, epileptologists have been deeply involved in the understanding of human behavior, and epilepsy has been historically considered a privileged window into the complex world of human emotions. The rapid expansion of neurosciences, during the twentieth century, forced the separation between neurology and psychiatry, but such findings and progresses in reality made the boundaries between neurology and psychiatry even more indistinct with a progressive need for transdisciplinary integration. In fact, the use of "neurological" techniques (e.g., neurophysiology and neuroimaging) in psychiatry, and the careful observation of psychopathological states and behavioral symptoms in patients with neurological disorders, enriched the neuroscientific literature with new data, shedding light on the neurobiology of human behavior.

It is now becoming evident that epilepsy, more than other neurological disorders, needs to be approached by a multidisciplinary team with multiple skills and different specialists. The need for a multidisciplinary approach obviously requires that the different health professionals speak the same language and are aware of problems and diagnostic and therapeutic options. The aim of this book is to give an up-to-date review of psychiatric problems in epilepsy with special attention to clinical aspects. I'm very grateful to all colleagues that contributed so enthusiastically to this project, sharing their tremendous expertise. This is a book written by clinicians for clinicians, bearing in mind the contribution of basic science to the understanding of human behavior.

London, UK Marco Mula, MD, PhD

Foreword I

Neuropsychiatric Symptoms of Epilepsy addresses a highly relevant topic which impacts on the life of many people with epilepsy and their families and requires constant consideration by all professionals involved in epilepsy care as well as scientists engaged in research on the mechanisms of the epilepsies and the search for new treatments.

Psychiatric comorbidities occur overall in about one-third of people with epilepsy during lifetime, and their incidence is much greater in high-risk groups such as individuals with seizures resistant to treatment. These comorbidities exhibit a variety of clinical manifestations, prognostic features, and pathophysiological mechanisms – accordingly, they require diversified management strategies. Psychiatric disorders, particularly mood disorders, have been repeatedly found to adversely affect quality of life of people with epilepsy to a greater extent compared with seizures themselves. Yet, not uncommonly, these disorders are underdiagnosed, and their clinical importance is often underestimated, particularly by primary care physicians but also by neurologists.

Marco Mula deserves praise for assembling a team of internationally recognized experts and producing a publication which, for its peculiarities, fills a gap in the epilepsy literature. *Neuropsychiatric Symptoms of Epilepsy* provides a comprehensive, analytical, up-to-date review of the wide range of psychiatric disorders that can occur in people with epilepsy and of the complex and at times bidirectional relationships between these disorders, the underlying causes of epilepsy, the effects of seizures themselves, and the role of pharmacological and surgical treatments. Throughout the chapters, emphasis is placed on those aspects which are most relevant for clinical management – from the value and indications of screening instruments to the challenges with differential diagnosis and from the rational approach to prevention and treatment to extensive discussion of potential benefits, limitations, and risks associated with available therapeutic options. The inclusion of authors with long-standing experience in the care of people with epilepsy and psychiatric disorders provides a clinically oriented perspective which is a special asset of this book. Appropriate emphasis is made on limitations of current tools, gaps in knowledge, and priority for future research, so that this book is also useful for researchers who have an interest in this area. All aspects are dealt with in considerable detail, but inclusion of summary boxes also helps in conveying the most relevant key messages.

Neuropsychiatric Symptoms of Epilepsy is a valuable resource for everyone involved in the care of people with epilepsy, and also for physicians who specialize in the management of psychiatric disorders. Specifically, this book should be especially useful to neurologists, geriatricians, psychiatrists, neuropsychiatrists, neuropsychologists, specialized nurses, as well as scientists engaged in basic and clinical research on epilepsy and its comorbidities.

Prof Emilio Perucca, MD, PhD
C. Mondino National Neurological Institute and
Department of Internal Medicine and Therapeutics,
University of Pavia, Pavia, Italy
President, International League Against Epilepsy

Foreword II

This book is a contribution to a series titled *Neuropsychiatric Symptoms of Neurological Disease* and forms a pivotal contribution to the very meaning and understanding of today's neuropsychiatry. The specialty of neuropsychiatry has a long and a shorter history. The hint of a brain basis for behavioral disorders stretches back to the times of Hippocrates, but really did not develop until the Renaissance and the later Enlightenment epochs. These times gave us early pioneers of the exploration of brain anatomy and more careful description of what we may refer to as neuropsychiatric disorders. These ideas burgeoned in the later nineteenth century, but there was more interest in mystical experiences, memory, and dreams, and in the brain as a creative organ, not just a passive receptor of sensory stimuli to be responded to in a reflex fashion. Then came the psychological insights of Sigmund Freud (1856–1939) exploring the unconscious palimpsest of behavior and its disorders. This had the unfortunate consequence of pulling a psychologically based neuroscience-free psychiatry away from the "new" discipline of neurology as we know it today. Into the void fell many patients, whose clinical signs and symptoms were poorly embraced by such a division. Of those falling, seizures were a particularly florid example of the conceptual muddles which arose, as more and more people with epilepsy came solely under a neurological purview, which had become divorced from any broader perspective on the associated comorbidities. The latter were occasioned by several factors, including social and educational limitations, stigma, the failure in a significant proportion of people to stop seizures, and the adverse effects of antiseizure medications.

Further there was scant regards to the neuroanatomical and neurophysiological substrates of epilepsy. It was considered that the seizure was all that demanded attention, and if they went away, then the patient would need no more help and also go away. Yet it was obvious that the seizure itself was but one expression of the underlying cerebral abnormalities, which are continuous and persist and continue to disrupt the organization of the brain. Since many people with epilepsy have such changes in the medial temporal cortex, and since it has been known for over a century that structures there are intimately linked with emotional regulation and expression, it is hardly surprising, unless ignorant of neuroanatomy, that there would be behavioral consequences beyond the seizures.

The psychoses associated with epilepsy have been well described since the mid-nineteenth century, as were the personality styles and the longer-term cognitive changes. Interest in them fell into abeyance for the better part of the twentieth century, but the introduction of the EEG in clinical practice provided a linchpin for recognizing the inter-ictal abnormalities and the association between temporal lobe epilepsy (as it was appropriately called) and associated cognitive and psychiatric disorders. Interestingly, it was not the traditional neurologists who embraced these findings, but lay organizations, parents, and carers, who had long known about such problems, but did not find a sympathetic ear for explanation or understanding.

Things have now changed considerably, and there are many people actively studying comorbidities of epilepsy, examining the effects of treatment for seizures on the mental state and behavior, and grappling with the ever-present problem of diagnostic challenges distinguishing epileptic from non-epileptic attacks.

The modern era of clinical neuropsychiatry began perhaps around the 1980s. My own *Neuropsychiatry* was published in 1981, and Jeff Cummings' *Clinical Neuropsychiatry* in 1985. The British Neuropsychiatric Association was established in 1987, the American Neuropsychiatric Association in 1988, and the Japanese Neuropsychiatric Association in 1996. The International Neuropsychiatric Association (INA) was formed in 1998 – neuropsychiatry is now a well-recognized discipline in many countries.

In *Neuropsychiatry,* I had ventured the following definition: Neuropsychiatry is a discipline which references certain disorders "which, on account of their presentation and pathogenesis, do not fall neatly into one category, and require multidisciplinary ideas for their full understanding." The clinical aspects of the subject matter were central and cover a spectrum of disorders. Yet, neuropsychiatry is not only interested in clinical abnormalities that are explained by our understanding of brain-behavior relationships, it is concerned with the "meaning" of abnormal behavior. This requires consideration of content as well as form, and the various life contingencies which impinge on patients which may influence their signs and symptoms. This recognizes the distinction between disease (pathology) and illness (what patients present with), and a propensity to tolerate diagnostic uncertainty. Alwyn Lishman in his paper *What is Neuropsychiatry*? explained that neuropsychiatry was not an "all-exclusive domain" embracing only the neurosciences, but "Social, developmental, psychodynamic and interpersonal forces must also be considered."

Neuropsychiatry is not simply an offshoot of psychiatry. It is a discipline which has arisen out of a clinical need for patients who have fallen badly between the cracks engendered by the developments of the clinical neurosciences in the twentieth century. Neuropsychiatrists must understand the signs and symptoms of a range of central nervous system disorders, as well as the psychology behind human motivation and desire. Nowhere is this more apparent than in dealing with epilepsy. In the nineteenth century, those most interested in the neurospychiatry of epilepsy were from France and Germany. The tradition in England is to be found in the writings of Hughlings Jackson (1835–1911), whose contributions to understanding the way the workings of the damaged brain are profound, and should form essential reading for any budding neuropsychiatrist.

In England after the Second World War, a strong tradition for managing epilepsy developed at the Maudsley Hospital, covering not only the use of the EEG, and the recognition of comorbidities, but also noting the effects of treatments on the mental state including temporal lobectomy. The legacy of this era has remained strong to the present day, and can be felt through this current text devoted to the neuropsychiatry of epilepsy. It is encouraging to read such a wide range of up-to-date information from colleagues from many different countries, with Marco Mula as conductor of the orchestra. This book is a substantial contribution, covering all of the important areas of the neuropsychiatry of epilepsy, one of the most interesting and absorbing disorders in clinical medicine.

UCL Institute of Neurology
Queen Square, London, United Kingdom

Prof. Michael R Trimble
MD FRCP FRCPsych

Contents

Contributors

Naoto Adachi, MD Adachi Mental Clinic, Kitano, Kiyota, Sapporo, Japan

Niruj Agrawal, MBBS, MD, MSc, Dip CBT, FRCPsych Department of Neuropsychiatry, St. George's University Hospitals NHS Foundation Trust, London, UK

Nozomi Akanuma, MD, PhD Lambeth Assessment, Liaison and Treatment Team, South London & Maudsley NHS Foundation Trust, London, UK

Ettore Beghi, MD Laboratory of Neurological Disorders, Department of Neuroscience, IRCCS-Mario Negri Institute, Milan, Italy

Massimiliano Beghi, MD Department of Mental Health, Medicine and Surgery, Department of Psychiatry, G. Salvini Hospital, Milan, Italy

Francesca Bisulli, MD, PhD IRCCS Institute of Neurological Sciences and Department of Biomedical and Neuromotor Sciences, Bellaria Hospital, University of Bologna, Bologna, Italy

Christian Brandt, MD Department of General Epileptology, Bethel Epilepsy Centre, Bielefeld, Germany

Andrea E. Cavanna, MD, PhD, FRCP Michael Trimble Neuropsychiatry Research Group, BSMHFT and University of Birmingham, Birmingham, UK

School of Life and Health SciencesAston University, Birmingham, UK

Sobell Department of Motor Neuroscience and Movement DisordersUCL and Institute of Neurology, London, UK

Department of NeuropsychiatryNational Centre for Mental Health25 Vincent Drive, BirminghamB152FG, UK

Hannah R. Cock, BSc, MD, MBBS, FRCP Epilepsy Group, Atkinson Morley Regional Neuroscience Centre, St. George's University Hospitals NHS Foundation Trust, St George's University of London, London, UK

Institute of Medical and Biomedical Education, St. George's University of London, London, UK

Cesare Maria Cornaggia, MD Department of Surgery and Interdisciplinary Medicine, University of Milano Bicocca, Monza, Italy

David W. Dunn, MD Departments of Psychiatry and Neurology, Indiana University School of Medicine, Riley Child and Adolescent Psychiatry Clinic, Indianapolis, IN, USA

Hesham Yousry Elnazer, MBBch, MRCPsych Department of Neuropsychiatry, St. George's University Hospitals NHS Foundation Trust, London, UK

Clare M. Galtrey, MA, PhD, MB BChir, MRCP Epilepsy Group, Atkinson Morley Regional Neuroscience Centre, St. George's University Hospitals NHS Foundation Trust, London, UK

Alla Guekht, MD, PhD Department of Neurology, Neurosurgery and Genetics, Russian National Research Medical University and Moscow Research and Clinical Center for Neuropsychiatry, Moscow, Russia

Andres M. Kanner, MD, FANA Epilepsy Section, Department of Neurology, Comprehensive Epilepsy Center, University of Miami, Miller School of Medicine, Miami, FL, USA

William G. Kronenberger, PhD Section of Psychology, Department of Psychiatry, Indiana University School of Medicine, Riley Child and Adolescent Psychiatry Clinic, Indianapolis, IN, USA

Andrey Mazarati, MD, PhD Neurology Division, Department of Pediatrics, David Geffen School of Medicine, University of California Los Angeles, Los Angeles, CA, USA

Stefano Meletti, MD, PhD Department of Biomedical, Metabolic, and Neural Science, University of Modena e Reggio Emilia, Modena, Italy

Neurology UnitNOCSAE Hospital – AUSL, Modena, Italy

Marco Mula, MD, PhD Epilepsy Group, Atkinson Morley Regional Neuroscience Centre, St. George's University Hospitals NHS Foundation Trust, St George's University of London, London, UK

Institute of Medical and Biomedical Sciences, St George's University of London, London, UK

Emilio Perucca, MD, PhD, FRCP(Edin) Department of Internal Medicine and Therapeutics, C. Mondino National Neurological Institute, University of Pavia, Pavia, Italy

Bruce Hermann PhD Department of Neurology, University of Wisconsin School of Medicine and Public Health, Madison, WI, USA

Federica Provini, MD, PhD IRCCS Institute of Neurological Sciences and Department of Biomedical and Neuromotor Sciences, Bellaria Hospital, University of Bologna, Bologna, Italy

Genevieve Rayner, PhD Melbourne School of Psychological Sciences, The University of Melbourne, Parkville, VIC, Australia

The Florey Institute of Neuroscience and Mental Health, Melbourne, VIC, Australia

Ramses Ribot, MD EEG Monitoring Unit, University of Miami Hospital, University of Miami, Miller School of Medicine, Miami, FL, USA

Howard Ring, MD Department of Psychiatry, University of Cambridge, Cambridge, UK

Anagha A. Sardesai, MBBS, MRCPsych Department of Learning Disability Psychiatry, Ida Darwin Hospital, Cambridgeshire and Peterborough NHS Foundation Trust, Fulbourn, UK

Steven C. Schachter, MD Departments of Neurology, Consortia for Improving Medicine with Innovation and Technology, Beth Israel Deaconess Medical Center and Massachusetts General Hospital, Harvard Medical School, Boston, MA, USA

Matthias Schmutz, MA, PhD Department of Psychiatry/Psychotherapy, Swiss Epilepsy Center, Zurich, Switzerland

Paolo Tinuper, MD IRCCS Institute of Neurological Sciences and Department of Biomedical and Neuromotor Sciences, Bellaria Hospital, University of Bologna, Bologna, Italy

Sarah J. Wilson, PhD Melbourne School of Psychological Sciences, The University of Melbourne, Parkville, VIC, Australia

The Florey Institute of Neuroscience and Mental Health, Melbourne, VIC, Australia

Comprehensive Epilepsy ProgrammeAustin Health, Heidelberg, VIC, Australia

Mahinda Yogarajah, BSc, MBBS, MRCP, PhD Epilepsy Group, Atkinson Morley Regional Neuroscience Centre, St. George's University Hospitals NHS Foundation Trust, London, UK

Chapter 1
Neurobehavioral Comorbidities of Epilepsy: Lessons from Animal Models

Andrey Mazarati

Abstract Animal models can afford useful insights into the mechanisms of neurobehavioral comorbidities of epilepsy. However, clinical relevance and value of the information that can be extracted from animal studies depend on many factors, including choice of proper models of epilepsy, choice of proper behavioral tasks, and accounting for the presence of multiple concurrent neurobehavioral disorders in the same epileptic animal. This chapter offers an overview of approaches used to examine selected neurobehavioral comorbidities in animal models of epilepsy. Assays used to study spatial and object memory, depression, anxiety, attention deficit/hyperactivity disorder, psychosis, and autism are described. First, the approaches are presented from a standpoint of single comorbidity, and mechanisms underlying respective epilepsy-associated neurobehavioral abnormalities are discussed. Further, examples are given as to how concurrent neurobehavioral perturbations may influence one another, and therefore how this may affect outcome measures and interpretation of the obtained data. It is suggested that systemic approach, rather than more commonly used isolated approach, offers more clinical-relevant and complete description of multifactorial systems that underlie neurobehavioral comorbidities of epilepsy.

Keywords Epilepsy • Behavior • Animal models • Cognition • Memory • Depression • Anxiety • Attention deficit/hyperactivity disorder • Psychosis • Autism

Do We Need Animal Models of Epilepsy Comorbidities?

Recent technological advances have contributed to a remarkable progress into understanding mechanisms of neurobehavioral disorders in epilepsy patients. Yet, clinical systems have inherent limitations which hinder both mechanistic studies

---

A. Mazarati, MD, PhD
Neurology Division, Department of Pediatrics,
David Geffen School of Medicine, University of California Los Angeles,
10833 LeConte Avenue, MDCC 220474,
Los Angeles, CA 90095, USA
e-mail: mazarati@ucla.edu

M. Mula (ed.), *Neuropsychiatric Symptoms of Epilepsy*, Neuropsychiatric Symptoms of Neurological Disease, DOI 10.1007/978-3-319-22159-5_1

and clinical trials. Among such limitations, to name a few, are medications which interfere with natural evolution of the disease, and in addition may themselves produce neurobehavioral side effects; difficulties with enrolling homogenous and quantitatively sound cohorts amenable to statistical analysis; psychosocial factors which can exacerbate biological aspects of the disease (e.g., stigma can further exacerbate mood disorders); unaccountable environmental factors; ethical concerns; and, particularly when it comes to clinical trials, compliance and safety considerations.

Most if not all of these limitations can be overcome, or at least substantially mitigated, through the employment of animal systems. Indeed, in experimental animals, the disease can be allowed to take its natural course without treatment interference, thus facilitating mechanistic insights; sample size is only limited by regulatory requirements (such as refinement, reduction, replacement, known as "3R" [1, 2], by the capacity of the laboratory and by the costs; the subjects are generally genetically homogenous and can be enrolled on demand by age and gender; biological aspects of the comorbidities are not contaminated by psychosocial factors (such as stigma, work environment, etc.); environmental and compliance concerns are limited or nonexistent.

Therefore, the questions are not whether animal models are needed, but how closely they reflect real-life scenarios and to what extent the information extracted in the laboratory setting is clinically relevant. With this regard, a long-standing skepticism has persisted in clinical milieu, which is particularly understandable when it comes to animal models of neuropsychiatric disorders. The liability lies with both sides. On the one hand, there is certain misconception as to the purpose of animal models, which by design is not expected to replicate a real-life system, but rather to facilitate its comprehension through simulation and visualization. On the other hand, for laboratory scientists, animal experiments frequently become a self-serving activity, when research is performed for the sake of the research, and clinical considerations are not factored into the study design and goals.

The purpose of this chapter is not to merely recite literature on neurobehavioral comorbidities of epilepsy, but to attempt narrowing the gap between clinicians and laboratory researchers through analysis of approaches used to model neuropsychiatric comorbidities of epilepsy.

Animal Assays Used to Examine Neurobehavioral Comorbidities of Epilepsy

In laboratory animals, the information cannot be obtained through self-reporting questionnaires of interviews. Hence, behavioral assays for neuropsychiatric disorders frequently have to rely on anthropomorphism; that is, the experimenter poses a question of how he or she would have behaved adequately under certain conditions and projects such apparent behavior on the animal. The expected responses are corrected to factor in the knowledge about species-specific behaviors (e.g., sociability of rodents, their preference toward dark vs. lit areas, etc.). Any deviation from a behavior deemed adequate by the researcher is then interpreted as pathological. Admittedly, there is always a strong subjective component in interpreting an animal's response. This bias can be mitigated by subjecting an animal to more than one behavioral test to examine a disorder of interest.

When validating behavioral tests and models for studying neuropsychiatric disorders, two principles are attempted to be abided by face validity and construct validity [3]. Face validity means resemblance of animals' behavior to behavior in humans, under similar conditions (but corrected for species-specifics). For example, avoiding the engagement with other animals of the same species would suggest good face validity for animal models of autism. Construct validity means resemblance of known underlying mechanisms. For example, the dysfunction of serotonergic transmission suggests good construct validity of a system for reproducing major depressive disorder. Better models would offer both good face validity and construct validity, although this is not always the case. For example, spontaneously hypertensive rats (SHR) present with symptoms of attention deficit and hyperimpulsivity and are deemed having good face validity for modeling attention deficit/hyperactivity disorder (ADHD) [4, 5]; construct validity of the system however is poor, as hypertension, which is inherent to the strain, is not a symptom of ADHD. When it comes to preclinical trials, predictive validity also comes in play, as the one reflecting the ability of a medication tested in an animal model to correctly predict the efficacy of this drug in a homologous human disorder [3]. Here, reverse translation is often applied. For example, if in a given animal model of depression, clinically available selective serotonin reuptake inhibitors (SSRI), fluoxetine and citalopram, effectively improve depressive behavior, then it is assumed that the model has good predictive validity, as novel investigational drugs effective in this model would also have therapeutic effects in patients.

Here, due to space restrictions, only most commonly used behavioral assays are discussed. Furthermore, the discussion is limited to rats and mice as most commonly used species in epilepsy and behavioral research. Finally, as mechanisms which drive various behaviors are complex and multifaceted, only select mechanisms are addressed.

Spatial Recognition and Memory

Morris water maze (MWM) is a common way to test animal's spatial recognition and memory [6–8]. The test relies on the fact that rodents are good, but not keen swimmers, and thus would avoid swimming if possible. The apparatus is a large cylindrical tank filled with water with a submerged escape platform placed in one of the virtual quadrants. When the animal is first placed in the tank, it swims aimlessly, eventually stumbles upon the platform and climbs on it (Fig. 1.1a; if exploratory swimming exceeds the set duration, the animal is manually guided to the platform). During the learning phase, as the task is repeated several times a day, normal

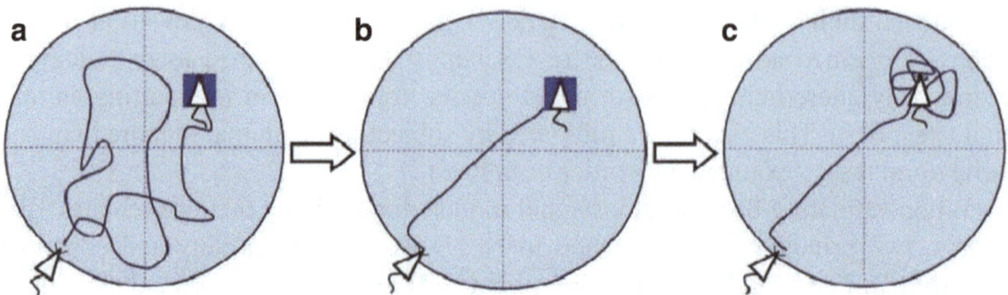

Fig. 1.1 Morris water maze (MWM) test for spatial learning and memory. Schematic rendering of spatial learning and memory in the MWM. Animal's movements around the tank are outlined by trace lines. (**a**, **b**) Spatial learning. (**a**) During the initial trials, upon placement in the tank, the animal swims around aimlessly, finds the platform (represented by the *blue square*) by accident, and climbs on it. (**b**) As the trials are repeated for several days, the animal learns the location of the platform and swims to it directly. (**c**) Spatial memory. After training, the platform is removed. Nevertheless, the animal spends more time swimming in the quadrant where the platform used to be, than in the other three quadrants of the tank

animals learn the placement of the platform, and the latency to the escape gradually declines. The training successfully culminates, when, after placing in the water, the animal swims directly to the platform and climbs on it, rather than explores various areas of the tank (Fig. 1.1b). The number of trials needed for the animal to learn the placement of the platform serves as a measure of spatial learning. During the retrieval phase, after initial training, the platform is removed. Normal animals spend more time swimming in the quadrant where the platforms used to be than in the other three quadrants of the tank (Fig. 1.1c). Total time spent in the relevant quadrant serves as a measure of spatial memory. Therefore, animals for which it takes longer to learn the platform location during the learning phase, and those which divide time equally among the four quadrants of the tank during the retrieval phase, are interpreted to have spatial cognitive impairments.

Among various mechanisms determining spatial cognition and memory, one can be singled out as particularly important. The processes of spatial recognition and memory are driven by a subset of pyramidal cells in the hippocampus called, due to their function, place cells [9, 10]. Single place cell fires each time the animal enters a particular location in the environment (known as place field). In the confined environment (such as MWM), the activation of each place cell is typically associated with a single place field. As the animal moves around the area, different place cells are activated. Collectively, place cells act as a representation of a specific location in space, thus forming a cognitive map [11]. Cognitive maps can be built by recording from single place cells as the animal moves around the enclosure, typically a cylinder. On the first training day, fasting animal is placed inside the cylinder, where food pellets are scattered on the floor so as to ensure that the animal visits all parts of the cylinder. On subsequent days, single food pellets are dropped consecutively and randomly at various locations, so that the animal travels along various paths. While the animal moves around the enclosure, the activity of single place cell is recorded. The resulting firing field reflects the activity of the recorded place

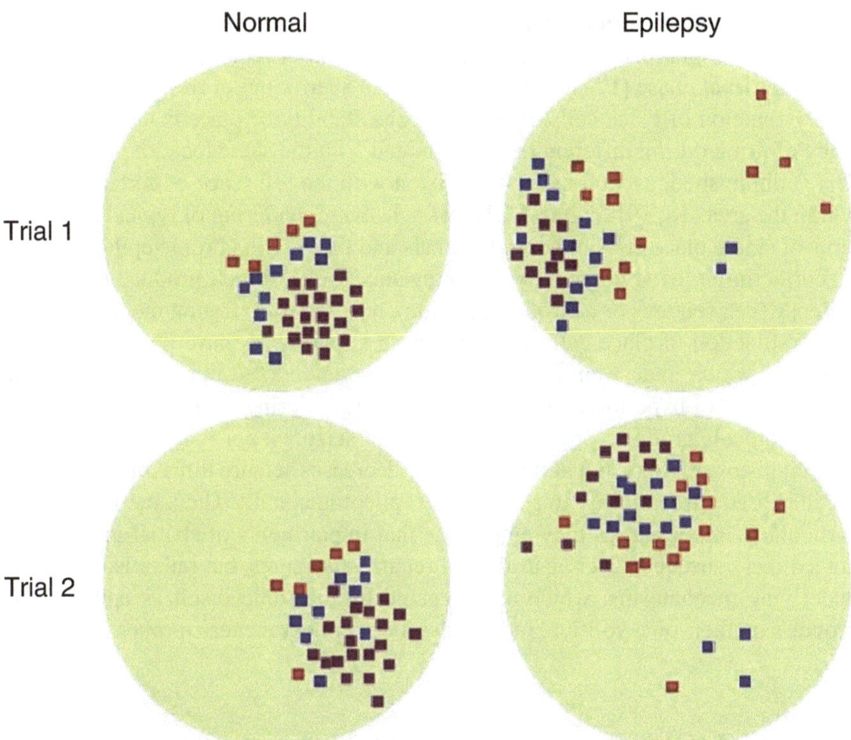

Fig. 1.2 Example of the stability of place cell firing patterns in a normal rat, and a rat with experimental MTLE. Schematic compilation of real-life place cell maps [18, 20–22], showing firing rate of a single place cell, while the animal is moving around the cylindrical enclosure, in two consecutive trials. Pixels reflect firing rates coded in the sequence, *yellow* (no firing)–*red*–*blue*–*purple* (highest firing rate) colors. In normal rats, the firing pattern is consistent between the trials 1 and 2. In animals with MTLE, the fields vary from one trial to another

cells with reference to different parts of the cylinder. In MWM, learning of the location of the platform and its retrieval is associated with firing of specific place cells, which "guide" the animal to the target area (these processes are known as place cell preplay and replay, applied to learning and memory, respectively) [12, 13] (Fig. 1.2).

Understandably, any dysfunction or loss of place cells, such as it occurs under conditions of mesial temporal lobe epilepsy (MTLE), is expected, and may in turn translate into deficits of spatial learning and memory.

Indeed, impaired performance in MWM and concurrent dysfunction of place cells has been reported in several experimental models of epilepsy. Status epilepticus (SE) induced in rodents by pilocarpine (or LiCl and pilocarpine combination) produces a variety of perturbations resembling human MTLE, such as spontaneous recurrent seizures developing after a brief "silent" period; extensive neurodegeneration and gliosis in the hippocampus; formation of aberrant excitatory hippocampal connections, etc. [14–16]. Interictally, epileptic animals present with profound deficits in MWM performance, including larger number of trials needed to learn the location of the platform during training, as well as poor recall of platform location during retrieval phase [17–19]. These behavioral aberrations correlate strongly with the dysfunction of place cells. Particularly, the stability of place cells (i.e., consistency of firing during different trials associated with the same location in the cylinder) is diminished, as well as their precision with the reference of certain location within the area [18, 19]. Figure 1.2 shows schematic rendering of typical firing patterns of single place cells in normal animals and those with chronic epilepsy.

Furthermore, even potentially epileptogenic insults, which produce no explicit epilepsy (i.e., seizures or neurodegeneration), result in long-lasting memory deficits and dysfunction of place cells. As such, these impairments have been observed in adult rats which underwent a series of primary generalized flurothyl-induced seizures [20, 21] or hyperthermia-induced seizures [22] during neonatal age; neither of these protocols produces spontaneous recurrent seizures, nor is it accompanied by explicit histopathology, but at the same time decreases seizure threshold, thus creating increased susceptibility to a secondary epileptogenic hit. The latter findings are particularly important, as they emphasize that impairments of spatial memory are not a direct consequence or an artifact of recurrent seizures, but rather have specific underlying mechanisms, which are triggered by the same insult as epilepsy, but progress on their own volition, independently of epileptogenesis proper.

Nonspatial (Object) Learning and Memory

Object memory is examined in the novel object recognition test, which is based on visual discriminative ability coupled with the natural curiosity, typical for rodents [23].

During the learning phase, the animal is placed in the confined environment, where it is presented for the exploration with two objects of distinct shapes (e.g., cube and pyramid). Normally, animals spend about similar time exploring each of the objects. After a period of exploration, the animal is removed, and after some time (generally 6–24 h), it is returned to the task area, where one of the objects is now replaced with a different one (e.g., the cube is replaced with a cylinder). During this phase, normal animals spend more time exploring the new object as compared with an already familiar one, while animals with impaired object memory treat both objects as novel and thus equally divide their time between the two. The proportion of time spent exploring novel versus familiar object is used to measure object memory.

Short-term object memory is primarily driven by the activity of rhinal and perirhinal cortices [24, 25], while long-term memory involves hippocampus as well [26], so that both short-term and long-term object memory can be affected in MTLE.

Impaired object memory has been reported in rats with pilocarpine SE-induced chronic epilepsy [27], although this has not been universally accepted [17]. Similar to spatial memory, potentially epileptogenic factors, such as cortical dysplasia induced by in utero irradiation [28], or a single primary generalized seizure induced by pentylenetetrazole, resulted [29] in the long-lasting impairments in object memory, even in the absence of recurrent seizure activity. Importantly, epilepsy-associated deficits in spatial and object memory are not redundant, as model-specific differences have been reported; thus, while single seizure episode resulted in the prolonged object memory disruption, while spatial memory was not compromised [30], animals with post-SE MTLE have been reported to present with spatial memory impairments, while object memory was spared [17].

Depression

Most commonly examined symptoms of depression are hopelessness/despair and anhedonia (i.e., inability to experience pleasure). Examination of the state of despair/hopelessness is performed using variations of the forced swimming test (FST) [31–33]. The test is designed to gauge animals' ability (or inability) to effectively cope with an inescapable stressful situation. The latter is created by placing the animal in a cylindrical tank filled with water, with no possibility to escape (e.g., platform, rope, etc.). Animals display several behavioral patterns, with two types prevailing. Active escaping behavior is characterized by climbing on, or swimming along the walls, or diving, and it is interpreted as effective coping. This behavior intermits with periods of immobility, where the animal passively floats, and movements are limited to maintaining the head above water so as to avoid drowning; when immobile, animals are thought to give up in their attempts to escape (Fig. 1.3). While both normal animals and those with experimentally induced depression display both types of behavior, in models of depression, such as depression-prone inbred strains of rats [33], mice with targeted mutations relevant to depression (e.g., overexpression of serotonin [5-HT] type 1A autoreceptors [34]), olfactory deprivation achieved by surgical removal of olfactory bulbs [35], chronic mild stress (e.g., repeated immobilization) [36], or Gram-negative bacterial infection mimicked by lipopolysaccharide (LPS, a state known as LPS sickness) [37], the immobility time significantly increases, whereby animals may spend most of the time immobile, rather than attempting to escape. Such exacerbated immobility is interpreted as a state of hopelessness/despair, and the state can be quantified by calculating the immobility to active swimming ratio. Indeed, the duration of immobility is effectively reduced by chronic treatment with antidepressants (such as SSRI and MAO inhibitors) [31, 32].

In mice, tail suspension test (TST) is frequently performed in lieu of FST [39]. In the TST, an inescapable stressful situation is created by suspending the mouse by the tail and quantifying active behavior (i.e., struggling attempts to free up) and immobility. These behaviors parallel respective patterns in the FST and are also amenable to standard antidepressant medications.

Another core symptom of depression, anhedonia, is examined using taste preference test. The test relies on innate affinity of rodents toward sweets [40]. When

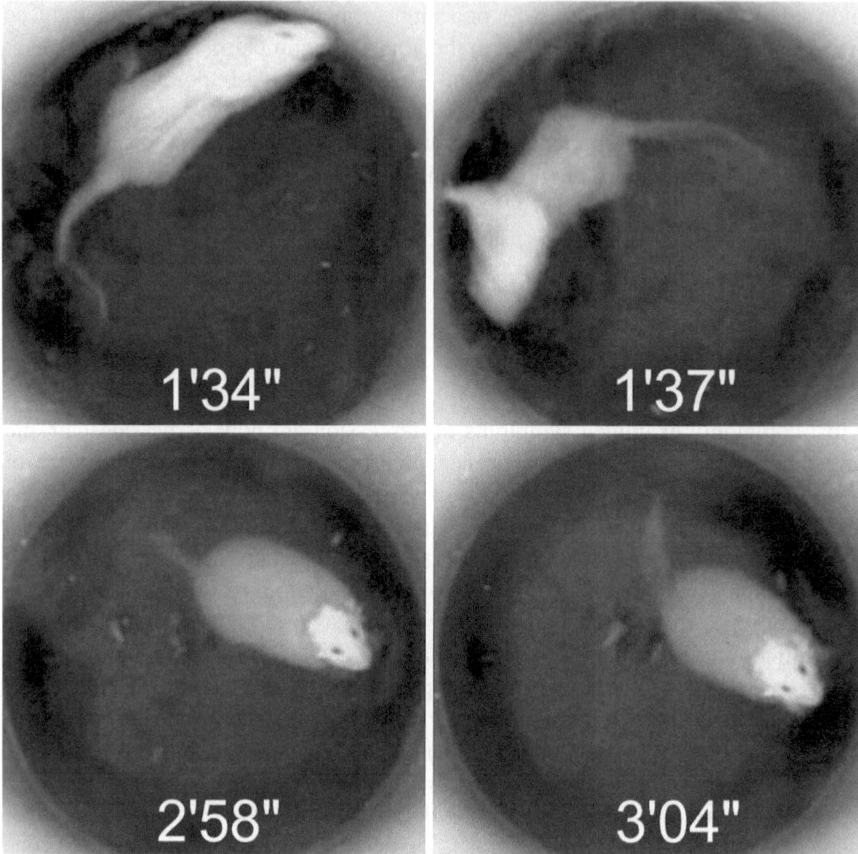

Fig. 1.3 Behavioral patterns in the forced swimming test (FST) for depression. Sample snapshots taken from pre-recorded video during FST. Time after the start of the test is indicated on each image. Examples of active swimming, which reflects active escape strategies, are presented at 1 min 34 s and 1 min 37 s. Note the change in the rat's position in the tank, which occurred during the 3-s period, and the fuzziness of images due to the animal's movement. Examples of immobility when animals move only enough to avoid drowning are presented at 2 min 58 s and 3 min 04 s. Note that the animal's position in the tank did not change during 6 s of recording and that the body is positioned vertically in the water [38] (Reprinted from Mazarati et al. [38], with permission from Elsevier)

presented with the choice of two bottles, one filled with water and another with sweet solution (e.g., low percent saccharin or sucrose), normal animals preferentially consume the latter. "Anhedonic" animals show no drink preference, but consume statistically equal volumes of water and saccharin. The presence of anhedonic state is thus measured by the consumed saccharin (sucrose) to water ratio.

Among the factors regulating behavior in depression tests, ascending serotonergic pathways (i.e., those emanating from raphe nuclei, and projecting to prefrontal cortex [PFC] and hippocampus) play a critical role [41, 42]. In turn, the release of serotonin from raphe into target areas has complex regulatory mechanism, but two are most notable: short feedback autoinhibitory loop involving 5-HT1A raphe autoreceptors [43–45] and descending glutamatergic (i.e., excitatory pathway) from PFC into the raphe [46]. Hence, such perturbations, as the upregulation of 5-HT1A autoreceptors or a diminished excitatory drive from PFC in the raphe, will translate into the diminished 5-HT output, and consequently, into depression.

Another important mechanism is the dysregulation of hypothalamo-pituitary-adrenocortical (HPA) axis. The HPA axis dysregulation occurs because of the compromised negative feedback mechanism, whereby cortisol (or corticosterone in rodents) released from adrenal cortex fails to suppress corticotrophin-releasing hormone (CRH) release from hypothalamus and/or adrenocorticotropic hormone (ACTH) release from the anterior pituitary. As a result, the response of the HPA axis to stressors becomes unabated and maladaptive [47, 48]. This has many central and peripheral consequences. One of such consequences, particularly relevant to depression, is the upregulation of raphe 5-HT1A autoreceptors [48–50], which, as discussed earlier, would lead in turn to the increased autoinhibition of serotonin release and its insufficient delivery into forebrain structures. The dysregulation of the HPA axis can be revealed using either dexamethasone (DEX) suppression test or the combined DEX/CRH test (both are also used in patients). The latter consists of measuring corticosterone plasma levels in response to the administration of DEX (which normally suppresses plasma corticosterone), followed by the administration of CRH (which normally increases plasma corticosterone). Blunted response to DEX and exacerbated response to CRH represent objective measures of the HPA axis hyperactivity [51].

Increased immobility time in the FST in rats and mice, or in TST in mice, as well as anhedonia have been reported in several models of MTLE [52–54], as well as models of absence epilepsy [55, 56]. It has been suggested that epilepsy-associated depression develops as a result of cascade of events, starting with brain inflammation. Brain inflammation, and particularly, the increased signaling of a cytokine interleukin-1β (IL-1β) is triggered by a precipitating insult (e.g., status epilepticus or traumatic brain injury), and may be sustained by recurrent seizures [57, 58]. IL-1β had been reported to facilitate or even precipitate seizure activity through the phosphorylation of NR2B subunit of the NMDA receptor [59]. At the same time, chronic inflammation has been implicated in mechanisms of depressive disorders [60] (one remarkable observation is a high prevalence of depression among patients with rheumatoid arthritis [61]). In animal systems, chronic inflammation, induced by the administration of LPS (an endotoxin of Gram-negative bacteria), produced a spectrum of depressive impairments, including despair/hopelessness and anhedonia in respective tests [37, 62]. One of the consequences of the activation of IL-1β signaling in animals with chronic epilepsy is the dysregulation of the HPA axis [38, 53]. The resulting sustained high levels of circulating corticosterone in turn upregulate 5-HT1A autoreceptors in raphe nuclei [63]. Upon the 5-HT1A autoreceptor upregulation, the resulting increased autoinhibition of serotonin release culminates in the development of depressive behavioral abnormalities. Indeed, treatment of epileptic/depressed animals with an IL-1 receptor blocker (IL-1ra, also known as anakinra) disrupted both neuroendocrine and behavioral symptoms of depression [38].

It should be noted that the presence of symptoms of depression in epileptic animals has not been universally accepted. In fact, several studies have found that animals with post-SE chronic epilepsy display decreased, rather than increased, immobility in the FST and TST [64, 65]. Such findings can be interpreted in one of the following ways: either seizures produce a true antidepressant effect or other events interfere with the swimming ability of epileptic rats, thus rendering commonly used behavioral tests inappropriate for studying depression. One such scenario is discussed further below under Multiple Concurrent Comorbidities.

Anxiety

General anxiety is most commonly examined using elevated plus maze test (EPMT) or its variations [66, 67]. The apparatus is composed of two perpendicularly crossing walking beams (arms): one is open and exposed to the light, and the other is closed (i.e., covered, so as to create the dark tunnel, Fig. 1.4). The apparatus is elevated over the ground, so as to create an insecure environment in the open arms. The animal is able to travel along each of the arms freely. Behavioral pattern in the EPMT is a result of the balance between animal's curiosity (i.e., exploration of all arms) and insecurity (when traveling along the elevated open arms). In rodents with general anxiety, time spent in closed arms is significantly longer than in normal animals. Anxiolytic medications increase the presence in open arms.

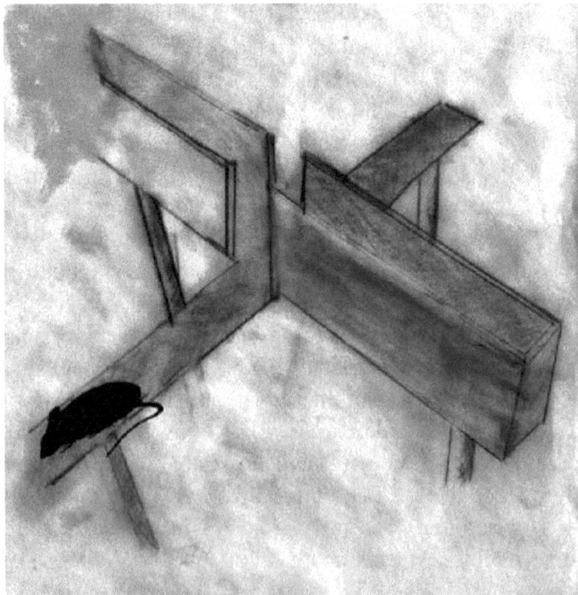

Fig. 1.4 Elevated plus maze test for general anxiety. Schematic rendering of the apparatus, with the test animals located in one of the open arms. For the description of the apparatus and the procedure, see text

The presence of general anxiety in epileptic animals has been controversial. Increased anxiety has been reported in several models of MTLE [65, 68] and absence epilepsy [69]. However, other studies reported the opposite effect of recurrent seizures, whereby epileptic animals exhibited decreased levels of anxiety in the EPMT [17, 70]. Such conflicting findings resemble those reported for depression, with two similar interpretations: either recurrent seizures produce anxiolytic effect or, for some reasons, tests for general anxiety, which work well in normal animals, become inappropriate in animals with chronic epilepsy. The latter possibility is also discussed later under Multiple Concurrent Comorbidities.

Social anxiety can be examined using a three-chamber sociability test, which is also commonly employed to study autism-like behavior (see below). Discerning between social anxiety as a stand-alone condition versus the one associated with autism may be complicated.

Attention Deficit Hyperactivity Disorder (ADHD)

The examination of ADHD relies on complex operant behavioral tasks with positive reinforcement (generally food pellets presented after a period of fasting). Commonly used variations include five-choice serial reaction time task (5-CSRT) [71] and lateralized reaction time task (LRTT) [4], but the principle is the same. In the LRTT, the operant chamber is equipped with five apertures on one side (Fig. 1.5). Each of the apertures can be lit up by a beam of light, which is delivered in an organized sequence. On the opposite side is the photocell-equipped food-pellet feeder. The animal is trained such that poking the nose in the aperture, which is about to light

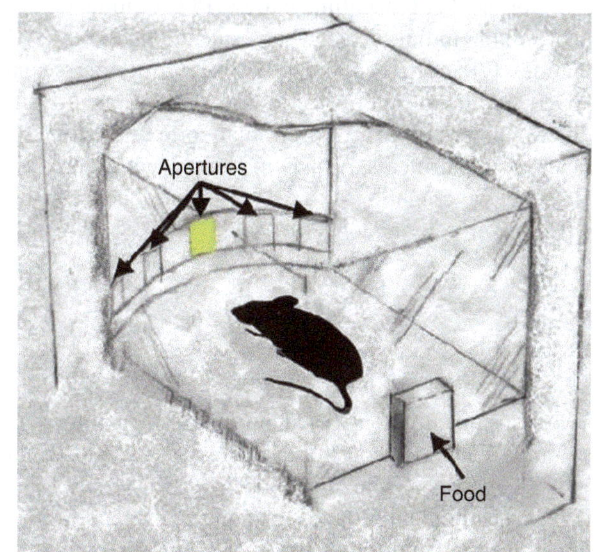

Fig. 1.5 Lateralized reaction time task (LRTT) for attention deficit/hyperactivity disorder. The chamber is soundproof. Five nose-poke apertures are in front of the rat; one of them is lit up. Photocell-equipped food pellet feeder is behind the animal. Poking the nose in the aperture which is about to light up is accompanied by the automated pellet delivery. During the test, the animal moves between the apertures and the feeder

up, is followed by the automated delivery of the food pellet. If the animal pokes the correct aperture at the correct time (e.g., 0.1, 0.5, 1 s, etc., before the light comes up), the food pellet is delivered from the feeder. Poking incorrect aperture reflects lack of attention; poking correct aperture prematurely reflects hyperimpulsivity. In neither of these cases, food reward is provided. Therefore, the numbers of incorrect and premature responses represent measurements of attention deficit and hyperimpulsivity, respectively.

Two neurotransmitter systems have been primarily implicated in the mechanisms of ADHD. Ascending dopaminergic projections from ventral tegmental area (VTA) into PFC (i.e., mesocortical pathway) and into nucleus accumbens (i.e., mesolimbic pathway), as well as noradrenergic projection from locus coeruleus (LC) into PFC play important roles in reward, impulsivity, and attention, and are compromised in ADHD [72–74]. Indeed, medications approved for the treatment of ADHD are dopamine-reuptake inhibitor methylphenidate and selective norepinephrine-reuptake inhibitor atomoxetine [75].

Animals with SE-induced MTLE present with both attention deficit and hyperimpulsivity. Real-time measurements of noradrenergic transmission by means of fast-scan cyclic voltammetry (FSCV) revealed that ADHD-like impairments develop due to the diminished norepinephrine output from LC into PFC. Furthermore, similar to epilepsy-associated depression, the observed noradrenergic deficit results from the increased autoinhibition of neurotransmitter release [76]. In case of norepinephrine, the upregulation of α2A adreno-autoreceptors in LC is responsible for the suppressed transmitter release I in the LC–PFC pathway.

Early-life primary generalized seizures produced in immature rodents by flurothyl result later in life in long-lasting ADHD-like abnormalities, even in the absence of explicit ictal events. In these animals, behavioral perturbations parallel the increased thickness of PFC [77]. Furthermore, direct administration of a GABA-A receptor blocker bicuculline into the PFC of immature rats results in transient interictal spiking in this area and subsequent long-lasting ADHD-like behavioral abnormalities [78]. These findings outline a different scenario of epilepsy-associated ADHD, which develops due to primary sustained dysfunction of PFC, rather than due to compromised LC–prefrontal cortex noradrenergic transmission. Similar to memory impairments, ADHD may represent either a true comorbidity of epilepsy (i.e., the two conditions coexist) or a consequence of early-life seizure event, even when seizures are no longer present.

Psychosis

Two tests are commonly used in rodents: locomotor activity in response to psychostimulants and the acoustic startle response (ASR; the latter is also used in patients in the diagnosis of schizophrenia).

Psychostimulant-induced locomotor response reflects the hypersensitivity of dopaminergic neurotransmission, which is a recognized mechanism of schizophrenia [79]. In turn, several variants are employed, such as amphetamine-induced hyperactivity in the "open field" and apomorhine-induced rearing and climbing [80]. In the amphetamine test, locomotor activity is quantified by counting the number of virtual squares crossed by the animal in the confined square area (known as "open field") over a set period of time, before versus after amphetamine administration. For the apomorhine test, the animal is placed in a small cylinder, with walls constructed as grid amenable to climbing; the climbing activity is scored before and after apomorhine injection. Animals with psychosis-like impairments display significantly steeper increase in locomotion upon amphetamine administration, and more climbing on the walls of the cylinder upon apomorhine administration than healthy controls.

The rationale for ASR in rodents is similar to that in patients with schizophrenia [81, 82]. It is based on the ability of the nervous system to adapt to a stronger sensory stimulus when a preceding signal is given as a warning. The test involves prepulse inhibition (PPI) protocol, and is performed in a startle chamber which detects whole-body mechanical reaction in response to an acoustic startle stimulus, which exceeds the background noise [83]. Acoustic prepulse stimulus is followed by a pulse stimulus after a set period, and the movement induced by the pulse is measured. In normal animals, the response to the pulse is inhibited when prepulse is presented; animals with psychosis-like impairments, in which sensory adaptation is compromised, show no inhibition of startle response in the prepulse–pulse sequence.

ASR has been extensively studied in the kindling model of MTLE. Repeated, initially subconvulsive electrical stimulations of limbic structures (e.g., hippocampus, amygdala, perirhinal cortex) lead to the occurrence and progressive development of complex partial seizures (hence, the kindling phenomenon) [84–87]. Kindled animals do not typically develop spontaneous seizures or profound histopathology associated with MTLE (although both may develop after very high number of stimulations). However, kindled animals respond with secondary generalized complex partial seizures in response to the stimulus, which is inconsequential in normal rats long after the kindling procedure has been completed (therefore, kindling can be described as a chronic epileptic state without spontaneous seizures). Kindled animals show exacerbated ASR, as well as exacerbated psychostimulant-induced locomotion [88–90]. Impaired ASR has been reported in other models of MTLE (e.g., SE induced by pilocarpine or kainic acid [91, 92]), as well as in a genetic model of absence epilepsy in rats (in Genetic Absence Epilepsy Rats from Strasbourg, GAERS) [93].

Autism

In rodents, most commonly examined symptoms of autism are impairments in sociability and repetitive behavior.

Animals' ability for social engagement is most commonly examined using the three-chamber sociability test [94–96]. The test is performed in a box divided into three connecting chambers. During the first (sociability) phase, one of the terminal chambers contains an unfamiliar rodent of the same species (conspecific), and the opposite terminal chamber – an unanimated object (Fig. 1.6). Both conspecific and the object are placed inside cylindrical wired cages, so as to isolate them from the rest of the space. The test animal is placed inside the box and is allowed to explore it freely. Animal's behavior is a result of the balance between general curiosity (manifested as exploration of both the object and the conspecific) and sociability (manifested as preferential engagement with conspecific over the object). Indeed, normal animals spend more time exploring/engaging with the conspecific, than with the object. In models of autism, however, animals show no conspecific versus object preference, and divide their time between the two equally. During the social novelty phase, which immediately follows the examination of sociability, the object is replaced with another novel conspecific, while the conspecific from the first phase remains in place, and the test is repeated. Now, normal animals spend more time engaging with the novel conspecific than with the already familiar one, while animals with autism-like impairments once again show no novel versus familiar conspecific preference.

In immature animals (between the time of birth and weaning), sociability is examined by assessing their interaction with the separated dame [96]. Pups, when separated from the dame, emit ultrasonic calls of certain modalities. In animal models of autism, the modality of ultrasonic vocalizations is altered in a specific fashion, presumably reflecting atypical vocalizations seen in autistic infants (e.g., the pups emit fewer harmonic, and more complex and short syllables [97, 98].

Self-directed repetitive behavior is analyzed by counting the duration of grooming during a set period (typically 10 min) [99]. In normal animals, grooming is episodic, while animals with autism-like abnormalities spend excessively long periods grooming, which is interpreted as the presence of self-directed repetitive behavior.

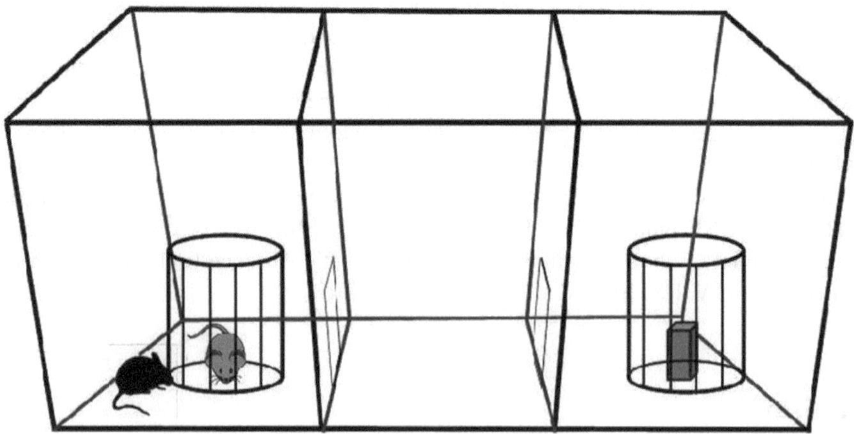

Fig. 1.6 Three-chamber sociability test for autism-like behavior. Shown is the sociability phase. Test mouse is shown in *black* in the left compartment. Conspecific mouse (in *gray*) is in the enclosure in the same compartment, and an unanimated object is inside the similar enclosure in the right compartment. Time spent exploring conspecific versus the unanimated object is counted. For the social novelty phase, the object is replaced with another conspecific, and the time spent exploring the familiar mouse (*left*) versus the novel one is calculated

Modeling autism in the laboratory reflects accepted views on the causes of the disease. Several inbred strains exist, which are characterized by behavioral and histopathological correlates of autism. BTBR mice are by far most commonly used [97, 99, 100]. These mice present with such core symptoms of autism as impaired sociability, repetitive and restricted behaviors, as well as impaired ultrasonic calls during neonatal age. Histopathologically, BTBR mice are characterized by missing corpus callosum, which reflects impaired long-range connectivity, typical of autism patients. Therefore, BTBR mice have generally good face and construct validity for modeling the disease. Other inbred strains with similar autism-like perturbations are represented by BALB/cByJ and C58/J mice [101]. Alongside inbred animals, multiple types of animals with targeted mutations are available, for example, Fmr1 knockout mice are used as a model of Fragile X syndrome [102]; Shank1 knockout mice [103] and oxytocin receptor knockout mice [104] reflect the implicated role of SHANK gene mutations and of oxytocin deficiency, respectively, in the mechanisms of autism. Finally, several models reflect the role of environmental factors in autism. The offspring of rats and mice which were treated with valproic acid during pregnancy presents with autism-like behavioral impairments [105]. Maternal immune activation (MIA) mimicked in pregnant rodents by either polyinosinic–polycytidylic acid (Poly I:C, a viral mimic) or LPS results in the offspring with impaired sociability, restricted and repetitive behaviors, and dysfunctional ultrasonic calls in neonates [98, 106].

Following the path of modeling autism proper, models of comorbidity between autism and epilepsy employ both genetic and environmental approaches. Dravet syndrome, which is caused by haploinsufficiency of the SCN1A gene encoding voltage-gated sodium channel NaV1.1, is characterized by recurrent intractable seizures and autism-like spectrum disorder [107, 108]. SCN1A (+/−) mice represent a model of Dravet syndrome with both good face validity (i.e., recurrent seizures and autism-like impairments) and construct validity [109]. Mice lacking adenomatous polyposis coli protein (APC) [110], as well as mice with triple repeat expansion of Aristaless-related homeobox (ARX) [111], present with infantile spasms during neonatal age and develop autism-like behavioral impairments later in life.

With regard to MIA (see above), the offspring of mice treated with either Poly I:C or LPS during pregnancy does not present with spontaneous seizures; however, these animals show increased propensity to MTLE upon the introduction of a second, otherwise inconsequential, postnatal hit to the hippocampus [112]. Signaling pathways involved in the development of autism alone versus autism+epilepsy prone phenotypes in the Poly I:C-induced MIA offspring have been identified: among many components of innate immunity induced by viral infection, an inflammatory cytokine interleukin-6 appears to be solely responsible for autism without increased propensity to epilepsy, whereas concurrent activation of interleukin-6 [113] and IL-1β is necessary and sufficient for producing autism+epilepsy prone phenotype [112].

Neonatal rats treated with the combination of LPS (to mimic Gram-negative infection), doxorubicin (an antineoplastic agent to produce diffuse brain damage), and p-chlorophenylalanine (a selective serotonin neurotoxin, thus used to mimic serotonin deficiency observed in patients with infantile spasms) produce infantile spasms, followed by severe cognitive and sociability deficits later in life [114]. This model therefore is deemed to reflect a combination of environmental influences (i.e., infection, nonspecific. and transmitter-specific neurotoxicity) as risk factors for the development of infantile spasms and autism.

Prerequisite Fitness Tests

Even before proceeding with the examination of comorbid disorders, it is important to establish that the animal's basic physiological functions and physical fitness are intact. Both excitotoxic neurodegeneration and recurrent seizures (even if infrequent and subtle) may affect the animal's ability to swim, maintain balance, consume food and fluids, taste, smell, see, etc. Therefore, the inclusion of basic fitness tests relevant to the employed behavioral assays should be a prerequisite for all such studies. Examples include Rotarod test to assess coordination and balance, swimming task with visible platform to assess appropriateness of MWM and FST, visual cliff test to assess visual perception, and quinine taste aversion test to assess anhedonia. Animals which fail in the basic tasks cannot be enrolled in behavioral studies of respective comorbidities. However, such prerequisite tests are not always performed, and thus the experiments proper may yield either false-negative or false-positive results.

Multiple Concurrent Comorbidities

Seventy years ago, Arturo Rosenblueth and Norbert Wiener described two types of scientific models – formal and material models [115]. Formal model approach, which is reductionist by nature, is most commonly employed for examining neurobehavioral comorbidities of epilepsy. In practical terms, it means that the experimental design focuses on one particular neurobehavioral disorder and its association with epilepsy, but either deliberately dismisses other variables or, when observing several concurrent disorders, does not regard them as dependent on, and connected to, one another. By virtue of being reductionist, such approach is far removed from real-life scenarios. As a result, clinical relevance of experimental findings, their proper interpretation, and applicability for preclinical trials, all become severely limited. Indeed, epilepsy patients often present with more than one neurobehavioral disorder (e.g., cognitive impairments frequently coexist with mood disorders, anxiety – with depression, etc.) [116–118]. Furthermore, epilepsy comorbidities may have complex relationships not only with seizures, but also among themselves, and thus are likely to influence each other's course and clinical manifestations.

On the upside, merely because an experimental study explores a specific comorbidity, it does not mean that this is the only neurobehavioral disorder that the animal has. On the contrary, as it has been discussed earlier, perturbations in mood, cognition, attention, social interaction, all have been reported within the framework of a single epilepsy model. The problem therefore is not a system-limitation proper, but the fact that typical experimental design simply ignores multiple neurobehavioral impairments in favor of a single disorder, which is the primary focus of the project.

Not only such simplification overlooks the complexity of real life, but it also can lead to faulty interpretations. Indeed, similar to clinical situations, in laboratory systems, coexisting neurobehavioral comorbidities may influence one another, and therefore may skew outcome measures (e.g., the presence of anxiety will likely affect the way epileptic animal performs in cognitive tasks, and the presence of depressive disorder – performance in attention tasks; Fig. 1.7).

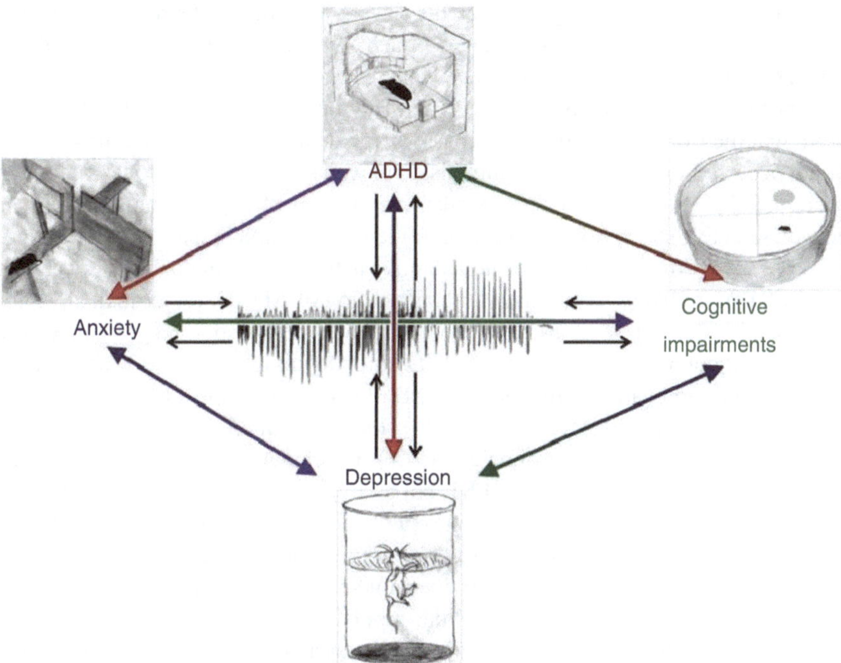

Fig. 1.7 Multiple interactions between seizures and neurobehavioral disorders in animal models of epilepsy comorbidities. Epilepsy proper (including both recurrent seizures and interictal events, such as interictal spikes) affects animal's behaviors and hence the performance in respective tests (examples given are lateralized reaction time task for ADHD, Morris water maze for spatial cognitive deficits, the forced swimming test for depression, and the elevated plus maze test for general anxiety). Furthermore, seizure–behavior interaction is often bidirectional (e.g., depression-associated suppression of serotonergic transmission or ADHD-associated compromised noradrenergic transmission may further exacerbate epilepsy). In addition, concurrent neurobehavioral disorders in animals with epilepsy interact with each other and thus may influence outcome measures. For example, the presence of depressive impairments may affect animal's performance in cognitive and memory tasks; the presence of ADHD may affect animal's ability to perform adequately in tests for depression, anxiety, etc. Such interactions emphasize the complexity of experimental animal systems and call for a systemic, rather than isolated, approach for studying neurobehavioral comorbidities of epilepsy in the laboratory

At the same time, when and if the interaction between different comorbidities is taken into account, animal studies may yield useful insights in human condition.

A case in point is comorbidity between depression and ADHD in animals with experimentally induced MTLE. Careful analysis of swimming behavior in epileptic rats during the FST has revealed complex behavioral patterns. While a majority of animals (approximately 2/3 in various experiments) show increased immobility time in the FST, thus pointing toward the presence of depressive disorder, a subset of epileptic rats exhibits increased active swimming, which was however different from the normal adaptive swimming behavior [76]. Unlike in normal rats, in the hyperactive epileptic animals, active swimming was nonadaptive: animals did not attempt to escape the tank, but rather trod water in the middle, without attempts to escape. On the surface, by merely looking at the passive-to-active swimming ratios, these animals could be categorized as the ones with reduced depressive behavior, with the conclusion that epilepsy may produce "antidepressant" effects [64, 65]. It turned out, however, that these animals, when examined in the LRTT, showed signs of hyperimpulsivity, that is, presented with symptoms of ADHD. Furthermore, looking at the biological substrate of passive versus nonadaptive swimming behaviors, it occurred that "depressed" animals displayed suppressed serotonergic tone in the raphe–PFC pathway, while "nonadaptive swimmers"/hyperimpulsive animals showed selective suppression of noradrenergic transmission in the LC–PFC ascending projection [76]. Therefore, the nonadaptive active swimming behavior observed in the FST more likely represented a manifestation of ADHD, rather than an "antidepressant" effect of seizures. This observation is also important, considering a well-known comorbidity between ADHD and depression, and the fact that in ADHD/depression patients, diagnosis of ADHD is often complicated as depression may mask symptoms of ADHD [119, 120]. Indeed, a small subpopulation of animals with chronic epilepsy (around 10–15 %), which acted only as depressed (i.e., having relevant impairments in the FST, but no hyperimpulsivity in the LRTT), was found to have compromised both raphe–PFC serotonergic transmission and LC–PFC noradrenergic transmission [76], thus suggesting that they may have ADHD alongside depression; only the former does not show up in behavioral tests [76].

The confounding contribution of hyperimpulsivity on animals' behavior can be extended to anxiety. As it has been mentioned earlier, several studies found that animals with MTLE present with reduced, rather than increased anxiety (with the interpretation that seizures may have anxiolytic effects) [17, 70]. However, the same animals that showed reduced anxiety in the EPMT presented with hyperimpulsivity in the LRTT [76]. It is thus more plausible that hyperimpulsivity impaired animals' ability to adequately perform in the EPMT for the examination of epilepsy-associated anxiety, thus rendering the test inappropriate under certain conditions.

These observations emphasize the importance of a broader approach in analyzing neurobehavioral disorders in animal epilepsy models. For example, it is not sufficient to merely claim that an animal has deficient spatial or object memory without objective confirmation of the substrate (e.g., dysfunction of place cells and neurodegeneration in perirhinal cortex, respectively). Indeed, if the same animal has depressive impairment (again correlating with the underlying neurobiological substrate, such as dysfunction of serotonergic transmission or dysregulation of the HPA axis), the lack of motivation may negatively affect its performance in memory tasks.

An effective way to improve clinical relevance of animal models of epilepsy comorbidities would be moving away from formal and toward material models. The latter attempts to account for many interconnected aspects and variables of an analyzed system, and to more closely approximate real-life situations (as Rosenblueth and Wiener put it, "the best material model for a cat is another, or preferably the same cat" [115]).

Material models are preferred even when only one single comorbidity is examined. On the one hand, this would allow accounting for whether and how comorbidities influence one another, and on the other hand, this may help explaining seemingly paradoxical findings by putting them in the context of a multifactorial system.

Acknowledgments The author wishes to thank Ms. Katherine Shin, Mr. Nathaniel Shin, and Mr. Don Shin for their creative assistance.

References

1. Baumans V. Science-based assessment of animal welfare: laboratory animals. Rev Sci Tech. 2005;24(2):503–13.
2. Scholz S, Sela E, Blaha L, Braunbeck T, Galay-Burgos M, Garcia-Franco M, et al. A European perspective on alternatives to animal testing for environmental hazard identification and risk assessment. Regul Toxicol Pharmacol. 2013;67(3):506–30.
3. van der Staay FJ, Arndt SS, Nordquist RE. Evaluation of animal models of neurobehavioral disorders. Behav Brain Funct. 2009;5:11.
4. Jentsch JD. Genetic vasopressin deficiency facilitates performance of a lateralized reaction-time task: altered attention and motor processes. J Neurosci. 2003;23(3):1066–71.
5. Jentsch JD. Impaired visuospatial divided attention in the spontaneously hypertensive rat. Behav Brain Res. 2005;157(2):323–30.
6. D'Hooge R, De Deyn PP. Applications of the Morris water maze in the study of learning and memory. Brain Res Brain Res Rev. 2001;36(1):60–90.
7. Brandeis R, Brandys Y, Yehuda S. The use of the Morris Water Maze in the study of memory and learning. Int J Neurosci. 1989;48(1–2):29–69.
8. Morris R. Developments of a water-maze procedure for studying spatial learning in the rat. J Neurosci Methods. 1984;11(1):47–60.
9. Bures J, Fenton AA, Kaminsky Y, Zinyuk L. Place cells and place navigation. Proc Natl Acad Sci U S A. 1997;94(1):343–50.
10. Fenton AA, Kao HY, Neymotin SA, Olypher A, Vayntrub Y, Lytton WW, et al. Unmasking the CA1 ensemble place code by exposures to small and large environments: more place cells and multiple, irregularly arranged, and expanded place fields in the larger space. J Neurosci. 2008;28(44):11250–62.
11. O'Keefe J, Nadel L. The hippocampus as a cognitive map. London: Oxford University Press; 1978. 584 p.
12. Dragoi G, Tonegawa S. Preplay of future place cell sequences by hippocampal cellular assemblies. Nature. 2011;469(7330):397–401.
13. Derdikman D, Moser MB. A dual role for hippocampal replay. Neuron. 2010;65(5):582–4.

14. Cavalheiro EA, Naffah-Mazzacoratti MG, Mello LE, Leite JP. The pilocarpine model of seizures. In: Pitkanen A, Schwartzkroin PA, Moshe SL, editors. Models of seizures and epilepsy. Amsterdam et al.: Elsevier; 2006. p. 433–48.
15. Dudek FE, Hellier JL, Williams PA, Ferraro DJ, Staley KJ. The course of cellular alterations associated with the development of spontaneous seizures after status epilepticus. Prog Brain Res. 2002;135:53–65.
16. Coulter DA, McIntyre DC, Loscher W. Animal models of limbic epilepsies: what can they tell us? Brain Pathol. 2002;12(2):240–56.
17. Detour J, Schroeder H, Desor D, Nehlig A. A 5-month period of epilepsy impairs spatial memory, decreases anxiety, but spares object recognition in the lithium-pilocarpine model in adult rats. Epilepsia. 2005;46(4):499–508.
18. Liu X, Muller RU, Huang LT, Kubie JL, Rotenberg A, Rivard B, et al. Seizure-induced changes in place cell physiology: relationship to spatial memory. J Neurosci. 2003;23(37):11505–15.
19. Titiz AS, Mahoney JM, Testorf ME, Holmes GL, Scott RC. Cognitive impairment in temporal lobe epilepsy: role of online and offline processing of single cell information. Hippocampus. 2014;24(9):1129–45.
20. Karnam HB, Zhou JL, Huang LT, Zhao Q, Shatskikh T, Holmes GL. Early life seizures cause long-standing impairment of the hippocampal map. Exp Neurol. 2009;217(2):378–87.
21. Zhou JL, Shatskikh TN, Liu X, Holmes GL. Impaired single cell firing and long-term potentiation parallels memory impairment following recurrent seizures. Eur J Neurosci. 2007;25(12):3667–77.
22. Dube CM, Zhou JL, Hamamura M, Zhao Q, Ring A, Abrahams J, et al. Cognitive dysfunction after experimental febrile seizures. Exp Neurol. 2009;215(1):167–77.
23. Ennaceur A, Delacour J. A new one-trial test for neurobiological studies of memory in rats. 1: behavioral data. Behav Brain Res. 1988;31(1):47–59.
24. Barker GR, Bird F, Alexander V, Warburton EC. Recognition memory for objects, place, and temporal order: a disconnection analysis of the role of the medial prefrontal cortex and perirhinal cortex. J Neurosci. 2007;27(11):2948–57.
25. Aggleton JP, Keen S, Warburton EC, Bussey TJ. Extensive cytotoxic lesions involving both the rhinal cortices and area TE impair recognition but spare spatial alternation in the rat. Brain Res Bull. 1997;43(3):279–87.
26. Hammond RS, Tull LE, Stackman RW. On the delay-dependent involvement of the hippocampus in object recognition memory. Neurobiol Learn Mem. 2004;82(1):26–34.
27. Brewster AL, Lugo JN, Patil VV, Lee WL, Qian Y, Vanegas F, et al. Rapamycin reverses status epilepticus-induced memory deficits and dendritic damage. PLoS One. 2013;8(3):e57808.
28. Zhou FW, Rani A, Martinez-Diaz H, Foster TC, Roper SN. Altered behavior in experimental cortical dysplasia. Epilepsia. 2011;52(12):2293–303.
29. Aniol VA, Ivanova-Dyatlova AY, Keren O, Guekht AB, Sarne Y, Gulyaeva NV. A single pentylenetetrazole-induced clonic-tonic seizure episode is accompanied by a slowly developing cognitive decline in rats. Epilepsy Behav. 2013;26(2):196–202.
30. Cornejo BJ, Mesches MH, Benke TA. A single early-life seizure impairs short-term memory but does not alter spatial learning, recognition memory, or anxiety. Epilepsy Behav. 2008;13(4):585–92.
31. Petit-Demouliere B, Chenu F, Bourin M. Forced swimming test in mice: a review of antidepressant activity. Psychopharmacology (Berl). 2005;177(3):245–55.
32. Porsolt RD, Le Pichon M, Jalfre M. Depression: a new animal model sensitive to antidepressant treatments. Nature. 1977;266(5604):730–2.
33. Overstreet DH, Wegener G. The flinders sensitive line rat model of depression – 25 years and still producing. Pharmacol Rev. 2013;65(1):143–55.
34. Richardson-Jones JW, Craige CP, Guiard BP, Stephen A, Metzger KL, Kung HF, et al. 5-HT1A autoreceptor levels determine vulnerability to stress and response to antidepressants. Neuron. 2010;65(1):40–52.

35. Song C, Leonard BE. The olfactory bulbectomised rat as a model of depression. Neurosci Biobehav Rev. 2005;29(4–5):627–47.
36. Willner P. Validity, reliability and utility of the chronic mild stress model of depression: a 10-year review and evaluation. Psychopharmacology (Berl). 1997;134(4):319–29.
37. Dantzer R. Cytokine, sickness behavior, and depression. Immunol Allergy Clin North Am. 2009;29(2):247–64.
38. Mazarati AM, Pineda E, Shin D, Tio D, Taylor AN, Sankar R. Comorbidity between epilepsy and depression: role of hippocampal interleukin-1beta. Neurobiol Dis. 2010;37(2): 461–7.
39. Cryan JF, Mombereau C, Vassout A. The tail suspension test as a model for assessing antidepressant activity: review of pharmacological and genetic studies in mice. Neurosci Biobehav Rev. 2005;29(4–5):571–625.
40. Willner P, Mitchell PJ. The validity of animal models of predisposition to depression. Behav Pharmacol. 2002;13(3):169–88.
41. Albert PR, Vahid-Ansari F, Luckhart C. Serotonin-prefrontal cortical circuitry in anxiety and depression phenotypes: pivotal role of pre- and post-synaptic 5-HT1A receptor expression. Front Behav Neurosci. 2014;8:199.
42. Hensler JG. Serotonergic modulation of the limbic system. Neurosci Biobehav Rev. 2006;30(2):203–14.
43. Aghajanian GK, Sprouse JS, Sheldon P, Rasmussen K. Electrophysiology of the central serotonin system: receptor subtypes and transducer mechanisms. Ann N Y Acad Sci. 1990;600:93–103; discussion.
44. Riad M, Garcia S, Watkins KC, Jodoin N, Doucet E, Langlois X, et al. Somatodendritic localization of 5-HT1A and preterminal axonal localization of 5-HT1B serotonin receptors in adult rat brain. J Comp Neurol. 2000;417(2):181–94.
45. Sprouse JS, Aghajanian GK. Electrophysiological responses of serotoninergic dorsal raphe neurons to 5-HT1A and 5-HT1B agonists. Synapse. 1987;1(1):3–9.
46. Warden MR, Selimbeyoglu A, Mirzabekov JJ, Lo M, Thompson KR, Kim SY, et al. A prefrontal cortex-brainstem neuronal projection that controls response to behavioural challenge. Nature. 2012;492(7429):428–32.
47. Herman JP, Cullinan WE. Neurocircuitry of stress: central control of the hypothalamo-pituitary-adrenocortical axis. Trends Neurosci. 1997;20(2):78–84.
48. Yu S, Holsboer F, Almeida OF. Neuronal actions of glucocorticoids: focus on depression. J Steroid Biochem Mol Biol. 2008;108(3–5):300–9.
49. Judge SJ, Ingram CD, Gartside SE. Moderate differences in circulating corticosterone alter receptor-mediated regulation of 5-hydroxytryptamine neuronal activity. J Psychopharmacol. 2004;18(4):475–83.
50. Chaouloff F. Serotonin, stress and corticoids. J Psychopharmacol. 2000;14(2):139–51.
51. Watson S, Gallagher P, Smith MS, Ferrier IN, Young AH. The DEX/CRH test-is it better than the DST? Psychoneuroendocrinology. 2006;31(7):889–94.
52. Mazarati A, Siddarth P, Baldwin RA, Shin D, Caplan R, Sankar R. Depression after status epilepticus: behavioural and biochemical deficits and effects of fluoxetine. Brain. 2008; 131(Pt 8):2071–83.
53. Mazarati A, Shin D, Auvin S, Caplan R, Sankar R. Kindling epileptogenesis in immature rats leads to persistent depressive behavior. Epilepsy Behav. 2007;10(3):377–83.
54. Mazarati AM, Shin D, Kwon YS, Bragin A, Pineda E, Tio D, et al. Elevated plasma corticosterone level and depressive behavior in experimental temporal lobe epilepsy. Neurobiol Dis. 2009;34(3):457–61.
55. Sarkisova K, van Luijtelaar G. The WAG/Rij strain: a genetic animal model of absence epilepsy with comorbidity of depression [corrected]. Prog Neuropsychopharmacol Biol Psychiatry. 2011;35(4):854–76.
56. Shaw FZ, Chuang SH, Shieh KR, Wang YJ. Depression- and anxiety-like behaviors of a rat model with absence epileptic discharges. Neuroscience. 2009;160(2):382–93.

57. Vezzani A, French J, Bartfai T, Baram TZ. The role of inflammation in epilepsy. Nat Rev Neurol. 2011;7(1):31–40.
58. Maroso M, Balosso S, Ravizza T, Liu J, Bianchi ME, Vezzani A. Interleukin-1 type 1 receptor/toll-like receptor signalling in epilepsy: the importance of IL-1beta and high-mobility group box 1. J Intern Med. 2011;270(4):319–26.
59. Viviani B, Bartesaghi S, Gardoni F, Vezzani A, Behrens MM, Bartfai T, et al. Interleukin-1beta enhances NMDA receptor-mediated intracellular calcium increase through activation of the Src family of kinases. J Neurosci. 2003;23(25):8692–700.
60. Krishnadas R, Cavanagh J. Depression: an inflammatory illness? J Neurol Neurosurg Psychiatr. 2012;83(5):495–502.
61. Bruce TO. Comorbid depression in rheumatoid arthritis: pathophysiology and clinical implications. Curr Psychiatr Rep. 2008;10(3):258–64.
62. Dantzer R, Kelley KW. Stress and immunity: an integrated view of relationships between the brain and the immune system. Life Sci. 1989;44(26):1995–2008.
63. Pineda EA, Hensler JG, Sankar R, Shin D, Burke TF, Mazarati AM. Interleukin-1beta causes fluoxetine resistance in an animal model of epilepsy-associated depression. Neurotherapeutics J Am Soc Exp Neurotherap. 2012;9(2):477–85.
64. Groticke I, Hoffmann K, Loscher W. Behavioral alterations in the pilocarpine model of temporal lobe epilepsy in mice. Exp Neurol. 2007;207(2):329–49.
65. Muller CJ, Groticke I, Bankstahl M, Loscher W. Behavioral and cognitive alterations, spontaneous seizures, and neuropathology developing after a pilocarpine-induced status epilepticus in C57BL/6 mice. Exp Neurol. 2009;219(1):284–97.
66. Carobrez AP, Bertoglio LJ. Ethological and temporal analyses of anxiety-like behavior: the elevated plus-maze model 20 years on. Neurosci Biobehav Rev. 2005;29(8):1193–205.
67. Pellow S, Chopin P, File SE, Briley M. Validation of open: closed arm entries in an elevated plus-maze as a measure of anxiety in the rat. J Neurosci Methods. 1985;14(3):149–67.
68. Helfer V, Deransart C, Marescaux C, Depaulis A. Amygdala kindling in the rat: anxiogenic-like consequences. Neuroscience. 1996;73(4):971–8.
69. Powell KL, Tang H, Ng C, Guillemain I, Dieuset G, Dezsi G, et al. Seizure expression, behavior, and brain morphology differences in colonies of Genetic Absence Epilepsy Rats from Strasbourg. Epilepsia. 2014;55(12):1959–68.
70. Jones NC, Kumar G, O'Brien TJ, Morris MJ, Rees SM, Salzberg MR. Anxiolytic effects of rapid amygdala kindling, and the influence of early life experience in rats. Behav Brain Res. 2009;203(1):81–7.
71. Robbins TW. The 5-choice serial reaction time task: behavioural pharmacology and functional neurochemistry. Psychopharmacology (Berl). 2002;163(3–4):362–80.
72. Russell VA. The nucleus accumbens motor-limbic interface of the spontaneously hypertensive rat as studied in vitro by the superfusion slice technique. Neurosci Biobehav Rev. 2000;24(1):133–6.
73. Aston-Jones G, Rajkowski J, Cohen J. Role of locus coeruleus in attention and behavioral flexibility. Biol Psychiatr. 1999;46(9):1309–20.
74. Viggiano D, Vallone D, Ruocco LA, Sadile AG. Behavioural, pharmacological, morpho-functional molecular studies reveal a hyperfunctioning mesocortical dopamine system in an animal model of attention deficit and hyperactivity disorder. Neurosci Biobehav Rev. 2003;27(7):683–9.
75. Reddy DS. Current pharmacotherapy of attention deficit hyperactivity disorder. Drugs Today. 2013;49(10):647–65.
76. Pineda E, Jentsch JD, Shin D, Griesbach G, Sankar R, Mazarati A. Behavioral impairments in rats with chronic epilepsy suggest comorbidity between epilepsy and attention deficit/hyperactivity disorder. Epilepsy Behav. 2014;31:267–75.
77. Kleen JK, Sesque A, Wu EX, Miller FA, Hernan AE, Holmes GL, et al. Early-life seizures produce lasting alterations in the structure and function of the prefrontal cortex. Epilepsy Behav. 2011;22(2):214–9.

78. Hernan AE, Alexander A, Jenks KR, Barry J, Lenck-Santini PP, Isaeva E, et al. Focal epileptiform activity in the prefrontal cortex is associated with long-term attention and sociability deficits. Neurobiol Dis. 2014;63:25–34.
79. Brisch R, Saniotis A, Wolf R, Bielau H, Bernstein HG, Steiner J, et al. The role of dopamine in schizophrenia from a neurobiological and evolutionary perspective: old fashioned, but still in vogue. Front Psychiatr. 2014;5:47.
80. Jones CA, Watson DJ, Fone KC. Animal models of schizophrenia. Br J Pharmacol. 2011;164(4):1162–94.
81. Braff DL, Geyer MA, Swerdlow NR. Human studies of prepulse inhibition of startle: normal subjects, patient groups, and pharmacological studies. Psychopharmacology (Berl). 2001; 156(2–3):234–58.
82. Swerdlow NR, Braff DL, Geyer MA. Animal models of deficient sensorimotor gating: what we know, what we think we know, and what we hope to know soon. Behav Pharmacol. 2000;11(3–4):185–204.
83. Geyer MA, Swerdlow NR, Mansbach RS, Braff DL. Startle response models of sensorimotor gating and habituation deficits in schizophrenia. Brain Res Bull. 1990;25(3):485–98.
84. Bertram E. The relevance of kindling for human epilepsy. Epilepsia. 2007;48 Suppl 2:65–74.
85. Morimoto K, Fahnestock M, Racine RJ. Kindling and status epilepticus models of epilepsy: rewiring the brain. Prog Neurobiol. 2004;73(1):1–60.
86. Sutula TP. Secondary epileptogenesis, kindling, and intractable epilepsy: a reappraisal from the perspective of neural plasticity. Int Rev Neurobiol. 2001;45:355–86.
87. Sutula TP, Ockuly J. Kindling, spontaneous seizures and the consequences of epilepsy: more than a model. In: Pitkanen A, Schwartzkroin PA, Moshe SL, editors. Models of seizures and epilepsy. Amsterdam et al.: Elsevier; 2006. p. 395–406.
88. Ma J, Leung LS. Kindled seizure in the prefrontal cortex activated behavioral hyperactivity and increase in accumbens gamma oscillations through the hippocampus. Behav Brain Res. 2010;206(1):68–77.
89. Howland JG, Hannesson DK, Barnes SJ, Phillips AG. Kindling of basolateral amygdala but not ventral hippocampus or perirhinal cortex disrupts sensorimotor gating in rats. Behav Brain Res. 2007;177(1):30–6.
90. Ma J, Leung LS. Schizophrenia-like behavioral changes after partial hippocampal kindling. Brain Res. 2004;997(1):111–8.
91. Koch M, Ebert U. Deficient sensorimotor gating following seizures in amygdala-kindled rats. Biol Psychiatry. 1998;44(4):290–7.
92. Labbate GP, da Silva AV, Barbosa-Silva RC. Effect of severe neonatal seizures on prepulse inhibition and hippocampal volume of rats tested in early adulthood. Neurosci Lett. 2014;568:62–6.
93. Jones NC, Martin S, Megatia I, Hakami T, Salzberg MR, Pinault D, et al. A genetic epilepsy rat model displays endophenotypes of psychosis. Neurobiol Dis. 2010;39(1):116–25.
94. Moy SS, Nadler JJ, Perez A, Barbaro RP, Johns JM, Magnuson TR, et al. Sociability and preference for social novelty in five inbred strains: an approach to assess autistic-like behavior in mice. Genes Brain Behav. 2004;3(5):287–302.
95. Nadler JJ, Moy SS, Dold G, Trang D, Simmons N, Perez A, et al. Automated apparatus for quantitation of social approach behaviors in mice. Genes Brain Behav. 2004;3(5):303–14.
96. Crawley JN. Chapter 9: Social behaviors. In: Craige CP, editor. What's wrong with my mouse? Hoboken: Wiley Interscience; 2007. p. 206–24.
97. Scattoni ML, Gandhy SU, Ricceri L, Crawley JN. Unusual repertoire of vocalizations in the BTBR T+tf/J mouse model of autism. PLoS One. 2008;3(8):e3067.
98. Malkova NV, Yu CZ, Hsiao EY, Moore MJ, Patterson PH. Maternal immune activation yields offspring displaying mouse versions of the three core symptoms of autism. Brain Behav Immun. 2012;26(4):607–16.
99. McFarlane HG, Kusek GK, Yang M, Phoenix JL, Bolivar VJ, Crawley JN. Autism-like behavioral phenotypes in BTBR T+tf/J mice. Genes Brain Behav. 2008;7(2):152–63.

100. Meyza KZ, Defensor EB, Jensen AL, Corley MJ, Pearson BL, Pobbe RL, et al. The BTBR T+ tf/J mouse model for autism spectrum disorders-in search of biomarkers. Behav Brain Res. 2013;251:25–34.
101. Teng BL, Nonneman RJ, Agster KL, Nikolova VD, Davis TT, Riddick NV, et al. Prosocial effects of oxytocin in two mouse models of autism spectrum disorders. Neuropharmacology. 2013;72:187–96.
102. Bernardet M, Crusio WE. Fmr1 KO mice as a possible model of autistic features. Sci World J. 2006;6:1164–76.
103. Wohr M, Roullet FI, Hung AY, Sheng M, Crawley JN. Communication impairments in mice lacking Shank1: reduced levels of ultrasonic vocalizations and scent marking behavior. PLoS One. 2011;6(6):e20631.
104. Pobbe RL, Pearson BL, Defensor EB, Bolivar VJ, Young 3rd WS, Lee HJ, et al. Oxytocin receptor knockout mice display deficits in the expression of autism-related behaviors. Horm Behav. 2012;61(3):436–44.
105. Roullet FI, Lai JK, Foster JA. In utero exposure to valproic acid and autism – a current review of clinical and animal studies. Neurotoxicol Teratol. 2013;36:47–56.
106. Le Belle JE, Sperry J, Ngo A, Ghochani Y, Laks DR, Lopez-Aranda M, et al. Maternal inflammation contributes to brain overgrowth and autism-associated behaviors through altered redox signaling in stem and progenitor cells. Stem Cell Rep. 2014;3(5):725–34.
107. Scheffer IE, Zhang YH, Jansen FE, Dibbens L. Dravet syndrome or genetic (generalized) epilepsy with febrile seizures plus? Brain Dev. 2009;31(5):394–400.
108. Li BM, Liu XR, Yi YH, Deng YH, Su T, Zou X, et al. Autism in Dravet syndrome: prevalence, features, and relationship to the clinical characteristics of epilepsy and mental retardation. Epilepsy Behav. 2011;21(3):291–5.
109. Han S, Tai C, Westenbroek RE, Yu FH, Cheah CS, Potter GB, et al. Autistic-like behaviour in Scn1a+/– mice and rescue by enhanced GABA-mediated neurotransmission. Nature. 2012;489(7416):385–90.
110. Mohn JL, Alexander J, Pirone A, Palka CD, Lee SY, Mebane L, et al. Adenomatous polyposis coli protein deletion leads to cognitive and autism-like disabilities. Mol Psychiatry. 2014;19(10):1133–42.
111. Sherr EH. The ARX, story (epilepsy, mental retardation, autism, and cerebral malformations): one gene leads to many phenotypes. Curr Op Ped. 2003;15(6):567–71.
112. Pineda E, Shin D, You SJ, Auvin S, Sankar R, Mazarati A. Maternal immune activation promotes hippocampal kindling epileptogenesis in mice. Ann Neurol. 2013;74(1):11–9.
113. Smith SE, Li J, Garbett K, Mirnics K, Patterson PH. Maternal immune activation alters fetal brain development through interleukin-6. J Neurosci. 2007;27(40):10695–702.
114. Scantlebury MH, Galanopoulou AS, Chudomelova L, Raffo E, Betancourth D, Moshe SL. A model of symptomatic infantile spasms syndrome. Neurobiol Dis. 2010;37(3):604–12.
115. Rosenblueth A, Wiener N. The role of models in science. Philos Sci. 1945;12(4):316–21.
116. Dulay MF, Schefft BK, Fargo JD, Privitera MD, Yeh HS. Severity of depressive symptoms, hippocampal sclerosis, auditory memory, and side of seizure focus in temporal lobe epilepsy. Epilepsy Behav. 2004;5(4):522–31.
117. Helmstaedter C, Sonntag-Dillender M, Hoppe C, Elger CE. Depressed mood and memory impairment in temporal lobe epilepsy as a function of focus lateralization and localization. Epilepsy Behav. 2004;5(5):696–701.
118. Kanner AM, Barry JJ, Gilliam F, Hermann B, Meador KJ. Depressive and anxiety disorders in epilepsy: do they differ in their potential to worsen common antiepileptic drug-related adverse events? Epilepsia. 2012;53(6):1104–8.
119. McIntosh D, Kutcher S, Binder C, Levitt A, Fallu A, Rosenbluth M. Adult ADHD and comorbid depression: a consensus-derived diagnostic algorithm for ADHD. Neuropsychiatr Dis Treat. 2009;5:137–50.
120. Daviss WB. A review of co-morbid depression in pediatric ADHD: etiology, phenomenology, and treatment. J Child Adolesc Psychopharmacol. 2008;18(6):565–71.

Chapter 2
Depression

Andres M. Kanner and Ramses Ribot

Abstract Depressive disorders are the most frequent psychiatric comorbidity in people with epilepsy, with lifetime prevalence rates of 30–35 %. Their prevalence is also higher than in the general population, and in particular, in people with poorly controlled seizures. In addition, there is a complex relation between epilepsy and depressive disorders, whereby not only are patients with epilepsy at greater risk of developing depressive disorders, but patients with primary depressive disorders are at greater risk of developing epilepsy. In this chapter, we review the salient aspects of depressive disorders in epilepsy that any clinician treating people with epilepsy must know.

Keywords Major Depressive Disorder • Postictal Depression • Ictal Depression • Suicidality • Antidepressant Drugs

Introduction

Depressive disorders are the most frequent psychiatric comorbidity in people with epilepsy (PWE), with lifetime prevalence rates ranging from 30 to 35 % [1]. Higher prevalence rates (21–33 %) have been also found in patients with persistent seizures when compared to seizure-free patients (4–6 %) in several cross-sectional studies [2–4]. Furthermore, a population-based survey of 185,000 households, which screened for lifetime symptoms of depression yielded higher rates in PWE than those with other chronic conditions [5], with at least one episode of symptoms of depression reported by 32 % of PWE, compared to 16 % of patients with asthma, 13 % with diabetes, and 8.6 % of healthy respondents. Similar prevalence rates have been identified in children and adolescents with epilepsy [6].

A.M. Kanner, MD, FANA (✉) • R. Ribot, MD
Epilepsy Section, Department of Neurology, Comprehensive Epilepsy Center, University of Miami, Miller School of Medicine, 1120 NW 14th Street, Room 1324, Miami, FL, 33136, USA

EEG Monitoring Unit, University of Miami Hospital, University of Miami, Miller School of Medicine, 1120 NW 14th Street, Room 1324, Miami, FL, 33136, USA
e-mail: a.kanner@med.miami.edu

M. Mula (ed.), *Neuropsychiatric Symptoms of Epilepsy*, Neuropsychiatric Symptoms of Neurological Disease, DOI 10.1007/978-3-319-22159-5_2

Despite this high occurrence of depressive disorders in PWE, they remain underrecognized and undertreated. For example, among 97 PWE with depressive episodes severe enough to warrant the use of psychotropic drugs, more than 1 year elapsed before 63 % of patients with spontaneous and 54 % with iatrogenic depressive episodes were referred for treatment [7], while in a study carried out in children with epilepsy, 26 % of 44 children with depressive symptoms had never been previously evaluated or treated [8].

Depressive disorders are easy to identify in a face-to-face evaluation in the office and/or with the use of self-report screening instruments that detect the presence of symptoms of depression (e.g., Beck Depression Inventory) and major depressive episodes (MDE)—its most severe clinical expression—e.g., Neurologic Depressive Disorders Inventory in Epilepsy (NDDI-E) [9, 10]. In fact, these instruments can be given to patients to fill out in the clinic while waiting to be seen by their doctor. What accounts for the failure to identify this comorbidity then? One of the principal reasons appears to be the failure by clinicians to enquire about them.

Depression and Epilepsy: A Complex Relation

The concept that depressive disorders are a "complication" of epilepsy reflects the common view of the relation between the two conditions. Yet, data from population-based studies have revealed a more complex, bidirectional relation between the two disorders, whereby not only are people with epilepsy at greater risk of developing depression, but people with depression are at greater risk of developing epilepsy. Furthermore, a lifetime history of depression has been associated with a worse response to the therapy of the seizure disorder.

Depression as a Risk Factor for Epilepsy

Twenty-six centuries ago, Hippocrates wrote*:* "melancholics become epileptics and epileptics melancholics," suggesting that "depression increases the risk of developing epilepsy and vice-versa." This observation has been confirmed with data from several population-based studies. Hesdorffer et al. (2012) used the United Kingdom's General Practice Research Database, which included a total of 3,773 PWE and 14,025 controls 10–60 years old [11]. Compared to controls, the incidence rate ratio of depression was significantly higher among patients who went on to develop epilepsy during the 3 years *preceding* its onset, and in PWE during the 3 years *that followed* the diagnosis of epilepsy; for suicidality, there was a higher incidence rate ratio during the 3 years before and 1 year after the diagnosis of epilepsy. In a second population-based study conducted in Sweden, investigators compared the risk of developing unprovoked seizures or epilepsy among patients who had been hospitalized for a psychiatric disorder ($n = 1885$) to a group of controls, matched for gender, and year of diagnosis selected randomly from the register of the Stockholm County population [12]. The age-adjusted odds ratio for development of unprovoked seizures was 2.5 for people with major depressive disorder, 2.7 for patients with bipolar illness, 2.7 for anxiety disorder, and 2.6 for suicide attempt. Three other population-based studies published between 1990 and 2006 demonstrated that patients with a depressive disorder had a threefold to sevenfold higher risk of developing epilepsy [13–15].

The above findings cannot be attributed to the use of psychotropic drugs despite the long-held belief that antidepressants have proconvulsive properties. In fact, there is increasing data from experimental animal studies that this type of medications may have a protective effect against the development of seizures. In humans with primary mood disorders, one study suggested that antidepressants (with two exceptions) may have a protective effect against seizure occurrence. This study investigated the incidence of seizures in patients with primary major depressive and obsessive compulsive disorders during the course of multicenter-randomized placebo-controlled trials of antidepressants carried out for regulatory purposes in the United States and compared the incidence of seizures between those randomized to a psychotropic drug and those given placebo [16]. Data for this study included Phase II and III multicenter-randomized placebo-controlled trials that encompassed 75,873 patients between 1985 and 2004. The trials included antidepressants of the tricyclic, selective serotonin-reuptake inhibitor (SSRI) and serotonin-norepinephrine reuptake inhibitor (SNRI) families as well as bupropion. The investigators found a *higher* incidence of seizures in patients randomized to clomipramine and bupropion in its immediate release form. On the other hand, subjects randomized to the other antidepressants were 52 % *less likely* (69 % less likely when excluding bupropion immediate release formulation) to develop seizures compared to those randomized to placebo. In addition, patients randomized to placebo were 19 times more likely to experience a seizure, compared to the expected incidence in the general population.

As indicated above, antidepressant drugs of the SSRI and tricyclic families have been found to display antiepileptic effects in several animal models of epilepsy [17], while reduction in seizure frequency has been suggested in three open trials with SSRIs in patients with treatment-resistant epilepsy [18–20]. In fact, the long-held belief of a proconvulsant effect of antidepressant drugs is derived from observations of seizures resulting from their use at very high doses (e.g., in overdoses). The only four antidepressants with known proconvulsant properties at therapeutic doses are amoxapine, clomipramine, maprotiline, and bupropion. Furthermore, since a psychiatric history has been associated with an increased risk of the development of epilepsy, seizure occurrence during their pharmacologic management may in fact reflect the “natural course” of the psychiatric disorder and not an iatrogenic effect of the psychotropic drug.

Common Pathogenic Operant in Depression and Epilepsy

The data presented in the preceding section might be explained by the existence of common neurobiologic pathogenic mechanisms shared by depressive disorders and epilepsy, including: (a) Neurotransmitter disturbances in the central nervous system such as serotonin, norepinephrine, dopamine, glutamate, and gamma-aminobutyric acid (GABA); (b) endocrine disturbances such as hyperactive hypothalamic-pituitary-adrenal axis, resulting in high serum concentrations of cortisol; (c) inflammatory mechanisms [21]. Here are some examples:

(a) Disturbances of serotonin transmission in the CNS have been identified as pivotal pathogenic mechanisms of completed suicide and of major depression and anxiety disorders. Similarly, decreased secretion of serotonin has been identified in several animal models of epilepsy, including the genetically epilepsy-prone rat [22], the pilocarpine status epilepticus model in the Wistar rat [23], as well as in cats, rabbits, and rhesus monkeys [22].
(b) High cortisol levels have become one of the neurobiologic markers of major depressive disorders. Likewise, several studies of animal models of epilepsy have confirmed that pretreatment with corticosterone accelerates the kindling process in rats [24].
(c) Glutamate is the excitatory neurotransmitter "par excellence," and high glutamatergic activity is the pivotal abnormality of the epileptogenic process. By the same token, patients with primary mood disorders have been found to have high glutamate in plasma and CSF, while magnetic resonance spectroscopy studies have revealed high cortical concentrations [25]. In addition, there are data suggesting that NMDA antagonists may exert an antidepressant effect in animal models of depression as well as in humans with treatment-resistant major depressive disorders [26]. In the case of GABA, an inhibitory neurotransmitter, which also plays a pivotal role in the epileptogenic process, low CSF, plasma, and intracortical concentrations have been found in humans with mood disorders [27].
(d) With respect to inflammatory disturbances, proinflammatory cytokines, in particular, interleukin-1β (IL-1β), have been found to play a pathogenic role in patients with mood disorders. In animal models of epilepsy, IL-1β has been shown to have proconvulsant properties, which are blocked by its naturally occurring antagonist (IL-1RA). The proconvulsant mechanism has been associated to a reduction in glutamate uptake by glial cells or an enhanced release of glutamate from these cells [28–30].

Clinical Manifestations

Depressive disorders in PWE may be identical to primary depressive disorders (e.g., major depression, bipolar disorder, cyclothymia, dysthymia, and minor depression). Nonetheless, in approximately 30–50 % of PWE, depressive episodes can present atypical clinical manifestations and fail to meet the diagnostic criteria included in the *Diagnostic and Statistical Manual of Mental Disorders-IV* (*DSM-IV*) [31]. They consist of symptoms of depression intermixed with brief euphoric mood, irritability, anxiety, paranoid feelings, and somatic symptoms (anergia, atypical pain, and insomnia). They tend to follow a chronic course with recurrent symptom-free periods. This type of depression had been recognized since the beginning of the twentieth century [32], and in later years was referred as "Interictal Dysphoric Disorder of Epilepsy" [33]. Yet, Mula et al. demonstrated that this form of depression was not specific to PWE [34].

Depressive and anxiety disorders often occur together. For example, in a study of 188 consecutive PWE, 31 met *DSM-IV* criteria of a current major depressive episode. Twenty-one of these patients had a mixed MDE and an anxiety disorder [35]. Recognition of such comorbidity is of the essence, as failure to target the anxiety symptomatology in the treatment plan can result in the recurrence of the depressive disorder. In addition, comorbid depressive and anxiety disorders in patients with and without epilepsy are associated with a worse course of the depressive disorder and a worse quality of life than in patients with only the depressive disorder [35].

Clinical Manifestations of Depressive Episodes Particular to Epilepsy

Depressive episodes and symptoms of depression in PWE can follow a temporal relation to the occurrence of seizures and present before (pre-ictal), as an expression of the ictus (ictal), after the seizure (postictal), or may be independent of the timing of the seizure occurrence (interictal). In addition, depressive episodes can be the expression of a "para-ictal" disorder, which occurs upon the sudden remission of seizures in patients with treatment-resistant epilepsy.

Pre-ictal symptoms of depression and depressive episodes typically present as a dysphoric mood in which the prodromal symptoms may extend for hours or even 1–3 days prior to the onset of a seizure. This was exemplified by Blanchet and Frommer [36] who assessed mood changes during the course of 56 days in 27 PWE, who rated their mood on a daily basis. Mood ratings pointed to a dysphoric state 3 days prior to a seizure in 22 (81 %) patients. This change in mood was greatest during the 24 h preceding the seizure. Patients or parents of children with epilepsy often report that dysphoric symptoms completely resolve the day after the ictus.

Ictal symptoms of depression are the clinical expression of a focal seizure without loss of consciousness in which the depressive symptoms are the sole (or predominant) semiology and in which the symptomatogenic zone involves limbic structures, in particular, in mesial temporal regions. The actual prevalence of ictal symptoms of depression is yet to be established in larger studies. Symptoms of depression ranked second after symptoms of anxiety/fear as the most common type of ictal affect in one study [37]. This presentation occurred in 21 % of 100 PWE who reported auras consisting of psychiatric symptoms [38, 39]. The most frequent symptoms include feelings of anhedonia, guilt, and suicidal ideation. Such mood changes are typically brief, stereotypical, occur out of context, and are associated with other ictal phenomena. More typically, however, ictal symptoms of depression are followed by an alteration of consciousness, as the ictus evolves from a focal seizure without loss of consciousness to a seizure with loss of consciousness.

Postictal symptoms of depression and depressive episodes have been recognized for decades, but have been investigated in a systematic manner in only one study [40]. Postictal symptoms of depression were identified in 43 of 100 consecutive patients with refractory partial seizure disorders. These symptoms occurred after in more than 50 % of seizures, and their duration ranged from 0.5 to 108 h, with a median duration of 24 h. However, postictal symptoms of depression can outlast the ictus for up to 2 weeks.

Of note, PWE may experience interictal depressive episodes with postictal exacerbation in severity of these symptoms [40]. Furthermore, in patients with interictal depressive episodes in remission, postictal symptoms of depression can occur despite the presence of adequate doses of antidepressant medication (Kanner AM, unpublished data). This observation suggests a different pathogenic mechanism operant in postictal and interictal depressive symptoms.

Depressive Episodes as an Expression of a Para-Ictal Disorder

The sudden remission of epileptic seizures in patients with treatment-resistant epilepsy can be followed by the occurrence of psychopathology presenting as a MDE or a psychotic episode. This phenomenon has been known as "forced normalization" [41], because the EEG recordings of these patients failed to reveal any epileptiform activity concurrent with the psychopathology. In later years, this phenomenon was referred as "alternating psychopathology" [42]. While this phenomenon is more often identified in the setting of a psychotic episode, depressive episodes are more frequent but often go unrecognized. Remission and/or improvement of psychiatric symptoms follow the recurrence of seizures, though symptomatic treatment can at times be effective.

Depressive Episodes as an Iatrogenic Effect

Caused by Antiepileptic Drugs

All antiepileptic drugs (AEDs) can potentially cause psychiatric symptoms, particularly when used at high doses [43]. However, AEDs with GABAergic properties, primarily phenobarbital, primidone, the benzodiazepines, tiagabine, and vigabatrin, are more likely to cause depression [44–47]. Other AEDs that have been associated with the development of depression include felbamate, topiramate, levetiracetam, zonisamide and more recently perampanel [7, 48, 49]. Psychiatric adverse events are more likely to be identified in patients susceptible to develop psychiatric disorders, such as those with a past psychiatric history or with a family psychiatric history [50]. Accordingly, obtaining a good personal (current and past) and family psychiatric history is of the essence to identify patients that may be at risk of developing iatrogenic depressive episodes.

The addition of AEDs with mood-stabilizing properties, such as carbamazepine, valproic acid, and lamotrigine, can occasionally cause depressive episodes, albeit with a significantly lower frequency than other AEDs. More often than not, these AEDs are associated with the occurrence of depression *upon their discontinuation* in patients with a prior history of depression or panic disorder, which had been kept in remission by these AEDs [51].

The Food and Drug Administration (FDA) announced in 2008 that it would require manufacturers of AEDs to add a warning to their labeling indicating that the use of these drugs increases the risk by a twofold of suicidal thoughts and behaviors [52]. The decision was based on an FDA meta-analysis of 199 clinical multicenter-randomized, double-blind placebo-controlled and parallel trials of 11 AEDs. The FDA data were carefully reviewed by a task force of the American Epilepsy Society, which identified several methodological flaws including: (1) grouping of all AEDs (which have different mechanisms of action) into one class; (2) basing the recommendation on spontaneously reported adverse events, rather than on systematically acquired data [53]. Furthermore, attempts to replicate the data from the FDA meta-analysis in five large studies yielded contradictory findings. Thus, it is possible that certain *but not every* AED can cause psychiatric adverse events that can lead to suicidal ideation and behavior, but this is likely to occur in patients with a predisposition for psychiatric illness. Accordingly, before starting an AED, like topiramate, zonisamide, vigabatrin, barbiturates, or levetiracetam, it is essential to inquire about a prior personal or psychiatric history.

Depression Following Epilepsy Surgery

It is not unusual to see "mood lability" within the initial 6 weeks to 3 months after surgery. Often, these symptoms subside, but in up to 30 % of patients, major depressive episodes may become apparent within the first 6 months [54]. Characteristically, symptoms vary from mild to very severe, including suicidal attempts. In most instances, these depressive disorders respond readily to pharmacologic treatment with antidepressant drugs (see below).

Patients with a prior history of depression are at greater risk. A German study found that patients with personality disorders are at higher risk of suffering from postoperative psychiatric complications, as compared with patients with other preoperative psychiatric conditions (such as depression) or with patients with no preoperative psychiatric diagnosis whatsoever [55]. While some studies have not found a relation between depression and the postsurgical control of seizures, others have [54]. All patients undergoing epilepsy surgery, therefore, should be advised of this potential complication, *prior to surgery*.

Impact of Depressive Disorders in PWE

Impact on Mortality Risk

Depressive disorders have a negative impact on the mortality of PWE. A recent population-based study from Sweden found premature mortality to be 11-fold higher in PWE than controls, with the mean age of death being at 34 years of age [56]. Close to 16 % of all deaths were attributed to external causes, which included death by suicide and accidents (in a motor vehicle, drug poisoning, falls, drowning, assault, and others). In fact, PWE had a greater than threefold higher risk of premature death from these causes than the control groups. Furthermore, among PWE who died from external causes, comorbid psychiatric disorders were identified in 75.2 %, the majority of which included depression and substance misuse. It is worth noticing that the lifetime prevalence of psychiatric disorders in PWE was 40.7 %, compared to 10.3 % in controls. In a separate population-based study conducted in Denmark, the presence of mood disorders increased the risk of suicide by 32-fold [57]. In a review of 21 studies, suicide accounted for 12 % of all deaths in PWE [58].

Impact on the Management of the Seizure Disorder

Worse Tolerance of Antiepileptic Drugs

The concomitant presence of MDE in PWE is associated with the endorsement of more severe adverse events and worse tolerability of AEDs [59, 60]. The study by Kanner et al. [60] demonstrated that the worse tolerance was not limited to MDE, but was of comparable magnitude in patients with less severe forms of depression such as subsyndromic depressive episodes. Tolerance was also worse among PWE who experienced anxiety disorders in addition to MDE [17].

Worse Response to the Pharmacologic and Surgical Treatment of the Seizure Disorder

Two studies have suggested a worse response of the seizure disorder to pharmacotherapy with AEDs. In a prospective study of 138 patients with new onset epilepsy, those with symptoms of depression and anxiety at the time of diagnosis of epilepsy were significantly less likely to be seizure-free at the 1-year follow-up evaluation [61]. The second study included 780 patients with new onset epilepsy; individuals with a history of psychiatric disorders preceding the onset of the epilepsy, and particularly depression, were twofold less likely to be seizure-free with AEDs, after a median follow-up period of 79 months, compared to patients without a psychiatric history [62].

Likewise, a lifetime history of psychiatric disorders and in particular depression has been associated with a worse postsurgical seizure outcome following an anterotemporal lobectomy. For example, in a study of 100 consecutive patients, only 12 % of patients who reached complete seizure freedom after surgery (mean follow-up period 8.3 ± 3.3 years) had a lifetime history of depression, while such history was identified in 67 % of patients who had auras, but no complex partial and/or secondarily generalized tonic-clonic seizures, and in 79 % of patients with persistent disabling seizures [63]. These data were confirmed in two other studies that included patients with mesial temporal sclerosis (MTS): in one study of 280 patients, those with a preoperative psychiatric diagnosis (38 % of the entire cohort) were significantly less likely to remain seizure-free [64], while in the second study of 115 patients, a presurgical history of major depressive disorders was a risk factor for persistent postsurgical seizures [65].

Impact on the Quality of Life

Several studies of patients with treatment-resistant epilepsy demonstrated that depressive disorders are strong predictors of poor quality of life, even after controlling for seizure frequency, severity, and other psychosocial variables [35, 66–69]. In one of these studies, depression was significantly associated with poor quality of life, independently of seizure type, but seizure freedom for the last 3 months improved the quality-of-life ratings [66]. Of note, comorbid depressive and anxiety disorders have a worse impact on the quality of life of PWE than the depressive or anxiety disorders occurring alone, and particularly when a major depressive episode is comorbid with more than one anxiety disorder [35].

Impact on Health-Care Costs

Patients with untreated depression were found to use significantly more health resources of all types, independent of seizure type or duration [70]. Mild-to-moderate depression was associated with a twofold increase in medical visits compared with nondepressed controls, while severe depression was associated with a fourfold increase. This could be in part due to the above reported increased risk of poor tolerance of AEDs and worse response to pharmacological and surgical treatments. The presence and severity of depression was also a predictor of lower disability scores, irrespective of the duration of the seizure disorder.

Identification of Depressive and Anxiety Disorders in the Outpatient Clinic

Providing clinicians with user-friendly self-reported screening instruments of depressive and anxiety disorders is probably the best solution to facilitate their identification in PWE in a busy outpatient clinic. Several self-reported instruments have been developed to identify and quantify the severity of symptoms of depression and anxiety; these include the Beck Depression Inventory (BDI-II) [9] and the Center of Epidemiologic Studies—Depression (CES-D), which have been validated for PWE [71]. Clinicians can use the Neurological Disorders Depression Inventory for Epilepsy, a six-item instrument which was validated to screen for MDE in PWE specifically [10]. This instrument has the advantage of having been constructed specifically to minimize confounding symptoms that plague other instruments, such as somatic symptoms, which may also be the expression of adverse events of AEDs, or of cognitive problems associated with epilepsy. Patients can fill out the instrument in less than 3 min. A score of >15 is suggestive of a MDE. These instruments are *not diagnostic* by themselves, and a subsequent more detailed evaluation is necessary. Once the diagnosis of a mood disorder has been confirmed with a psychiatric evaluation, the self-rating screening instruments can be given at every visit to document symptom remission.

As already discussed, comorbid anxiety disorders or symptoms of anxiety are a common occurrence, and their identification and effective treatment is of the essence. The seven-item Patient's Health Questionnaire Generalized Anxiety Disorder–7 (GAD-7) is an ideal self-rating instrument to screen for generalized anxiety disorder (GAD) [72]. It takes 2–3 min for patients to complete; a score of >10 is suggestive of a GAD.

Treatment of Depressive Disorders in PWE

The management of depressive disorders consists of pharmacotherapy and/or psychotherapy, and is similar to the one provided to patients with primary depressive disorders. Given the relatively high comorbid occurrence of depressive and anxiety disorders, we will include treatment strategies that encompass the management of the latter.

With respect to pharmacologic therapy, the selective serotonin-reuptake inhibitor (SSRI) and serotonin-norepinephrine reuptake inhibitors (SNRI) have become the first line of treatment of primary depressive and anxiety disorders, and have replaced the tricyclic antidepressants (TCA) because of their lower toxicity. To date, there are no published double-blind placebo-controlled trials that have tested the efficacy of these two families of antidepressants in PWE. In their absence, two consensus statements have been published outlining pharmacological and psychotherapeutic approaches for PWE with mood and anxiety disorders using data from the management of primary mood disorders and from open trials with SSRIs in PWE [73, 74]. Both documents recommend the use of these antidepressant drugs in PWE. However, their use remains empirical given the absence of controlled trials.

Before starting pharmacotherapy, it is important to determine if the depressive episodes resulted from an iatrogenic process, which may result from the following:

- The introduction of an AED with negative psychotropic properties (e.g., barbiturates, topiramate, benzodiazepines, zonisamide, vigabatrin, levetiracetam), particularly in PWE at risk of developing psychiatric disorders (e.g., patients with a prior psychiatric history and/or family history).

- The discontinuation of an AED with mood-stabilizing properties (e.g., carbamazepine, oxcarbazepine, valproic acid, lamotrigine) in patients with a personal (or family) history of mood disorder, which was in remission and/or masked by one of these AEDs.
- The addition of an AED with enzyme-inducing properties (carbamazepine, phenytoin, barbiturates) in PWE taking an SSRI, which had resulted in remission of the depressive episode. In these patients, these AEDs will increase the clearance of the antidepressant, lower its serum concentration, and limit its efficacy.

Another cautionary consideration before starting an antidepressant drug is to rule out a history of a manic or hypomanic episode that may be suggestive of a bipolar disorder, as these drugs can potentially trigger a manic or hypomanic episode in the short term, while it may worsen the course of the bipolar disorder in the long term, particularly in the case of rapid-cycling bipolar disease. In such cases, an AED with mood-stabilizing and antidepressant properties such as lamotrigine, carbamazepine, oxcarbazepine, and valproic acid should be considered.

Pharmacokinetic Interaction Between Antidepressant Drugs and AEDs

Most antidepressant drugs are metabolized in the liver, and their metabolism is accelerated in the presence of AEDs with enzyme-inducing properties (e.g., carbamazepine, phenytoin, barbiturates, and oxcarbazepine at doses of >900 mg/day and topiramate at doses >200 mg/day). This pharmacokinetic effect is not observed with the new AEDs, gabapentin, lamotrigine, tiagabine, levetiracetam, zonisamide, pregabalin, vigabatrin, and ezogabine.

Conversely, some of the SSRIs are inhibitors of one or more isoenzymes of the Cytochrome P450 (CYP 450) system. These antidepressants include fluoxetine, paroxetine, fluvoxamine, and, to a lesser degree, sertraline [75–77]. Escitalopram and citalopram, on the other hand, do not have pharmacokinetic interactions with AEDs. Sertraline has been shown rarely to increase phenytoin levels, and this is thought to be associated with displacement by tight protein binding, or by inhibition of the CYP 450 system [78].

Choice of Antidepressant

The criteria used to choose an antidepressant must be based on the following criteria:

1. The type of depressive episode: retarded versus agitated. In the former, SNRIs may be more effective, given their noradrenergic effect. In the latter, SSRIs should be considered first.

2. Depending on the presence of comorbid anxiety disorder(s) and their type. In such cases, the clinician must identify the SSRI or SNRI, which can cover the symptoms of both conditions.
3. The adverse event profile of the antidepressant drug, in particular, those drugs with a propensity to cause weight gain.

Dosing of the antidepressant must be the same as in the treatment of primary mood disorders. The aim is to achieve complete symptom remission, as persistence of symptoms is associated with an increased risk of recurrence of a MDE. Furthermore, clinicians must adjust the dose in the presence of enzyme-inducing AEDs, by increasing it by 30 %.

Are AEDs with Mood-Stabilizing Properties Sufficient to Treat Depressive Disorders?

The use of AEDs in primary mood disorders has become common practice, particularly in patients with bipolar disorders in a manic state. Lamotrigine has been used as an augmenting agent to concomitant antidepressants in refractory depressive disorders. Most AEDs with positive psychotropic properties have mood-stabilizing and antimanic properties (e.g., carbamazepine, oxcarbazepine, valproic acid), while lamotrigine is the only one which has been found to yield mood-stabilizing and antidepressant properties in patients with depressive episodes occurring in the context of bipolar disorders. Pregabalin has been found to yield anxiolytic properties, and has an indication for the treatment of generalized anxiety disorders in Europe, but not in the United States, while gabapentin has been found to be effective for the treatment of social phobia.

To date, no study has suggested that an AED with positive psychotropic properties alone can cause the remission of a MDE in PWE. As indicated earlier, discontinuation of these AEDs has been associated with the development of depressive and/or anxiety disorders in patients at risk of depressive and/or anxiety disorders. These observations imply a mood-stabilizing role of these drugs, but not an antidepressant effect per se.

Psychotherapy

In addition to pharmacological intervention, the value of psychotherapy for the treatment of depression in PWE should not be overlooked. Counseling and psychotherapy, in particular, cognitive behavior therapy, can be useful in helping the patient deal with the stressors and limitations of living with epilepsy. In addition, cognitive behavior therapy has been found to be an effective treatment modality for depressive and anxiety disorders in patients with primary mood and anxiety disorders as well as in PWE. Often, a combination of CBT and pharmacotherapy is necessary.

Other Types of Psychiatric Treatments

Electroconvulsive therapy (ECT) is *not* contraindicated in depressed PWE [79, 80]. It is a well-tolerated treatment and is worth considering in PWE with very severe depression that fails to respond to antidepressant drugs. Furthermore, there is no evidence that ECT increases the risk of epilepsy [81], and, in fact, it has been used in the treatment of refractory status epilepticus.

Vagal nerve stimulation (VNS) is used as an adjunctive treatment for epilepsy and has also shown long-term mood effects [82]. The impact of other neurostimulation interventions, such as deep brain stimulation (DBS) or transcranial magnetic stimulation, on mood in PWE has not been studied in controlled trials.

Concluding Remarks

We reviewed data that highlight the importance of an early recognition and treatment of depressive disorders in PWE. Physicians who treat PWE do not have any further excuse for ignoring the existence of this psychiatric comorbidity, as it has a negative impact on the response to pharmacologic treatment of the seizure disorders, the quality of life of PWE, and the associated increased risk of death by external causes which can be prevented or at least minimized with a timely identification and intervention. The long-held belief that antidepressant drugs lower the seizure threshold does not appear to apply to the use of SSRIs and SNRIs at therapeutic doses.

References

1. Tellez-Zenteno JF, Patten SB, Jette N, Williams J, Wiebe S. Psychiatric comorbidity in epilepsy: a population-based analysis. Epilepsia. 2007;48(12):2336–44.
2. Edeh J, Toone B. Relationship between interictal psychopathology and the type of epilepsy. Results of a survey in general practice. Br J Psychiatry. 1987;151:95–101.
3. Jacoby A, Baker GA, Steen N, Potts P, Chadwick DW. The clinical course of epilepsy and its psychosocial correlates: findings from a U.K. Community study. Epilepsia. 1996;37(2):148–61.
4. O'Donoghue MF, Goodridge DM, Redhead K, Sander JW, Duncan JS. Assessing the psychosocial consequences of epilepsy: a community-based study. Br J Gen Pract. 1999;49(440):211–4.
5. Ettinger A, Reed M, Cramer J. Depression and comorbidity in community-based patients with epilepsy or asthma. Neurology. 2004;63(6):1008–14.
6. Caplan R, Siddarth P, Gurbani S, Hanson R, Sankar R, Shields WD. Depression and anxiety disorders in pediatric epilepsy. Epilepsia. 2005;46(5):720–30.
7. Kanner AM, Kozak AM, Frey M. The use of sertraline in patients with epilepsy: is it safe? Epilepsy Behav. 2000;1(2):100–5.
8. Ettinger AB, Weisbrot DM, Nolan EE, Gadow KD, Vitale SA, Andriola MR, et al. Symptoms of depression and anxiety in pediatric epilepsy patients. Epilepsia. 1998;39(6):595–9.

9. Beck AT, Ward CH, Mendelson M, Mock J, Erbaugh J. An inventory for measuring depression. Arch Gen Psychiatry. 1961;4:561–71.
10. Gilliam FG, Barry JJ, Hermann BP, Meador KJ, Vahle V, Kanner AM. Rapid detection of major depression in epilepsy: a multicentre study. Lancet Neurol. 2006;5(5):399–405.
11. Hesdorffer DC, Ishihara L, Mynepalli L, Webb DJ, Weil J, Hauser WA. Epilepsy, suicidality, and psychiatric disorders: a bidirectional association. Ann Neurol. 2012;72:184–91.
12. Adelow C, Anderson T, Ahlbom A, Tomson T. Hospitalization for psychiatric disorders before and after onset of unprovoked seizures/epilepsy. Neurology. 2012;78:396–401.
13. Forsgren L, Nystrom L. An incident case-referent study of epileptic seizures in adults. Epilepsy Res. 1990;6(1):66–81.
14. Dc H, Hauser WA, Annegers JF, Cascino G. Major depression is a risk factor for seizures in older adults. Ann Neurol. 2000;47(2):246–9.
15. Hesdorffer DC, Hauser WA, Olafsson E, Ludvigsson P, Kjartansson O. Depression and suicide attempt as risk factors for incident unprovoked seizures. Ann Neurol. 2006;59(1):35–41.
16. Alper K, Schwartz KA, Kolts RL, Khan A. Seizure incidence in psychopharmacological clinical trials: an analysis of Food and Drug Administration (FDA) summary basis of approval reports. Biol Psychiatry. 2007;62(4):345–54.
17. Kanner AM. Depression and epilepsy: how can we explain their bidirectional relation? Epilepsia. 2011;52 Suppl 1:21–7.
18. Specchio LM, Iudice A, Specchio N, La Neve A, Spinelli A, Galli R, et al. Citalopram as treatment of depression in patients with epilepsy. Clin Neuropharmacol. 2004;27(3):133–6.
19. Favale E, Rubino V, Mainardi P, Lunardi G, Albano C. The anticonvulsant effect of fluoxetine in humans. Neurology. 1995;45:1926.
20. Favale E, Audenino D, Cocito L, Albano C. The anticonvulsant effect of citalopram as an indirect evidence of serotonergic impairment in human epileptogenesis. Seizure. 2003;12(5):316–8.
21. Kanner AM. Can neurobiological pathogenic mechanisms of depression facilitate the development of seizure disorders? Lancet Neurol. 2012;11(12):1093–102.
22. Jobe PC. Affective disorder and epilepsy comorbidity in the genetically epilepsy prone-rat (GEPR). In: Gilliam FG, Kanner AM, Sheline YI, editors. Depression and brain dysfunction. London: Taylor & Francis; 2006. p. 121–57.
23. Mazarati AM, Siddarth P, Baldwin RA, et al. Depression after status epilepticus: behavioural and biochemical deficits and effects of fluoxetine. Brain. 2008;131:2071–83.
24. Kumar G, Couper A, O'Brien TJ, Salzberg MR, Jones NC, Rees SM, Morris MJ. The acceleration of amygdala kindling epileptogenesis by chronic low-dose corticosterone involves both mineralocorticoid and glucocorticoid receptors. Psychoneuroendocrinology. 2007;32(7):834–42.
25. Sanacora G, Mason GF, Rothman DL, Krystal JH. Increased occipital cortex GABA concentrations in depressed patients after therapy with selective serotonin reuptake inhibitors. Am J Psychiatry. 2002;159:663–5.
26. Zarate Jr CA, Singh JB, Carlson PJ, et al. A randomized trial of an N-methyl-D-aspartate antagonist in treatment-resistant major depression. Arch Gen Psychiatry. 2006;63(8):856–64.
27. Rajkowska G, O'Dwyer G, Teleki Z, Stockmeier CA, Miguel-Hidalgo JJ. GABAergic neurons immunoreactive for calcium binding proteins are reduced in the prefrontal cortex in major depression. Neuropsychopharmacology. 2007;32:471–82.
28. Vezzani A, Conti M, De Luigi A, Ravizza T, Moneta D, Marchesi F, De Simoni MG. Interleukin-1beta immunoreactivity and microglia are enhanced in the rat hippocampus by focal kainate application: functional evidence for enhancement of electrographic seizures. J Neurosci. 1999;19:5054–65.
29. Vezzani A, Moneta D, Conti M, Richichi C, Ravizza T, De Luigi A, et al. Powerful anticonvulsant action of IL-1 receptor antagonist on intracerebral injection and astrocytic overexpression in mice. Proc Natl Acad Sci U S A. 2000;97:11534–9.
30. Vezzani A, Balosso S, Ravizza T. The role of cytokines in the pathophysiology of epilepsy. Brain Behav Immun. 2008;22:797–803.

31. Mendez MF, Cummings JL, Benson DF. Depression in epilepsy. Significance and phenomenology. Arch Neurol. 1986;43(8):766–70.
32. Kraepelin E. Psychiatrie, vol. 3. Leipzig: Barth; 1923.
33. Blumer D, Zielinksi J. Pharmacologic treatment of psychiatric disorders associated with epilepsy. J Epilepsy. 1988;1:135–50.
34. Mula M, Jauch R, Cavanna A, Collimedaglia L, Barbagli D, Gaus V, et al. Clinical and psychopathological definition of the interictal dysphoric disorder of epilepsy. Epilepsia. 2008;49(4):650–6.
35. Kanner AM, Barry JJ, Gilliam F, Hermann B, Meador KJ. Anxiety disorders, subsyndromic depressive episodes, and major depressive episodes: do they differ on their impact on the quality of life of patients with epilepsy? Epilepsia. 2010;51(7):1152–8.
36. Blanchet P, Frommer GP. Mood change preceding epileptic seizures. J Nerv Ment Dis. 1986;174(8):471–6.
37. Williams D. The structure of emotions reflected in epileptic experiences. Brain. 1956;79(1):29–67.
38. Daly D. Ictal affect. Am J Psychiatry. 1958;115(2):97–108.
39. Weil A. Depressive reactions associated with temporal lobe uncinate seizures. J Nerv Ment Dis. 1955;121:505–10.
40. Kanner AM, Soto A, Gross-Kanner H. Prevalence and clinical characteristics of postictal psychiatric symptoms in partial epilepsy. Neurology. 2004;62(5):708–13.
41. Landoldt H. Some clinical electroencephalographical correlations in epileptic psychosis (twilight states). Electroencephalogr Clin Neurophysiol. 1953;5:121 (abstract).
42. Savard G, Andermann LF, Reutens D, Andermann F. Epilepsy, surgical treatment and postoperative psychiatric complications: A re-evaluation of the evidence. In: Trimble M, Schmitz B, editors. Forced normalization and alternative psychosis of epilepsy. Petersfield: Writson Biomedical Publishing Ltd.; 1998. p. 179–92.
43. McConnell H, Duncan D. Chapter 10: Treatment of psychiatric comorbidity in epilepsy. In: McConnell H, Snyder P, editors. Psychiatric comorbidity in epilepsy. Washington: American Psychiatric Press; 1998. p. 245–361.
44. Barabas G, Matthews WS. Barbiturate anticonvulsants as a cause of severe depression. Pediatrics. 1988;82(2):284–5.
45. Brent DA, Crumrine PK, Varma RR, Allan M, Allman C. Phenobarbital treatment and major depressive disorder in children with epilepsy. Pediatrics. 1987;80(6):909–17.
46. Ferrari M, Barabas G, Matthews WS. Psychologic and behavioral disturbance among epileptic children treated with barbiturate anticonvulsants. Am J Psychiatry. 1983;140(1):112–3.
47. Ring HA, Reynolds EH. Vigabatrin and behaviour disturbance. Lancet. 1990;335(8695):970.
48. McConnell H, Snyder PJ, Duffy JD, Weilburg J, Valeriano J, Brillman J, et al. Neuropsychiatric side effects to treatment with Felbamate. J Neuropsych Clin Neurosci. 1996;8(3):341–6.
49. Mula M, Trimble MR, Yuen A, Liu RS, Sander JW. Psychiatric adverse events during levetiracetam therapy. Neurology. 2003;61:704–6.
50. Trimble RM, Rösch N, Betts T, Crawford PM. Psychiatric symptoms after therapy with new antiepileptic drugs: psychopathological and seizure related variables. Seizure. 2000;9:249–54.
51. Ketter TA, Malow BA, Flamini R, White SR, Post RM, Theodore WH. Anticonvulsant withdrawal-emergent psychopathology. Neurology. 1994;44(1):55–61.
52. Barclay L. FDA requires warnings about suicidality risk with antiepileptic drugs. Medscape Medical News. 2008. http://www.medscape.com/viewarticle/585541.
53. Hesdorffer DC, Kanner AM. The FDA alert on suicidality and antiepileptic drugs: fire or false alarm? Epilepsia. 2009;50(5):978–86.
54. Kanner AM, Balabanov AJ. Chapter 133a: Psychiatric outcome of epilepsy surgery. In: Lüders HO, Bongaman W, Najim IM, editors. Textbook of epilepsy surgery. 3rd ed. London: Informa Healthcare; 2008. p. 1254–62.
55. Koch-Stoecker S. Psychiatric effects of surgery for temporal lobe epilepsy. In: Trimble M, Schmitz B, editors. The neuropsychiatry of epilepsy. Cambridge: Cambridge University Press; 2002. p. 266–82.

56. Fazel S, Wolf A, Långström N, Newton CR, Lichtenstein P. Premature mortality in epilepsy and the role of psychiatric comorbidity: a total population study. Lancet. 2013;382(9905):1646–54.
57. Christensen J, Vestergaard M, Mortensen PB, Sidenius P, Agerbo E. Epilepsy and risk of suicide: a population-based case-control study. Lancet Neurol. 2007;6(8):693–8.
58. Jones JE, Hermann BP, Barry JJ, Gilliam FG, Kanner AM, Meador KJ. Rates and risk factors for suicide, suicidal ideation, and suicide attempts in chronic epilepsy. Epilepsy Behav. 2003;4(3):31–8.
59. Perucca P, Jacoby A, Marson AG, Baker GA, Lane S, Benn EK, Thurman DJ, et al. Adverse antiepileptic drug effects in new-onset seizures: a case-control study. Neurology. 2011;76(3):273–9.
60. Kanner AM, Barry JJ, Gilliam F, Hermann B, Meador KJ. Depressive and anxiety disorders in epilepsy: do they differ in their potential to worsen common antiepileptic drug-related adverse events? Epilepsia. 2012;53(6):1104–8.
61. Petrovski S, Szoeke CE, Jones NC, Salzberg MR, Sheffield LJ, Huggins RM, O'Brien TJ. Neuropsychiatric symptomatology predicts seizure recurrence in newly treated patients. Neurology. 2010;75(11):1015–21.
62. Hitiris N, Mohanraj R, Norrie J, Sills GJ, Brodie MJ. Predictors of pharmacoresistant epilepsy. Epilepsy Res. 2007;75(2–3):192–6.
63. Kanner AM, Byrne R, Chicharro A, Wuu J, Frey M. A lifetime psychiatric history predicts a worse seizure outcome following temporal lobectomy. Neurology. 2009;72(9):793–9.
64. Cleary RA, Thompson PJ, Fox Z, Foong J. Predictors of psychiatric and seizure outcome following temporal lobe epilepsy surgery. Epilepsia. 2012;53(10):1705–12.
65. de Araújo Filho GM, Gomes FL, Mazetto L, Marinho MM, Tavares IM, Caboclo LO, et al. Major depressive disorder as a predictor of a worse seizure outcome one year after surgery in patients with temporal lobe epilepsy and mesial temporal sclerosis. Seizure. 2012;8:619–23.
66. Cramer JA, Blum M, Reed M, Fanning K, Project EI. The influence of comorbid depression on quality of life for people with epilepsy. Epilepsy Behav. 2003;4:515–21.
67. Lehrner J, Kalchmayr R, Serles W, Olbrich A, Pataraia E, Aull S, et al. Health-related quality of life (HRQOL), activity of daily living (ADL) and depressive mood disorder in temporal lobe epilepsy patients. Seizure. 1999;8(2):88–92.
68. Gilliam F, Kuzniecky R, Faught E, Black L, Carpenter G, Schrodt R. Patient-validated content of epilepsy-specific quality-of-life measurement. Epilepsia. 1997;38(2):233–6.
69. Perrine K, Hermann BP, Meador KJ, Vickrey BG, Cramer JA, Hays RD, Devinsky O. The relationship of neuropsychological functioning to quality of life in epilepsy [see comments]. Arch Neurol. 1995;52(10):997–1003.
70. Cramer JA, Blum D, Fanning K, Reed M, Epilepsy Impact Project Group. The impact of comorbid depression on health resource utilization in a community sample of people with epilepsy. Epilepsy Behav. 2004;5:337–42.
71. Jones JE, Watson R, Sheth R, Caplan R, Koehn M, Seidenberg M, Hermann B. Psychiatric comorbidity in children with new onset epilepsy. Dev Med Child Neurol. 2007;49(7):493–7.
72. Kroenke K, Spitzer RL, Williams JB, Monahan PO, Löwe B. Anxiety disorders in primary care: prevalence, impairment, comorbidity, and detection. Ann Intern Med. 2007;146:317–25.
73. Barry JJ, Ettinger AB, Friel P, Gilliam FG, Harden CL, Hermann B, et al. Consensus statement: the evaluation and treatment of people with epilepsy and affective disorders. Epilepsy Behav. 2008;13(Suppl1):S1–29.
74. Kerr MP, Mensah S, Besag F, de Toffol B, Ettinger A, Kanemoto K, et al. International consensus clinical practice statements for the treatment of neuropsychiatric conditions associated with epilepsy. Epilepsia. 2011;52(11):2133–8.
75. Fritze J, Unsorg B, Lanczik M. Interaction between carbamazepine and fluvoxamine. Acta Psychiatr Scand. 1991;84(6):583–4.

76. Grimsley SR, Jann MW, Carter JG, D'Mello AP, D'SouzaM J. Increased carbamazepine plasma concentrations after fluoxetine coadministration. Clin Pharmacol Ther. 1991;50(1):10–5.
77. Pearson HJ. Interaction of fluoxetine with carbamazepine. J Clin Psychiatry. 1990;51(3):126.
78. Haselberger MB, Freedman LS, Tolbert S. Elevated serum phenytoin concentrations associated with coadministration of sertraline. J Clin Psychopharmacol. 1997;17(2):107–9.
79. Fink M, Kellner CH, Sackeim HA. Intractable seizures, status epilepticus, and ECT. J ECT. 1999;15(4):282–4.
80. Regenold WT, Weintraub D, Taller A. Electroconvulsive therapy for epilepsy and major depression. Am J Geriatr Psychiatry. 1998;6(2):180–3.
81. Blackwood DH, Cull RE, Freeman CP, Evans JI, Mawdsley C. A study of the incidence of epilepsy following ECT. J Neurol Neurosurg Psychiatry. 1980;43(12):1098–102.
82. Marangell LB, Rush AJ, George MS, Sackeim HA, Johnson CR, Husain MM, et al. Vagus nerve stimulation (VNS) for major depressive episodes: one year outcomes. Biol Psychiatry. 2002;51(4):280–7.

Chapter 3
Mania and Elation

Marco Mula

Abstract Despite the substantial literature on mood disorders in epilepsy, the majority of authors focused on depression with limited data on manic symptoms. Historically, this was due to the general impression that both psychomotor excitation and overt mania were rarely encountered in epilepsy. However, recent studies demonstrated that manic symptoms can be occasionally seen in the context of epilepsy, either as seizure-based phenomena or as treatment-emergent adverse events.

This chapter briefly describes the evolution of the concept of bipolar disorders and covers the main symptom clusters usually described in manic episodes. In the epilepsy setting, peri-ictal manic symptoms are described post-ictally and are often associated with psychotic symptoms. Inter-ictal manic symptoms are definitely rare. Specific clinical entities, such as the inter-ictal dysphoric disorder of epilepsy, present some overlaps with the more unstable form of rapid cycling bipolar type II patients, but main psychopathological features are different. Manic symptoms as treatment-emergent adverse events of antiepileptic drugs are anecdotally described as well as after epilepsy surgery. Finally, major treatment options for mania in patients with epilepsy and the use of lithium are discussed.

Keywords Epilepsy • Bipolar Disorder • Mania • Antiepileptic Drugs • Lithium • Adverse Events • Inter-ictal Dysphoric Disorder • Epilepsy Surgery

Introduction

The relationship between epilepsy and depression has a long story. Around 400 BC, the Greek physician Hippocrates observed that "melancholics ordinarily become epileptics, and epileptics, melancholics: what determines the preference is the

M. Mula, MD, PhD
Epilepsy Group, Atkinson Morley Regional Neuroscience Centre, St. George's University Hospitals NHS Foundation Trust, Blackshaw Road, London SW17 0QT, UK

Institute of Medical and Biomedical Sciences, St George's University of London, London, UK
e-mail: mmula@sgul.ac.uk

M. Mula (ed.), *Neuropsychiatric Symptoms of Epilepsy*, Neuropsychiatric Symptoms of Neurological Disease, DOI 10.1007/978-3-319-22159-5_3

direction the malady takes; if it bears upon the body, epilepsy, if upon the intelligence, melancholy" [1]. Nowadays, it seems well established that reasons for such a close link are both biological and psychosocial [2]. However, manic symptoms in epilepsy have been traditionally considered less common as compared to depression. Nevertheless, epilepsy and bipolar disorders have many similarities. First, both of them are episodic conditions with a time course of the disease that can become chronic. Second, both of them have similar rates of drug-refractory patients, namely about 30 % in epilepsy [3] and 40 % in bipolar patients [4]. Still, without treatment, the rate of episodes in bipolar disorder increases, and the symptom-free intervals become shorter [5], a progression of the disease very similar to that described for epilepsy [3]. Finally, both conditions respond to antiepileptic drugs and seem to share a number of biochemical and neurobiological underpinnings, such as the kindling phenomenon, changes in neurotransmitters (i.e., GABA, excitatory aminoacids, dopamine, serotonin), modifications in voltage-opened ion channels (i.e., sodium, calcium, potassium), and changes in second messenger systems (i.e., G-proteins, phosphatidylinositol, protein kinase C, myristoylated alanine-rich C kinase substrate) [6, 7]. All these evidences taken together clearly suggest a common underlying pathophysiology or better a close link between the neurobiology of seizures and that of mood polarity.

The aim of this chapter is to review the possible clinical scenarios where manic symptoms can potentially occur in patients with epilepsy. Treatment options are also discussed.

What Is Mania?

The contemporary conceptualization of the manic-depressive illness is traced back to 1854, when Jules Baillarger described to the French Imperial Academy of Medicine, a biphasic mental illness causing recurrent oscillations between mania and depression [8]. The same year, Jean-Pierre Falret presented a case description on what was essentially the same disorder. This illness was named "folie circulaire" (circular insanity) by Falret, and "folie à double forme" (dual-form insanity) by Baillarger [9]. After that, Emil Kraepelin categorized and studied the natural course of untreated bipolar patients and coined the term "manic depressive psychosis" [10]. He noted that intervals of acute illness, manic or depressive, were generally punctuated by relatively symptom-free intervals in which the patient was able to function normally. More recently, in 1968, both the newly revised classification systems ICD-8 and DSM-II introduced the term "manic-depressive illness," subsequently substituted by "bipolar disorder" in subsequent DSM and ICD editions.

Epidemiological studies suggest that bipolar disorders, considering the whole spectrum, affect up to 5 % of the general population [11, 12]. A manic episode is not a disorder in itself, but rather a part of a disorder. If symptoms are not the result of substance use or abuse (e.g., alcohol, drugs, medications), or are not caused by a general medical condition, they are usually part of a bipolar disorder.

A manic episode is characterized by a period of at least 1 week, where an elevated, expansive, or unusually irritable mood, as well as notably persistent goal-directed activity is present. The mood disturbance associated with manic symptoms should be observable by others (e.g., friends or relatives of the individual) and must be uncharacteristic of the individual's usual state. These feelings must be sufficiently severe to cause difficulty or impairment in occupational, social, educational, or other important functioning. Typical symptoms include: inflated self-esteem or grandiosity, decreased need for sleep (e.g., one feels rested after only 3 h of sleep), being more talkative than usual or pressure to keep talking, flight of ideas or subjective experience that thoughts are racing, attention easily drawn to unimportant or irrelevant items, increase in goal-directed activity (either socially, at work or school, or sexually) or psychomotor agitation, and excessive involvement in pleasurable activities that have a high potential for painful consequences (e.g., engaging in unrestrained buying sprees, sexual indiscretions, or foolish business investments). A hypomanic episode has the same symptoms as a manic episode, with a few important differences: the mood usually is not severe enough to cause problems with the person working or socializing with others; never require hospitalization; there are never any psychotic features.

However, apart from this general framework, the phenomenology of mania is quite complex, as manic symptoms can sometimes occur as isolated symptoms, as subtle temperamental features, or even in the context of depression (i.e., mixed episodes). For this reason, a number of authors investigated the "factor" structure of mania and hypomania in order to identify specific symptom clusters. In hypomania, most of the authors agree that two groups of symptoms can be easily identified, namely positive-productive symptoms and problem-causing symptoms [13], also defined as the "sunny" and "dark" side of hypomania [14]. Basically, increased energy levels, elation, and psychomotor activation belong to the first group, while irritability and risk-taking behaviors to the latter. In the case of mania, current studies suggest a more diversified factor structure, with hyperactivity, decreased sleep, rapid/pressured speech, and hyperverbosity representing the core symptoms of mania, while other dimensions, such as hypersexuality, extravagance, religiosity/mystical experiences, and violent and assaultive behaviors, can be considered linked to the core, maybe reflecting specific clinical endophenotypes [15].

Do Manic Symptoms Occur in Epilepsy?

As already mentioned, data on manic symptoms in epilepsy are more than scant. However, a rational approach to the problem is always to identify elements that may potentially contribute, such as seizures or the epileptic disorder (Table 3.1). In fact, patients with epilepsy may experience a number of psychiatric manifestations around the ictus that have to be clearly differentiated from true psychiatric comorbidities. The practicality of classifying such symptoms according to their temporal relation to seizure occurrence (peri-ictal/para-ictal symptoms vs. inter-ictal

Table 3.1 Manic symptoms in epilepsy

Seizure/epilepsy	Peri-ictal	Pre-ictal dysphoria
		Ictal mania (nonconvulsive focal status epilepticus – extratemporal, nondominant hemisphere)
		Post-ictal mania (frontal, nondominant hemisphere)
	Para-ictal	*Alternative mania* (forced normalization phenomenon)
	Inter-ictal	*Inter-ictal mania* (bipolar disorder, inter-ictal dysphoric disorder)
Treatment	*Antiepileptic drugs or vagus nerve stimulation*	*Secondary mania* (toxic encephalopathy)
		Seizure worsening (*postictal mania*)
		Seizure control (*alternative mania*)
	Surgery	*Postoperative mania* (nondominant temporal lobectomy)

symptoms) is well established. Peri-ictal phenomena have been well described by Gowers [16] and Jackson [17], and also by Kraepelin [10] and Bleuler [18]. The differentiation between peri-ictal and inter-ictal psychiatric symptoms has relevant implications in terms of prognosis and treatment. Finally, epilepsy treatment plays another important role in the occurrence of psychiatric symptoms and, for this reason, the role of antiepileptic drugs and epilepsy surgery will be discussed.

Data on pre-ictal symptoms are limited. However, around one-third of patients with temporal lobe epilepsy report premonitory symptoms, usually preceding secondarily generalized tonic-clonic seizures [19]. Most of the times, these symptoms are focal seizures (i.e., auras), but sometimes patients clearly describe prodromal mood swings with depressed mood and irritability that occur hours to days before a seizure, and these symptoms are typically relieved by the convulsion itself [20]. Among pre-ictal symptoms, behavioral changes are those most frequently reported [21]. In our case series, around 13 % of patients with temporal lobe epilepsy experience irritability, dysphoria, or depressed mood preceding seizures [22]. Such feelings are almost indistinguishable from inter-ictal ones, apart from the duration and the close relation with seizure occurrence. It seems, therefore, important for clinicians to enquire about these phenomena, because they cannot be detected by rating scales or questionnaires [23].

Ictal mania has been very rarely reported in isolation, as it can be occasionally observed in the context of a focal nonconvulsive status, usually accompanied also by hallucinations [24]. However, negativism, anxiety/fear, irritability, and aggression are classic behavioral manifestations described in nonconvulsive status of temporal lobe origin [25], while indifference, perplexity, mutism, or poverty and slowness of speech are described in extratemporal status, especially in frontal polar cases. In this regard, it is important to point out that, in some cases, the continuous epileptic activity is restricted to deep limbic areas, and the scalp EEG may be even normal [26, 27]. The association between ictal manic symptoms and the nondominant hemisphere, as suggested by Flor-Henry [28], has been matter of debate, with some authors clearly pointing on the right hemisphere [29], while others the left [24]. However, EEG and SPECT findings in post-ictal mania clearly show functional changes in right-hemisphere structures, mainly the frontal, temporal, and paralimbic areas [30].

Post-ictal mood changes are less recognized in clinical practice, but are frequently reported by patients and their relatives. Manic/hypomanic symptoms are reported post-ictally in 22 % of patients, often with associated psychotic phenomenology [31]. It seems that post-ictal mania has a distinct position among psychiatric manifestations observed in the post-ictal period. Such manic episodes last for a longer period and have a higher frequency of recurrence than post-ictal psychoses, being associated with an older age at onset, EEG frontal discharges, and nondominant hemisphere involvement [30].

Finally, inter-ictal manic symptoms may suggest a true comorbidity between epilepsy and bipolar disorders. However, also in this case, it seems evident that in a large proportion of cases, inter-ictal mania or dysphoria are related to phenotype copies of bipolar disorder, such as the inter-ictal dysphoric disorder [23]. Premodern psychiatrists, such as Kraepelin and Bleuler, observed that patients with epilepsy could develop a pleomorphic pattern of depressive symptoms intermixed with euphoric moods, irritability, fear, and anxiety, as well as anergia, pain, and insomnia [32, 33]. This concept has been revitalized during the twentieth century by Blumer who coined the term inter-ictal dysphoric disorder to refer to this type of somatoform-depressive disorder, claimed as typical of patients with epilepsy [34]. Since its introduction, the concept of inter-ictal dysphoric disorder has been matter of debate [35]. Recent data show that the inter-ictal dysphoric disorder can be diagnosed in a subgroup of patients with drug-refractory epilepsy, but does not seem to be a disease-specific syndrome, being observed also in patients with migraine. Further studies are needed to clarify whether this syndrome is an organic mood disorder typical of neurological disorders or an affective syndrome observed in subjects with chronic medical conditions.

Manic Symptoms as Treatment-Emergent Adverse Events

Organic mania, or better secondary mania, is a clinical syndrome which resembles a manic state, but is due to specific factors such as physical illnesses (e.g., hyperthyroidism) or drugs (e.g., L-dopa, decongestants, sympathomimetics, steroids, and others). This concept received little attention in neuropsychiatric literature, because it was thought to be relatively uncommon before the seminal paper by Krauthammer and Klerman [36].

Anecdotally, manic/hypomanic symptoms have been described as a treatment-emergent adverse event of almost all antiepileptic drugs [37]. In this regard, a case of hypomania driven by vagus nerve stimulation is of particular interest [38], because it suggests that the mechanism underlying the control of seizures could be interlinked with that of regulation of mood and the control of its polarity.

In patients with epilepsy, drug-related manic symptoms can be classified into three main groups: (1) due to a toxic effect of the drug; (2) in the context of post-ictal psychopathology; (3) due to the forced normalization phenomenon (Table 3.1). The first group resembles the concept of secondary mania, also described by Krauthammer and Klerman, while the others are completely different entities whose pathophysiology resides in the pathophysiology of the epilepsy itself and are, therefore, unique to patients with epilepsy [37]. Post-ictal mania and forced normalization are only indirectly related to the drug and do not depend on the specific mechanism of action of the compound [39]. These episodes may be misleadingly interpreted by the epileptologists as a side effect of the anticonvulsant, while they are strictly connected to seizure precipitation or control, and must be carefully noted because this differentiation has important implications regarding prognosis and treatment.

Another important scenario in epileptology is that of epilepsy surgery. Since the early series, the possibility that brain surgery could be associated with the development of psychiatric disorders, in particular, psychoses, has been discussed [40, 41]. A few centers, however, regularly include psychiatric screening as part of their preoperative assessment, but postoperative psychiatric follow-up is often excluded. Assessment of psychosocial adjustment is rarely performed, in contrast to the often scrupulous recording of neuropsychological deficits. In some patients, elevated mood can be detected a few days after surgery [42]. It may begin with an excessive feeling of gratefulness for the surgeon who is denoted as the savior and responsible for the patient's new life. While this affection is partly comprehensible, the mood may switch into a socially inappropriate euphoric state, including seeking emotional closeness to rather distant persons, and finally the development of classic manic symptoms (e.g., increased levels of energy, insomnia, pressured speech, flight of ideas, marked irritability, and increased sexual activity). Risk factors have included right temporal resection and bilateral electrographic ictal foci [43]. In most cases, hypomanic symptoms are identified in the early postsurgical period and typically are short-lived. Pharmacotherapy is rarely required, unless the patient does not respond to redirection over the euphoric mood and limit setting of inappropriate behavior. Low doses of atypical antipsychotic medication for a few days up to 2 weeks may be sufficient. Of note, postsurgical hypomanic episodes may herald an undetected bipolar disorder and should alert the clinician to the cautious use of antidepressant drugs [42].

Treatment of Mania in Epilepsy

Lithium has a significant wealth of literature supporting its utility as an antimanic agent, although it seems to be less effective for dysphoria, mixed states, or rapid cycling [44–46]. Valproate, carbamazepine, and, to a lesser extent, oxcarbazepine, have proven efficacy for manic symptoms. Atypical antipsychotics (olanzapine, quetiapine, risperidone, aripiprazole, ziprasidone) are also considered effective antimanic agents with less potential, compared to previous generation neuroleptics, to cause tardive dyskinesia and extrapyramidal symptoms [45, 46]. Olanzapine, quetiapine, and risperidone have been associated with weight gain and metabolic syndrome, being, therefore, not preferred in combination with valproate. Aripiprazole and ziprasidone seem to have a favorable metabolic profile, but akathisia remains an unfavorable side effect [45, 46]. All these agents are dopamine blockers and may, therefore, lower the seizure threshold. For this reason, antipsychotics need to be carefully used in patients with epilepsy.

In the acute treatment of mania, lithium still plays a major role. In patients with epilepsy, it is important to consider interactions with antiepileptic drugs and seizure risk. The concomitant prescription of lithium carbonate and carbamazepine, though possibly associated with a favorable pharmacodynamic interaction on mood stabilization, may increase lithium toxicity with the potential occurrence of severe hyponatremia when lithium alone is stopped [47] and a significant modification in thyroid function with reduction in T4 and free T4 [48]. Conversely, the combination of lithium and valproate has a better tolerability, but side effects such as weight gain, sedation, and tremor may become easily evident. The combination with lamotrigine seems to be the best option [49] in terms of tolerability. Conversely, co-therapy with topiramate may reduce lithium clearance, leading to lithium-toxic plasma levels [50].

Lithium may have proconvulsant properties, especially at high plasma levels (>3.0 mEq/L). At therapeutic levels, the effect of lithium on seizure frequency in individuals with epilepsy is inconsistent [51]. If the prescription of lithium is needed and medically indicated, lithium can be adopted, but vigilant monitoring of blood levels and careful clinical follow-up are needed.

References

1. Temkin N. The falling sickness. Baltimore: The John Hopkins Press; 1971.
2. Mula M, Schmitz B. Depression in epilepsy: mechanisms and therapeutic approach. Ther Adv Neurol Disord. 2009;2(5):337–44.
3. Kwan P, Sander JW. The natural history of epilepsy: an epidemiological view. J Neurol Neurosurg Psychiatry. 2004;75(10):1376–81.
4. Maj M, Pirozzi R, Magliano L, Bartoli L. Long-term outcome of lithium prophylaxis in bipolar disorder: a 5-year prospective study of 402 patients at a lithium clinic. Am J Psychiatry. 1998;155(1):30–5.
5. Angst J, Sellaro R. Historical perspectives and natural history of bipolar disorder. Biol Psychiatry. 2000;48(6):445–57.
6. Amann B, Grunze H. Neurochemical underpinnings in bipolar disorder and epilepsy. Epilepsia. 2005;46 Suppl 4:26–30.
7. Mazza M, Di Nicola M, Della Marca G, Janiri L, Bria P, Mazza S. Bipolar disorder and epilepsy: a bidirectional relation? Neurobiological underpinnings, current hypotheses, and future research directions. Neuroscientist: Rev J Bring Neurobiol Neurol Psychiatry. 2007;13(4):392–404.
8. Mula M, Marotta AE, Monaco F. Epilepsy and bipolar disorders. Expert Rev Neurother. 2010;10(1):13–23.

9. Sedler MJ. Falret's discovery: the origin of the concept of bipolar affective illness. Translated by M. J. Sedler and Eric C. Dessain. Am J Psychiatry. 1983;140(9):1127–33.
10. Kraepelin E, Johnstone T. Lectures on clinical psychiatry (3rd rev ed/by Thomas Johnstone. ed. [S.l.]). Bailliere Tindall and Cox; 1912.
11. Akiskal HS, Bourgeois ML, Angst J, Post R, Moller H, Hirschfeld R. Re-evaluating the prevalence of and diagnostic composition within the broad clinical spectrum of bipolar disorders. J Affect Disord. 2000;59 Suppl 1:S5–30.
12. Judd LL, Akiskal HS. The prevalence and disability of bipolar spectrum disorders in the US population: re-analysis of the ECA database taking into account subthreshold cases. J Affect Disord. 2003;73(1–2):123–31.
13. Hantouche EG, Angst J, Akiskal HS. Factor structure of hypomania: interrelationships with cyclothymia and the soft bipolar spectrum. J Affect Disord. 2003;73(1–2):39–47.
14. Akiskal HS, Hantouche EG, Allilaire JF. Bipolar II with and without cyclothymic temperament: "dark" and "sunny" expressions of soft bipolarity. J Affect Disord. 2003;73(1–2):49–57.
15. Cassano GB, Mula M, Rucci P, Miniati M, Frank E, Kupfer DJ, et al. The structure of lifetime manic-hypomanic spectrum. J Affect Disord. 2009;112(1–3):59–70.
16. Gowers WRS. Epilepsy, and other chronic convulsive diseases: their causes, symptoms & treatment. London: J & A Churchill; 1881. pp. xiv. 309.
17. Jackson JHD. On epilepsy; in answer to the question-What is the nature of the internal commotion which takes place during an epileptic paroxysm? Samuel Highley, London; 1850.
18. Bleuler E. Lehrbuch der Psychiatrie. Springer, Berlin; 1916. p. viii. 518.
19. Gaitatzis A, Trimble MR, Sander JW. The psychiatric comorbidity of epilepsy. Acta Neurol Scand. 2004;110(4):207–20.
20. Blanchet P, Frommer GP. Mood change preceding epileptic seizures. J Nerv Ment Dis. 1986;174(8):471–6.
21. Scaramelli A, Braga P, Avellanal A, Bogacz A, Camejo C, Rega I, et al. Prodromal symptoms in epileptic patients: clinical characterization of the pre-ictal phase. Seizure. 2009;18(4):246–50.
22. Mula M, Jauch R, Cavanna A, Gaus V, Kretz R, Collimedaglia L, et al. Interictal dysphoric disorder and periictal dysphoric symptoms in patients with epilepsy. Epilepsia. 2010;51(7):1139–45.
23. Mula M, Schmitz B, Jauch R, Cavanna A, Cantello R, Monaco F, et al. On the prevalence of bipolar disorder in epilepsy. Epilepsy Behav. 2008;13(4):658–61.
24. Guillem E, Plas J, Musa C, Notides C, Lepine JP, Chevalier JF. Ictal mania: a case report. Can J Psychiatry. 2000;45(5):493–4.
25. Rohr-Le Floch J, Gauthier G, Beaumanoir A. Confusional states of epileptic origin, value of emergency EEG. Rev Neurol (Paris). 1988;144(6–7):425–36.
26. Wieser HG. Temporal lobe or psychomotor status epilepticus. A case report. Electroencephalogr Clin Neurophysiol. 1980;48(5):558–72.
27. Trimble MR, Schmitz B. Forced normalization and alternative psychoses of epilepsy. Petersfield: Wrightson Biomedical Pub. Ltd.; 1998. xi, 235p p.
28. Flor-Henry P. Schizophrenic-like reactions and affective psychoses associated with temporal lobe epilepsy: etiological factors. Am J Psychiatry. 1969;126(3):400–4.
29. Gillig P, Sackellares JC, Greenberg HS. Right hemisphere partial complex seizures: mania, hallucinations, and speech disturbances during ictal events. Epilepsia. 1988;29(1):26–9.
30. Nishida T, Kudo T, Inoue Y, Nakamura F, Yoshimura M, Matsuda K, et al. Postictal mania versus postictal psychosis: differences in clinical features, epileptogenic zone, and brain functional changes during postictal period. Epilepsia. 2006;47(12):2104–14.
31. Kanner AM, Soto A, Gross-Kanner H. Prevalence and clinical characteristics of postictal psychiatric symptoms in partial epilepsy. Neurology. 2004;62(5):708–13.
32. Kraepelin E, Diefendorf AR. Clinical psychiatry (1907). Delmar: Scholars' Facsimiles and Reprints; 1981. xvii,562p p.
33. Bleuler E. Textbook of psychiatry. New York: The Macmillan Co; 1924.

34. Blumer D. Dysphoric disorders and paroxysmal affects: recognition and treatment of epilepsy-related psychiatric disorders. Harv Rev Psychiatry. 2000;8(1):8–17.
35. Mula M. The interictal dysphoric disorder of epilepsy: a still open debate. Curr Neurol Neurosci Rep. 2013;13(6):355.
36. Krauthammer C, Klerman GL. Secondary mania: manic syndromes associated with antecedent physical illness or drugs. Arch Gen Psychiatry. 1978;35(11):1333–9.
37. Mula M, Monaco F. Antiepileptic drug-induced mania in patients with epilepsy: what do we know? Epilepsy Behav. 2006;9(2):265–7.
38. Klein JP, Jean-Baptiste M, Thompson JL, Bowers Jr MB. A case report of hypomania following vagus nerve stimulation for refractory epilepsy. J Clin Psychiatry. 2003;64(4):485.
39. Mula M, Monaco F. Antiepileptic drugs and psychopathology of epilepsy: an update. Epileptic Disord. 2009;11(1):1–9.
40. Bruton CJ, Stevens JR, Frith CD. Epilepsy, psychosis, and schizophrenia: clinical and neuropathologic correlations. Neurology. 1994;44(1):34–42.
41. Taylor DC. Ontogenesis of chronic epileptic psychoses: a reanalysis. Psychol Med. 1971;1(3):247–53.
42. Koch-Stoecker S, Schmitz B, Kanner AM. Treatment of postsurgical psychiatric complications. Epilepsia. 2013;54 Suppl 1:46–52.
43. Carran MA, Kohler CG, O'Connor MJ, Bilker WB, Sperling MR. Mania following temporal lobectomy. Neurology. 2003;61(6):770–4.
44. Grunze H, Kasper S, Goodwin G, Bowden C, Baldwin D, Licht R, et al. World Federation of Societies of Biological Psychiatry (WFSBP) guidelines for biological treatment of bipolar disorders. Part I: treatment of bipolar depression. World J Biol Psychiatry. 2002;3(3):115–24.
45. Grunze H, Vieta E, Goodwin GM, Bowden C, Licht RW, Moller HJ, et al. The World Federation of Societies of Biological Psychiatry (WFSBP) Guidelines for the Biological Treatment of Bipolar Disorders: Update 2010 on the treatment of acute bipolar depression. World J Biol Psychiatry. 2010;11(2):81–109.
46. Grunze H, Vieta E, Goodwin GM, Bowden C, Licht RW, Moller HJ, et al. The World Federation of Societies of Biological Psychiatry (WFSBP) guidelines for the biological treatment of bipolar disorders: update 2009 on the treatment of acute mania. World J Biol Psychiatry. 2009;10(2):85–116.
47. Vieweg V, Shutty M, Hundley P, Leadbetter R. Combined treatment with lithium and carbamazepine. Am J Psychiatry. 1991;148(3):398–9.
48. Kramlinger KG, Post RM. Addition of lithium carbonate to carbamazepine: hematological and thyroid effects. Am J Psychiatry. 1990;147(5):615–20.
49. Chen C, Veronese L, Yin Y. The effects of lamotrigine on the pharmacokinetics of lithium. Br J Clin Pharmacol. 2000;50(3):193–5.
50. Abraham G, Owen J. Topiramate can cause lithium toxicity. J Clin Psychopharmacol. 2004;24(5):565–7.
51. Erwin CW, Gerber CJ, Morrison SD, James JF. Lithium carbonate and convulsive disorders. Arch Gen Psychiatry. 1973;28(5):646–8.

Chapter 4
Anxiety

Christian Brandt

Abstract Anxiety disorders constitute important, though for a long time, neglected comorbidities of epilepsy. They deserve attention, because they are frequent and negatively impact the quality of life of persons with epilepsy. This chapter covers aspects of the neurobiological and pathophysiological correlates of anxiety and anxiety disorders, classification and differential diagnosis of epilepsy-related anxiety, epidemiology, the relationship between anxiety and different forms of epilepsy, and the influence of epilepsy surgery on concomitant anxiety. The bidirectional relationship between epilepsy and anxiety deserves broad attention, as this extends to the different levels of this comorbidity from animal models (for instance, GAERS rats may show increased levels of anxiety when compared to healthy controls, already before the onset of epilepsy) to epidemiology (anxiety may be detected up to 3 years before epilepsy diagnosis). Treatment (drugs, psychotherapy, alternative treatments) is also covered. Selective serotonin-reuptake inhibitors and serotonin-noradrenalin reuptake inhibitors are established in the treatment of anxiety disorders. It would be of value in persons with epilepsy and a comorbid anxiety disorder to treat both conditions with a single drug, which leads to the issue of anxiolytic properties of antiepileptic drugs (AEDs). Strong evidence has been demonstrated for pregabalin in social phobia and generalized anxiety disorder, lamotrigine in posttraumatic stress disorder, and gabapentin in social anxiety. Anxiety may also be a side effect of AEDs. Case vignettes at the end of the chapter illustrate the issue.

Keywords Epilepsy • Anxiety • Epidemiology • Prevalence • Bidirectional Relationship • Antiepileptic Drugs • Pregabalin • Animal Models • Quality Of Life

---

C. Brandt, MD
Department of General Epileptology, Bethel Epilepsy Centre,
Maraweg 21, Bielefeld 33617, Germany
e-mail: christian.brandt@mara.de

M. Mula (ed.), *Neuropsychiatric Symptoms of Epilepsy*, Neuropsychiatric Symptoms of Neurological Disease, DOI 10.1007/978-3-319-22159-5_4

Introduction

Anxiety disorders constitute important, though for a long time, neglected comorbidities of epilepsy [1]. They deserve attention, because they are frequent and negatively impact the quality of life of persons with epilepsy. While stigma and social consequences of epilepsy may lead to consecutive anxiety, there is also a bidirectional relationship between both disorders. One aspect of this relationship is that an anxiety disorder may also precede the onset of epilepsy. Animal models mirror the relationship between both disorders.

Neurobiological Correlates of Anxiety

Activation of brain regions in anxiety in healthy subjects and in patients with different anxiety disorders has been studied extensively by means of fMRI. Different areas have been found to be involved in different subtypes of anxiety disorders: hyperactivity of amygdala and insula in posttraumatic stress disorder (PTSD), social phobia and specific phobia, hypoactivation in the dorsal and rostral anterior cingulate cortices, and the ventromedial prefrontal cortex structures linked to the experience and regulation of emotion in PTSD [2]. The serotonin system is crucially involved in the development of anxiety, and PET studies showed decreased 5-HT1A binding in persons with temporal lobe epilepsy (TLE), thus demonstrating that the serotonin system is disturbed in persons with TLE [3]. The hippocampus plays an important role in re-experiencing fear, and the mechanisms are similar to epileptic discharges [4]. Activation of fear circuits is a major hypothesis for explaining symptoms in anxiety disorders, and the reduction of an excessive output from these neurons may theoretically improve the clinical picture [4, 5]. GABAergic inhibition and modulation of Ca-channels work antiepileptic and anxiolytic, which may be an explanation for the efficacy of some antiepileptic drugs in anxiety disorders [6] that will be discussed below. Imbalances in the GABAergic system have been found in brain specimens of operated patients with refractory temporal lobe epilepsy and comorbid anxiety and/or depression [7].

Ictal, Postictal, and Interictal Anxiety

First of all, anxiety may be a seizure symptom, that is, a simple partial seizure may present with anxiety as part of the seizure semiology. It is a key issue for the clinician to clarify the differential diagnosis between ictal anxiety and an anxiety disorder. Several features have been described as helpful: ictal psychiatric symptoms are usually brief, stereotyped, occur out of the context, and are associated with other seizure-related phenomena such as subtle or overt automatisms or postictal confusion of variable duration [8].

Ictal anxiety is frequent in right temporal lobe epilepsy [9] and rare in extratemporal epilepsy [10]. It seems to be reported by 10–15 % patients with partial seizures [11], is more common in women than men [12, 13], and seems to have a poor prognostic value for surgery [14]. Ictal anxiety can be differentiated through a careful history-taking, with special attention to the association between the duration of the attacks and the presence of accompanying nonparoxysmal symptoms of an anxiety disorder like avoidance behavior or the "circle of fear." Linguistic methods may be helpful in the differential diagnostic process [15]. Although not in the narrow focus of this chapter, it should be mentioned that dissociative seizures also may go along with anxiety. Persons with dissociative seizures described a greater number of somatic symptoms of anxiety during the attacks when compared to persons with epilepsy [16].

Structured interviews are of value in establishing the diagnosis of an anxiety disorder [17]. They form a gold standard, but screening instruments that are easy and quick to administer are helpful in a busy clinic. A widely used screening instrument for anxiety disorders is the GAD-7 [18], which may also be used in the context of epilepsy. It is only recently that a Korean version of this instrument has been validated in persons with epilepsy [19].

Harter et al. reported on a patient who had had a few generalized tonic-clonic seizures in his youth and subsequently developed agoraphobia with panic disorder [20]. This man had had a couple of self-induced seizures, and sometime after refraining from inducing seizures, he developed anxiety that was first suspected to be of epileptic origin. EEG and MRI were normal, and thorough history-taking led to the correct diagnosis. Psychotherapy relieved the symptoms. One remarkable feature of this case is that the patient had only had a few seizures and that these were moreover self-induced, and that he, despite this, developed an anxiety disorder.

Postictal psychiatric symptoms have been studied thoroughly using a questionnaire of 42 items answered by 114 patients with regard to a period of 72 h after a seizure [21]. Anxiety was the most frequent postictal emotional symptom, experienced by 45 out of the 114 patients. This is not only of theoretical interest but has also therapeutic implications. It means that some patients deserve special attention during the first 3 days following a seizure, because of emotional disturbances.

Anxiety is high in patients who report stress – acute or chronic – as seizure-precipitant [22–24]. Many persons with epilepsy attribute seizures to stress, though it is not yet clear in how many of them this is a true seizure-precipitant, maybe mediated by high levels of anxiety, or a mere attribution that is driven by anxiety.

Epidemiology

Several studies have assessed the prevalence of comorbid anxiety in people with epilepsy, applying different methods (telephone interviews, mailed questionnaires, direct contact in the clinic as ways of approaching the patients, and self-assessment or psychological examination as ways of assessing symptoms resp.

diagnosis) and referring to different populations. Symptoms of anxiety and anxiety disorders are more frequent in patients with epilepsy than in the general population. According to Tellez-Zenteno et al. [25], people without epilepsy reported a lifetime incidence of 11.2 % for any anxiety disorder compared with 22.8 % in the group with epilepsy. With regard to the last 12 months, there was a prevalence of 4.6 % in the group without epilepsy compared to 12.8 % in the group with epilepsy. A major strength of the study is that it is a population-based one with a huge number of included subjects. A potential weakness of the study is how the diagnosis of epilepsy was asserted. In fact, this was done by asking the interviewees "do you have epilepsy diagnosed by a health professional?" This might have led to over-reporting or underreporting. According to an also nationwide study from England [26], using an approach similar to the Canadian one, the prevalence of any depressive or anxiety disorder in people with epilepsy was 30.6 %, which corresponded to an adjusted odds ratio (OR) of 1.9. The OR for social phobia was 5.2, for agoraphobia 3.2, and for generalized anxiety disorder (GAD) 2.6. Anxiety symptoms are – not surprisingly – also present in patients with epilepsy and depression [27].

Brandt et al. found the diagnosis of an anxiety disorder in 19.6 % of patients with refractory epilepsy, a figure that is well within the range reported for epilepsy in general [28]. This study also assessed prevalence rates for the subtypes of anxiety disorder, namely 7.2 % for social phobia, 6.2 % for specific phobia, 5.1 % for panic disorder, 3.1 % for generalized anxiety disorder, 2.1 % each for anxiety disorder not further specified and obsessive-compulsive disorder (OCD), and 1.0 % for posttraumatic stress disorder. A trend for people with shorter epilepsy duration ($P=0.084$) and younger age ($P=0.078$) being more likely to have a diagnosis of anxiety disorder was revealed. This could mean that people with epilepsy might be able to develop coping strategies with increasing age or with increasing duration of the disease. 34.2 % of the inpatients of the same center were found to suffer from an anxiety disorder, using a slightly different methodology [29]. The higher figure might be due to different methodology, but it is more likely that it reflects a higher morbidity in inpatients when compared to outpatients. Gandy et al. directly compared people with refractory epilepsy and with well-controlled epilepsy with respect to mood, and anxiety disorders and suicidality [30]. They did not find any significant difference between the groups. Over all patients, they found a rate of 29 % for an anxiety disorder. High prevalence of anxiety in people with epilepsy extends to different ethnic populations respectively of a variety of countries [31, 32]. Anxiety is also frequent in children and adolescents with epilepsy [33, 34]. A recent study applying the State Trait Anxiety Inventory (STAI) [35] to persons with epilepsy and to healthy controls found an increased prevalence of self-reported anxiety, both state and trait, in people with epilepsy compared to matched controls [36]. Poorer general health, worry about seizures, and self-reported antiepileptic drug (AED) side effects were contributory factors for anxiety; good social support was protective. Anxiety is also present during pregnancy in women with epilepsy (22.4 %), especially when taking antiepileptic drugs (AED) (26.3 %), further increasing with polytherapy (31.4 %) [37]. Comorbid anxiety in epilepsy in general has been found to be associated with a current history of depression, perceived side effects, lower educational attainment, chronic ill health, female gender, and unemployment [38]; high seizure frequency and female gender [39]; and higher scores relating to powerful others [40]. Increased levels of neuroticism have also been found to be a risk factor [41]. Stigma [42], higher escape-avoidance and decreased distancing [43], and increased use of wish-fulfilling fantasy [44] predicted higher levels of anxiety. The findings are, however, not necessarily consistent with each other [45]. Factors to influence anxiety are also social aspects of stigma, effectiveness of seizure control, employment status, and the number of different epilepsy drugs [46]. This is an important recent finding in a time, where it sometimes seems that neurobiological factors are the only ones finding attention and social factors do not find the attention they might deserve. There seems to be also a relationship between cardiorespiratory fitness and level of anxiety in persons with temporal lobe epilepsy [47]. A significant negative correlation was observed between the levels of tension-anxiety and maximal aerobic power. Persons with anxiety (and also depressive) disorders scored higher in the Adverse Events Profile [48]. Reports of adverse events should be evaluated in the light of comorbid depression or anxiety.

An anxiety disorder may not only accompany epilepsy but also precede its onset by 3 years [49]. This finding points already to the bidirectional relationship between epilepsy and anxiety that will be discussed further below.

Anxiety and Epilepsy Syndrome, Localization and Lateralization

A study from Hong Kong found a higher prevalence of anxiety in patients with frontal lobe epilepsy than in those with generalized epilepsy [50]. A limitation of the study might be that the authors combined idiopathic, cryptogenic, and symptomatic forms of generalized epilepsies (GE). Patients who were diagnosed as having GE after stroke or infection or trauma were included. There was also a high proportion of cryptogenic GE. It would be of interest to see the results for idiopathic GE, which might form a more homogeneous group.

A clear lateralization could not be demonstrated for psychopathology (including anxiety) in epilepsy patients by several studies [51, 52], nor could a clear localization (temporal lobe vs. extract temporal lobe epilepsy) be shown [53].

Bidirectional Relationship

An anxiety disorder may not only be the consequence of epilepsy but also precede the onset of epilepsy by 3 years [49]. Also, in a population-based study from Sweden, the incidence of seizure disorders was higher in persons with a history of several psychiatric disorders, one of which were anxiety disorders. One explanation for the bidirectional relationship between anxiety disorders and epilepsy may be in the role that serotonin plays for both diseases [54]. These findings are paralleled in a couple of animal studies: Genetic absence epilepsy rats of Strasbourg (GAERS), a genetic model of human generalized epilepsy, showed increased levels of anxiety when compared to healthy controls. The development of anxiety was already detectable before the onset of epilepsy [55]. Genetically epilepsy-prone rats (GEPR), another animal model for epilepsy, have serotonergic and noradrenalinergic abnormalities [56]. Status epilepticus in early life caused an increase in anxiety-like behavior in male Wistar rats. Behavioral change could be prevented by the administration of ketamine during the status [57]. Subconvulsive doses of pilocarpine led to anxiety-like behavior in male Wistar rats [58]. Plastic changes in amygdala and hippocampus induced by kainate injection in mice were associated with increased anxiety-like behavior [59]. In humans, a previous psychiatric history (and/or genetic predisposition for psychiatric disorder), neurobiologic changes associated with the underlying epilepsy, peri-ictal phenomena, and iatrogenic and reactive processes influence the development of a psychiatric comorbidity in persons with epilepsy [60].

Anxiety Pre and Post Epilepsy Surgery

In surgical patient collectives, between 0 and 45 % of patients had symptoms of anxiety, differences in assessment accounting for the different prevalence rates [61]. The majority of postsurgical evaluations showed – at least after a while – an amelioration of anxiety, but exaggeration and even de novo anxiety were possible. A bidirectional relationship between epilepsy and anxiety – as discussed above – has also been demonstrated by the fact that the presence of anxiety predicts a worse seizure outcome after epilepsy surgery [62, 63], and that epilepsy surgery, vice versa, may improve the pre-existing anxiety symptoms, especially when seizure freedom could be achieved [61, 64, 65]. Depression and anxiety influence quality of life after epilepsy surgery [66].

Impact of Anxiety on Quality of Life in Persons with Epilepsy

Comorbid anxiety disorders or anxiety symptoms have a negative impact on the subject's quality of life in adults and children, and adolescents, especially within the context of a combined comorbidity of anxiety and depression [48, 67, 68]. Patients who attribute the control over their illness to the so-called powerful others experience higher levels of anxiety [40]. Self-perception of seizure precipitants also increased the anxiety level [22]. It may be that patients attribute seizures to irrelevant factors and thus experience anxiety. Anxiety (and also depression) is associated with the presence of adverse events (AE) to antiepileptic drugs [69]. This is actually a finding that may have a major impact on clinical practice: it can be speculated that it might be necessary in patients who report a high number or severity of AE to focus on a comorbid anxiety or mood disorder rather than merely on changing the antiepileptic drug regimen. The causal relationship may, however, also be the other way, that is, a higher rate of AEs might lead to a mood or anxiety disorder. A comorbid anxiety disorder is a risk factor for suicidality in people with epilepsy [70]. High anxiety levels have been found to have a negative impact on memory performance measured by the California Verbal Learning Test, thus impairing its lateralizing value in presurgical diagnostics [71].

Drug-resistant epilepsy patients with anxiety and/or depression symptoms may be more likely to miss outpatient appointments, and – suffering from both comorbidities– may be admitted more frequently for inpatient services compared to controls [72].

Iatrogenic Anxiety

AEDs may cause anxiety as an adverse event (AE). Several AEDs have been associated with anxiety as an AE, but only a minority causes it frequently [73]. The newer AED lacosamide does not seem to lead to increased anxiety [74].

Treatment of Anxiety Disorders in Persons with Epilepsy

Selective serotonin-reuptake inhibitors (SSRI) and serotonin-noradrenalin reuptake inhibitors are established in the treatment of several subsyndromes of anxiety disorder [75, 76]. There is, however, a latency of 2–6 weeks [77] before they can show full efficacy. Benzodiazepines (BZD), mainly alprazolam, are advocated as treatment during that phase. As BZDs have also antiepileptic properties, treatment of both conditions with one drug should be possible. They are, however, only treatment option of further choice in epilepsy. There is data for anxiolytic properties of AEDs with varying degrees of evidence. Strong evidence (at least one randomized controlled trial) has been demonstrated for pregabalin in social phobia and generalized anxiety disorder, lamotrigine in posttraumatic stress disorder, and gabapentin in social anxiety [6]. This refers to the efficacy on anxiety disorders in general, not necessarily meaning comorbid anxiety disorders in persons with epilepsy. Pregabalin has been shown not only to improve seizure frequency but also to reduce effectively symptoms of anxiety in patients with refractory focal epilepsy and comorbid anxiety disorder in an open, uncontrolled study [78]. Efficacy on seizure frequency was especially high in persons with an anxiety disorder, leading to the speculation that an improvement of anxiety may lead to an improvement of epilepsy, which again touches the field of the bidirectional relationship between both diseases.

Epilepsy patients treated with add-on levetiracetam (LEV) for their seizure disorder showed significantly less anxiety after LEV was added [79]. This was, however, only true for the subgroup that had an improved seizure frequency and is thus not a specific anxiolytic effect of LEV. This finding is therefore in line with the above-mentioned studies showing improvements of anxiety symptoms after successful epilepsy surgery. Anxiety has – among other psychiatric conditions – also been reported as a side effect of LEV [80].

An important point is the collaboration between neurologists and psychiatrists, at least if the treating physician does not unify both specialties in one person. It has been hypothesized that neurologists and psychiatrists do not cooperate to the extent they should and in the way they used to previously [81]. It has been advocated to train neurologists in recognizing and treating psychiatric disorders, and to psychiatrists, vice versa [82]. An embedded psychiatrist within an epilepsy service may lead to amelioration of comorbid psychiatric symptoms by initiating or adjusting pharmacological treatment or by delivering time-limited psychotherapy [83]. Many European epilepsy centers have dedicated services for persons with epilepsy and comorbid psychiatric disorders (http://www.mara.de/fileadmin/Krankenhaus_Mara/downloads/ezb_verhaltensmed_u_psychoth_epileptologie_201408.pdf.pdf) [84]. These are wards, where neurologists, psychiatrists, specialized nurses, and other healthcare professionals, for instance, occupational therapists, work together in an interdisciplinary setting applying drug therapy and psychotherapy. These institutions take account of the high comorbidity, not only of epileptic and dissociative seizures but also of epilepsy and psychiatric disorders, for example, anxiety. This is in fact a paradigm of the concept of comprehensive care for people with epilepsy [85].

Psychotherapy

Cognitive-behavioral therapy (CBT) has been shown to improve anxiety in patients with epilepsy [86] in a noncontrolled study in a small group of patients and is regarded as the psychotherapeutic procedure with the highest evidence in favor [76]. Psychodynamic therapy is second-line [76]. It has, however, to be questioned that an approach with a standard manual is adequate. Probably, a specific program for people with epilepsy and anxiety symptoms should be designed. Combination of pharmacotherapy and psychotherapy has been advocated. Amygdala hyperactivation has been found to normalize after exposure therapy [87], which shows an organic correlate of the efficacy of this psychotherapeutic procedure.

Alternative Treatments

Bright light therapy for symptoms of anxiety and depression in patients with focal epilepsy has been examined in a randomized controlled trial [88], but the results are inconclusive.

Conclusion

Anxiety disorders are important comorbidities of epilepsy. Recent research has elucidated many aspects of this comorbidity. There is, however, still a major need for future research, and especially for such leading to improvement in clinical practice, for instance, the development of specific screening instruments and disorder-specific psychotherapeutic procedures. Care for persons with the comorbidity of epilepsy and anxiety – as well as other psychiatric diseases – is a constitutional part of comprehensive care for people with epilepsy. This issue should be subject to further research, especially, concerning efficacy, also concerning its economic aspects.

Case Vignettes

Case 4.1

This is a now 49-year-old lady who had developed epilepsy at age 10. She experiences simple partial seizures with a strange sensation rising from the stomach, anxiousness, nervousness, and visual hallucinations. These proceed to complex partial seizures of psychomotor semiology with oroalimentary and hand automatisms. She also had generalized tonic-clonic seizures 10 years before, but these do not occur any more. They seized after the introduction of carbamazepine into her therapeutic regimen. In addition, she has episodes during which her systolic blood pressure rises up to 200 mmHg, accompanied by anxiety, a tight chest and heat sensation, hyperventilation, and numbness of both legs. She avoids traveling in buses. MRI revealed a right-sided hippocampal sclerosis, and during EEG, she experienced an epigastric aura, accompanied by a right anterior-temporal seizure pattern (rhythmic theta activity). In conclusion, her epilepsy was classified as a right-sided temporal lobe epilepsy due to hippocampal sclerosis. Additionally, an anxiety disorder, not further specified, was diagnosed. It was recommended to change the antiepileptic drug regimen from carbamazepine to oxcarbazepine and to refer her to presurgical diagnostics. She refused, however. She was advised to continue psychotherapy, which she had already begun.

Case 4.2

This is a report on a 39-year-old female patient who suffers from epilepsy since the age of 29 years. Her first seizure had been a generalized tonic-clonic seizure during the ninth month of pregnancy with her third child. She was started on lamotrigine after her second grand mal seizure that occurred 3 years after the first one. She continued to have grand mal seizures with varying frequency. She also experiences absence-like seizures lasting a couple seconds and occurring two to ten times per day. When being among many people, for instance, in a supermarket, she gets sweat attacks, heart palpitations, dizziness, fear that an epileptic seizure might come, tremor, and hyperventilation. She would be ashamed to have a seizure in the public. On admission, she was under lamotrigine 200 mg b.d., valproic acid 450 mg b.d., oxazepam 40 mg o.d., and trimipramine 40 mg o.d. EEG revealed generalized 3-Hz spike-wave complexes lasting from 1 to 10 s. Psychological diagnostics: The Symptom Checklist revised (SCL-90-R) revealed high parameters in all domains as well as a high global severity index. A score of 24 in the Beck Depression Inventory (BDI) indicated a moderate depressive episode. The results of the State/Trait Inventory (STAI) showed an elevated situation-related anxiousness and a more-than-average disposition to show anxious reactions. Dissociative symptoms (FDS-20) were in the upper normal range, and the results of the Childhood Trauma Questionnaire (CTQ) indicated mild emotional and physical negligence. In conclusion, she has a diagnosis of an idiopathic generalized epilepsy (although the age of the first manifestation was atypical), a moderate depressive episode, and agoraphobia. She was admitted to the psychotherapeutic ward for combined antiepileptic drug treatment and psychotherapy. She is, however, reluctant to continue, showing avoiding tendencies, and will be discharged after a short stay, getting the offer to be re-admitted if desired.

Case 4.3

This 33-year-old male patient suffers from epilepsy since early infancy. According to his mother, he was seizure-free under phenobarbitone for 3 years and without any drug for another 22 years. He did not become seizure-free again, despite treatment with different AEDs. He describes a disgusting, strange feeling that is difficult to describe, accompanied by slowed thinking and anxiety. He also describes seizures with falls, lateral tongue-biting, and bilateral shaking of arms and legs with a duration of 2 min, followed by reorientation over 15 min. He would feel exhausted and have muscle pain after the seizures. These seizures would occur with a frequency of 6–8 per year. He feels depressed and lives in fear of further seizures. In addition, he experiences multiple symptoms since several months, including drowsiness, shivering, listlessness, irritability, a sensation of roaring noises, paraesthesia, cold feeling of the arms and legs, episodes of derealization, and depersonalization. 3-T MRI, several EEGs (including 24 h recording), and examination of the cerebrospinal fluid revealed normal results. He works full-term and lives alone. Neuropsychological examination showed slightly impaired concentration when exposed to multiple information under time pressure. The diagnostic process was difficult, as only episodes resembling auras could be captured by video-EEG recordings. These showed normal results – a fact that is not helpful, as auras may go without seizure patterns in surface EEG recording. Nevertheless, tonic seizures and one generalized tonic-clonic seizure were observed by experienced health professionals (nurses with long-standing experience in epileptology). In addition, the patient fulfilled the diagnostic criteria of a generalized anxiety disorder. He participated in an inpatient program consisting of individual sessions of cognitive-behavioral therapy and group sessions of body therapy, relaxation therapy, music and arts therapy, theater group, and occupational therapy. During the course of the therapy, he learned to overcome his avoiding tendencies and self-regulate panic attacks. He will continue psychotherapy on an outpatient basis. His AED regimen was switched from levetiracetam to oxcarbazepine. The efficacy of this is subject to observation.

Acknowledgments I would like to thank Michael Frauenheim, MD, and Kirsten Labudda, PhD, my co-heads at the ward for behavior medicine and psychotherapy in epileptology at Bethel Epilepsy Centre, for their valuable contributions to the pathophysiology part of the chapter and to the case reports.

References

1. Kanner AM. Anxiety disorders in epilepsy: the forgotten psychiatric comorbidity. Epilepsy Curr. 2011;11(3):90–1.
2. Etkin A, Wager TD. Functional neuroimaging of anxiety: a meta-analysis of emotional processing in PTSD, social anxiety disorder, and specific phobia. Am J Psychiatry. 2007;164(10):1476–88.
3. Toczek MT, Carson RE, Lang L, Ma Y, Spanaki MV, Der MG, et al. PET imaging of 5-HT1A receptor binding in patients with temporal lobe epilepsy. Neurology. 2003;60(5):749–56.
4. Stahl SM. Brainstorms: symptoms and circuits, part 2: anxiety disorders. J Clin Psychiatry. 2003;64(12):1408–9.
5. Rogawski MA, Löscher W. The neurobiology of antiepileptic drugs for the treatment of non-epileptic conditions. Nat Med. 2004;10:685–92.
6. Mula M, Pini S, Cassano GB. The role of anticonvulsant drugs in anxiety disorders: a critical review of the evidence. J Clin Psychopharmacol. 2007;27(3):263–72.
7. Rocha L, Alonso-Vanegas M, Martinez-Juarez IE, Orozco-Suarez S, Escalante-Santiago D, Feria-Romero IA, et al. GABAergic alterations in neocortex of patients with pharmacoresis-

tant temporal lobe epilepsy can explain the comorbidity of anxiety and depression: the potential impact of clinical factors. Front Cell Neurosci. 2014;8:442.
8. Mula M, Monaco F. Ictal and peri-ictal psychopathology. Behav Neurol. 2011;24(1):21–5.
9. Guimond A, Braun CM, Belanger E, Rouleau I. Ictal fear depends on the cerebral laterality of the epileptic activity. Epileptic Disord. 2008;10(2):101–12.
10. Oehl B, Schulze-Bonhage A, Lanz M, Brandt A, Altenmuller DM. Occipital lobe epilepsy with fear as leading ictal symptom. Epilepsy Behav. 2012;23(3):379–83.
11. Gaitatzis A, Trimble MR, Sander JW. The psychiatric comorbidity of epilepsy. Acta Neurol Scand. 2004;110(4):207–20.
12. Chiesa V, Gardella E, Tassi L, Canger R, Lo Russo G, Piazzini A, et al. Age-related gender differences in reporting ictal fear: analysis of case histories and review of the literature. Epilepsia. 2007;48(12):2361–4.
13. Toth V, Fogarasi A, Karadi K, Kovacs N, Ebner A, Janszky J. Ictal affective symptoms in temporal lobe epilepsy are related to gender and age. Epilepsia. 2010;51(7):1126–32.
14. Feichtinger M, Pauli E, Schafer I, Eberhardt KW, Tomandl B, Huk J, et al. Ictal fear in temporal lobe epilepsy: surgical outcome and focal hippocampal changes revealed by proton magnetic resonance spectroscopy imaging. Arch Neurol. 2001;58(5):771–7.
15. Schoendienst M, Reuber M. Epilepsy and anxiety. In: Schachter S, Holmes G, Kasteleijn-Nolst Trenité D, editors. Behavioral aspects of epilepsy. New York: Demos; 2008. p. 219–26.
16. Goldstein LH, Mellers JD. Ictal symptoms of anxiety, avoidance behaviour, and dissociation in patients with dissociative seizures. J Neurol Neurosurg Psychiatry. 2006;77(5):616–21.
17. Bragatti JA, Torres CM, Londero RG, Assmann JB, Fontana V, Martin KC, et al. Prevalence of psychiatric comorbidities in temporal lobe epilepsy: the value of structured psychiatric interviews. Epileptic Disord. 2010;12(4):283–91.
18. Spitzer RL, Kroenke K, Williams JB, Lowe B. A brief measure for assessing generalized anxiety disorder: the GAD-7. Archiv Intern Med. 2006;166(10):1092–7.
19. Seo JG, Cho YW, Lee SJ, Lee JJ, Kim JE, Moon HJ, et al. Validation of the generalized anxiety disorder-7 in people with epilepsy: a MEPSY study. Epilepsy Behav. 2014;35:59–63.
20. Harter C, Brandt C, Angenendt J. Agoraphobia with panic disorder or epilepsy? Differential diagnostic considerations in a case. Psychiatr Prax. 2000;27(5):252–4.
21. Kanner AM, Soto A, Gross-Kanner H. Prevalence and clinical characteristics of postictal psychiatric symptoms in partial epilepsy. Neurology. 2004;62(5):708–13.
22. Sperling MR, Schilling CA, Glosser D, Tracy JI, Asadi-Pooya AA. Self-perception of seizure precipitants and their relation to anxiety level, depression, and health locus of control in epilepsy. Seizure. 2008;17(4):302–7.
23. Haut SR, Hall CB, Borkowski T, Tennen H, Lipton RB. Clinical features of the pre-ictal state: mood changes and premonitory symptoms. Epilepsy Behav. 2012;23(4):415–21.
24. Privitera M, Walters M, Lee I, Polak E, Fleck A, Schwieterman D, et al. Characteristics of people with self-reported stress-precipitated seizures. Epilepsy Behav. 2014;41:74–7.
25. Tellez-Zenteno JF, Patten SB, Jette N, Williams J, Wiebe S. Psychiatric comorbidity in epilepsy: a population-based analysis. Epilepsia. 2007;48(12):2336–44.
26. Rai D, Kerr MP, McManus S, Jordanova V, Lewis G, Brugha TS. Epilepsy and psychiatric comorbidity: a nationally representative population-based study. Epilepsia. 2012;53(6):1095–103.
27. Robertson MM, Trimble MR, Townsend HR. Phenomenology of depression in epilepsy. Epilepsia. 1987;28(4):364–72.
28. Brandt C, Schoendienst M, Trentowska M, May TW, Pohlmann-Eden B, Tuschen-Caffier B, et al. Prevalence of anxiety disorders in patients with refractory focal epilepsy--a prospective clinic based survey. Epilepsy Behav. 2010;17(2):259–63.
29. Illies D, Herzig C, Schröder K, Schöndienst M, Brandt C, Neuner F, et al. Psychische Störungen bei Patienten mit fokalen und generalisierten Epilepsien. In: Vögele C, editor. 30 Symposium Klinische Psychologie und Psychotherapie der DGPs Fachgruppe Klinische Psychologie und Psychotherapie; Luxemburg. Luxemburg: University of Luxemburg; 2012. p. 113–4.

30. Gandy M, Sharpe L, Perry KN, Miller L, Thayer Z, Boserio J, et al. Rates of DSM-IV mood, anxiety disorders, and suicidality in Australian adult epilepsy outpatients: a comparison of well-controlled versus refractory epilepsy. Epilepsy Behav. 2013;26(1):29–35.
31. Maroufi A, Khomand P, Ahmadiani S, Alizadeh NS, Gharibi F. Prevalence and quality of anxiety in patients with epilepsy. Epilepsy Behav. 2014;32:34–7.
32. Al-Khateeb JM, Al-Khateeb AJ. Research on psychosocial aspects of epilepsy in Arab countries: a review of literature. Epilepsy Behav. 2014;31:256–62.
33. Reilly C, Agnew R, Neville BG. Depression and anxiety in childhood epilepsy: a review. Seizure. 2011;20(8):589–97.
34. Jones JE, Blocher JB, Jackson DC, Sung C, Fujikawa M. Social anxiety and self-concept in children with epilepsy: a pilot intervention study. Seizure. 2014;23(9):780–5.
35. Spielberger CD, Gorssuch RL, Lushene PR, Vagg PR, Jacobs GA. Manual for the state-trait anxiety inventory. Palo Alto: Consulting Psychologists Press; 1983.
36. Jacoby A, Snape D, Lane S, Baker GA. Self-reported anxiety and sleep problems in people with epilepsy and their association with quality of life. Epilepsy Behav. 2015;43:149–58.
37. Bjork MH, Veiby G, Reiter SC, Berle JO, Daltveit AK, Spigset O, et al. Depression and anxiety in women with epilepsy during pregnancy and after delivery: a prospective population-based cohort study on frequency, risk factors, medication, and prognosis. Epilepsia. 2015;56(1):28–39.
38. Mensah SA, Beavis JM, Thapar AK, Kerr MP. A community study of the presence of anxiety disorder in people with epilepsy. Epilepsy Behav. 2007;11(1):118–24.
39. Kimiskidis VK, Triantafyllou NI, Kararizou E, Gatzonis SS, Fountoulakis KN, Siatouni A, et al. Depression and anxiety in epilepsy: the association with demographic and seizure-related variables. Ann Gen Psychiatry. 2007;6:28.
40. Asadi-Pooya AA, Schilling CA, Glosser D, Tracy JI, Sperling MR. Health locus of control in patients with epilepsy and its relationship to anxiety, depression, and seizure control. Epilepsy Behav. 2007;11(3):347–50.
41. Endermann M, Zimmermann F. Factors associated with health-related quality of life, anxiety and depression among young adults with epilepsy and mild cognitive impairments in short-term residential care. Seizure. 2009;18(3):167–75.
42. McCagh J, Fisk JE, Baker GA. Epilepsy, psychosocial and cognitive functioning. Epilepsy Res. 2009;86(1):1–14.
43. Goldstein LH, Holland L, Soteriou H, Mellers JD. Illness representations, coping styles and mood in adults with epilepsy. Epilepsy Res. 2005;67(1–2):1–11.
44. Thompson PJ, Upton D. The impact of chronic epilepsy on the family. Seizure. 1992;1(1):43–8.
45. Gandy M, Sharpe L, Perry KN. Psychosocial predictors of depression and anxiety in patients with epilepsy: a systematic review. J Affect Disord. 2012;140(3):222–32.
46. Peterson CL, Walker C, Shears G. The social context of anxiety and depression: exploring the role of anxiety and depression in the lives of Australian adults with epilepsy. Epilepsy Behav. 2014;34:29–33.
47. Arida RM, Gomes da Silva S, de Almeida AA, Cavalheiro EA, Zavala-Tecuapetla C, Brand S, et al. Differential effects of exercise on brain opioid receptor binding and activation in rats. J Neurochem. 2015;132(2):206–17.
48. Kanner AM, Barry JJ, Gilliam F, Hermann B, Meador KJ. Anxiety disorders, subsyndromic depressive episodes, and major depressive episodes: do they differ on their impact on the quality of life of patients with epilepsy? Epilepsia. 2010;51(7):1152–8.
49. Hesdorffer DC, Ishihara L, Mynepalli L, Webb DJ, Weil J, Hauser WA. Epilepsy, suicidality, and psychiatric disorders: a bidirectional association. Ann Neurol. 2012;72(2):184–91.
50. Tang WK, Lu J, Ungvari GS, Wong KS, Kwan P. Anxiety symptoms in patients with frontal lobe epilepsy versus generalized epilepsy. Seizure. 2012;21(6):457–60.
51. Altshuler LL, Devinsky O, Post RM, Theodore W. Depression, anxiety, and temporal lobe epilepsy. Laterality of focus and symptoms. Arch Neurol. 1990;47(3):284–8.
52. Sperli F, Rentsch D, Despland PA, Foletti G, Jallon P, Picard F, et al. Psychiatric comorbidity in patients evaluated for chronic epilepsy: a differential role of the right hemisphere? Eur Neruol. 2009;61(6):350–7.

53. Swinkels WA, van Emde Boas W, Kuyk J, van Dyck R, Spinhoven P. Interictal depression, anxiety, personality traits, and psychological dissociation in patients with temporal lobe epilepsy (TLE) and extra-TLE. Epilepsia. 2006;47(12):2092–103.
54. Kanner AM. Psychiatric issues in epilepsy: the complex relation of mood, anxiety disorders, and epilepsy. Epilepsy Behav. 2009;15(1):83–7.
55. Jones NC, Salzberg MR, Kumar G, Couper A, Morris MJ, O'Brien TJ. Elevated anxiety and depressive-like behavior in a rat model of genetic generalized epilepsy suggesting common causation. Exp Neurol. 2008;209(1):254–60.
56. Dailey JW, Mishra PK, Ko KH, Penny JE, Jobe PC. Serotonergic abnormalities in the central nervous system of seizure-naive genetically epilepsy-prone rats. Life Sci. 1992;50(4):319–26.
57. Loss CM, Cordova SD, de Oliveira DL. Ketamine reduces neuronal degeneration and anxiety levels when administered during early life-induced status epilepticus in rats. Brain Res. 2012;1474:110–7.
58. Duarte FS, Duzzioni M, Hoeller AA, Silva NM, Ern AL, Piermartiri TC, et al. Anxiogenic-like profile of Wistar adult rats based on the pilocarpine model: an animal model for trait anxiety? Psychopharmacology (Berl). 2013;227(2):209–19.
59. O'Loughlin EK, Pakan JM, McDermott KW, Yilmazer-Hanke D. Expression of neuropeptide Y1 receptors in the amygdala and hippocampus and anxiety-like behavior associated with Ammon's horn sclerosis following intrahippocampal kainate injection in C57BL/6 J mice. Epilepsy Behav. 2014;37:175–83.
60. Kanner AM. Lennox-lombroso lecture, 2013: psychiatric comorbidities through the life of the seizure disorder: a complex relation with a not so complex solution. Epilepsy Curr. 2014;14(6):323–8.
61. Cleary RA, Baxendale SA, Thompson PJ, Foong J. Predicting and preventing psychopathology following temporal lobe epilepsy surgery. Epilepsy Behav. 2013;26(3):322–34.
62. Guarnieri R, Walz R, Hallak JE, Coimbra E, de Almeida E, Cescato MP, et al. Do psychiatric comorbidities predict postoperative seizure outcome in temporal lobe epilepsy surgery? Epilepsy Behav. 2009;14(3):529–34.
63. Kanner AM, Byrne R, Chicharro A, Wuu J, Frey M. A lifetime psychiatric history predicts a worse seizure outcome following temporal lobectomy. Neurology. 2009;72(9):793–9.
64. Meldolesi GN, Di Gennaro G, Quarato PP, Esposito V, Grammaldo LG, Morosini P, et al. Changes in depression, anxiety, anger, and personality after resective surgery for drug-resistant temporal lobe epilepsy: a 2-year follow-up study. Epilepsy Res. 2007;77(1):22–30.
65. Devinsky O, Barr WB, Vickrey BG, Berg AT, Bazil CW, Pacia SV, et al. Changes in depression and anxiety after resective surgery for epilepsy. Neurology. 2005;65(11):1744–9.
66. Hamid H, Blackmon K, Cong X, Dziura J, Atlas LY, Vickrey BG, et al. Mood, anxiety, and incomplete seizure control affect quality of life after epilepsy surgery. Neurology. 2014;82(10):887–94.
67. Kwan P, Yu E, Leung H, Leon T, Mychaskiw MA. Association of subjective anxiety, depression, and sleep disturbance with quality-of-life ratings in adults with epilepsy. Epilepsia. 2009;50(5):1059–66.
68. Stevanovic D, Jancic J, Lakic A. The impact of depression and anxiety disorder symptoms on the health-related quality of life of children and adolescents with epilepsy. Epilepsia. 2011;52(8):e75–8.
69. Gomez-Arias B, Crail-Melendez D, Lopez-Zapata R, Martinez-Juarez IE. Severity of anxiety and depression are related to a higher perception of adverse effects of antiepileptic drugs. Seizure. 2012;21(8):588–94.
70. Christensen J, Vestergaard M, Mortensen PB, Sidenius P, Agerbo E. Epilepsy and risk of suicide: a population-based case-control study. Lancet Neurol. 2007;6(8):693–8.
71. Brown FC, Westerveld M, Langfitt JT, Hamberger M, Hamid H, Shinnar S, et al. Influence of anxiety on memory performance in temporal lobe epilepsy. Epilepsy Behav. 2014;31:19–24.

72. Hamilton KT, Anderson CT, Dahodwala N, Lawler K, Hesdorffer D, French J, et al. Utilization of care among drug resistant epilepsy patients with symptoms of anxiety and depression. Seizure. 2014;23(3):196–200.
73. Piedad J, Rickards H, Besag FM, Cavanna AE. Beneficial and adverse psychotropic effects of antiepileptic drugs in patients with epilepsy: a summary of prevalence, underlying mechanisms and data limitations. CNS Drugs. 2012;26(4):319–35.
74. Moseley BD, Cole D, Iwuora O, Strawn JR, Privitera M. The effects of lacosamide on depression and anxiety in patients with epilepsy. Epilepsy Res. 2015;110:115–8.
75. Mula M. Treatment of anxiety disorders in epilepsy: an evidence-based approach. Epilepsia. 2013;54 Suppl 1:13–8.
76. Bandelow B, Lichte T, Rudolf S, Wiltink J, Beutel ME. The German guidelines for the treatment of anxiety disorders. Eur Arch Psychiatry Clin Neurosci. 2015;265(5):363–73.
77. Bandelow B, Boerner JR, Kasper S, Linden M, Wittchen HU, Moller HJ. The diagnosis and treatment of generalized anxiety disorder. Dtsch Arztebl Int. 2013;110(17):300–9; quiz 310.
78. Brandt C, Schoendienst M, Trentowska M, Schrecke M, Fueratsch N, Witte-Boelt K, et al. Efficacy and safety of pregabalin in refractory focal epilepsy with and without comorbid anxiety disorders – results of an open-label, parallel group, investigator-initiated, proof-of-concept study. Epilepsy Behav. 2013;29(2):298–304.
79. Hagemann A, May TW, Nieder E, Witte-Bolt K, Pohlmann-Eden B, Elger CE, et al. Quality of life, anxiety and depression in adult patients after add-on of levetiracetam and conversion to levetiracetam monotherapy. Epilepsy Res. 2013;104(1–2):140–50.
80. Mula M, Trimble MR, Yuen A, Liu RS, Sander JW. Psychiatric adverse events during levetiracetam therapy. Neurology. 2003;61(5):704–6.
81. Kanner AM. When did neurologists and psychiatrists stop talking to each other? Epilepsy Behav. 2003;4(6):597–601.
82. Kanner AM. Is it time to train neurologists in the management of mood and anxiety disorders? Epilepsy Behav. 2014;34:139–43.
83. Chen JJ, Caller TA, Mecchella JN, Thakur DS, Homa K, Finn CT, et al. Reducing severity of comorbid psychiatric symptoms in an epilepsy clinic using a colocation model: results of a pilot intervention. Epilepsy Behav. 2014;39:92–6.
84. http://www.mara.de/fileadmin/Krankenhaus_Mara/downloads/ezb_verhaltensmed_u_psychoth_epileptologie_201408.pdf.pdf.
85. Pfäfflin M, Fraser RT, Thorbecke R, Specht U, Wolf P (eds.) Comprehensive care for people with epilepsy. Eastleigh: John Libbey Eurotext; 2001.
86. Macrodimitris S, Wershler J, Hatfield M, Hamilton K, Backs-Dermott B, Mothersill K, et al. Group cognitive-behavioral therapy for patients with epilepsy and comorbid depression and anxiety. Epilepsy Behav. 2011;20(1):83–8.
87. Goossens L, Sunaert S, Peeters R, Griez EJ, Schruers KR. Amygdala hyperfunction in phobic fear normalizes after exposure. Biol Psychiatry. 2007;62(10):1119–25.
88. Baxendale S, O'Sullivan J, Heaney D. Bright light therapy for symptoms of anxiety and depression in focal epilepsy: randomised controlled trial. Br J Psychiatry. 2013; 202(5):352–6.

Chapter 5
Delusions and Hallucinations

Naoto Adachi and Nozomi Akanuma

Abstract Delusions and hallucinations are core symptoms of psychoses. The prevalence of psychoses in people with epilepsy is higher than in the general population. Links between psychoses and epilepsy have been observed since ancient times. Today, we are aware that not only epilepsy-related vulnerability factors but also individual-related (general) vulnerability factors make people with epilepsy more prone to psychoses. Bidirectional relationships between epilepsy and psychoses in their genesis are also recognized. Chronological relationships between the onset of the seizure and of the psychoses themselves are a feature unique to psychoses in epilepsy, which are classified as ictal, post-ictal, and inter-ictal accordingly. In this chapter, we have described delusions and hallucinations in people with epilepsy within the three subclassifications, since the manifestations are rather different among the three groups. We have summarized their treatment and prognosis, which again differ between the three types of epilepsy psychoses. We have then presented newer concepts on the genesis of these symptoms. Many characteristics are common between ictal (particularly during seizure status) and post-ictal phenomena; thus, there may be a practical value to have them unified and classed as peri-ictal phenomena. We have also reviewed accumulating evidence illustrating characteristics common between "epileptic" and "functional" psychoses. This highlights the importance of individual-related (general) vulnerability factors for the genesis of delusions and hallucinations in people with epilepsy.

Keywords Delusion • Hallucination • Psychosis • Epilepsy • Vulnerability • Ictal psychotic phenomenon • Post-ictal psychosis • Peri-ictal psychosis • Inter-ictal psychosis • Functional psychosis • Organic psychosis • Genesis of psychoses

N. Adachi, MD (✉)
Adachi Mental Clinic, Kitano 7-5-12, Kiyota, Sapporo 004-0867, Japan
e-mail: adacchan@tky2.3web.ne.jp

N. Akanuma, MD, PhD
Lambeth Assessment, Liaison and Treatment Team, South London & Maudsley NHS Foundation Trust, 380 Streatham High Road, London SW16 6HP, UK
e-mail: nozomi.akanuma@slam.nhs.uk

M. Mula (ed.), *Neuropsychiatric Symptoms of Epilepsy*, Neuropsychiatric Symptoms of Neurological Disease, DOI 10.1007/978-3-319-22159-5_5

Introduction

Links between psychoses and epilepsy have been recognized and documented since ancient times [1]. The position of epilepsy in the field of psychiatry has notably changed, as diagnosis and treatment for psychoses has advanced. Epilepsy was considered a mental disorder/insanity; therefore, no separate entity as "psychosis in epilepsy" was established until the early twentieth century [2]. Today, the *DSM-5* [3] includes specifics of psychoses in epilepsy with commonly used subclassifications under psychotic disorder due to another medical condition (code 293.8). We recognize that the prevalence of psychoses is higher in people with epilepsy than in the general population [4–6]. Their vulnerable factors are related to both epilepsy and generic features such as genetic predisposition to psychoses and intellectual functioning. Bidirectional relationships between epilepsy and psychoses in their genesis are also observed [7–9].

During the era before modern psychiatry, psychoses were conditions with anomalous behavior, including hallucinations, delusional ideas, elated mood, psychomotor excitement, impaired consciousness, dissociation, or dementia. In the middle of the nineteenth century, it became possible to recognize psychotic symptoms that occurred following obvious cerebral pathology or damage, such as neurosyphilis and wartime head injury [2]. These psychoses were called "organic psychosis" in contrast to "functional psychosis" (the condition without apparent brain damage or disorders), including what we now call schizophrenia. At around the same period of time, psychoses were defined as a condition occurring under clear consciousness, excluding symptoms and behavior under clouded consciousness (due to cerebral or systemic abnormalities), which were termed "delirium" [10, 11].

Understanding the psychopathology of psychoses was dramatically increased in the early twentieth century when German psychiatrists [12, 13] established a methodology for mental state examination and its description for patients treated in long-stay hospitals. Delusions and hallucinations were at the center of these studies. Classification of psychoses, together with other mental disorders, also progressed by using psychopathology, etiology, course of illnesses, and their prognosis: the foundation of modern classifications that we currently use [3, 14]. It was generally accepted that the psychopathology of the delusions or hallucinations *per se* did not have a diagnostic value for a specific condition, although certain symptoms tended to be observed more frequently in one condition than the others. It was also understood that both delusions and hallucinations could be seen in the nonclinical population [15].

Since the operational diagnostic criteria (e.g., DSM [3] and ICD [14]) became common for the use of research and clinical practice in 1980s, abnormal thoughts and perceptions, mainly delusions and hallucinations, were seen as the core symptoms of psychoses. These symptoms were coined by Crow [16] "positive symptoms" of psychoses, while other symptoms, including blunted affect and abulia, were called "negative symptoms." In the recently published *DSM-5* [3], a wider range of symptoms has been added to the diagnostic criteria for psychotic disorders, which include formal thought disorders, grossly disorganized or abnormal motor behavior (including catatonia), and negative symptoms.

Psychoses in people with epilepsy became distinguished from "functional psychoses" and even other "organic psychoses" in the middle of the twentieth century [17, 18]. There is a feature unique to epilepsy in observing psychotic episodes: chronological relationships between the onset of seizures and that of psychotic symptoms. The psychotic symptoms are classified as ictal, post-ictal, and inter-ictal phenomena, depending on the timing of the psychotic episodes emerging in association with the seizures.

In this chapter, we will first summarize the definition of delusions and hallucinations in general and raise issues relevant to these symptoms in epilepsy. We will then discuss characteristics of delusions and hallucinations in people with epilepsy with special reference to the unique characteristics within epilepsy. We will attempt to appraise some issues of current diagnostic criteria and classification. The last part of this chapter will cover treatment principles and prognosis of these symptoms in people with epilepsy.

General Psychopathology of Delusions, Hallucinations, and Related Symptoms

Delusions

Delusions are defined as false, uncorrectable convictions or judgments, out of keeping with reality and with socially shared beliefs of the individual's background and culture [19]. Jaspers [13] described three main criteria for delusions: (1) the belief is held with extraordinary conviction and with an incomparable subjective certainly (certainty); (2) the belief is maintained imperviously to other experiences and to compelling counterarguments (incorrigibility); and (3) the content of the belief is impossible or false (impossibility/falsity). Jaspars' criteria have long been used as a golden standard. In particular, incorrigibility may be the most essential for diagnosing the phenomena [20].

Delusions often manifest certain themes, for example, delusions of guilt, grandiosity, reference, or persecution [21]. The theme of the delusions may be congruent to the mood or incongruent to it. It is possible to have delusions with one specific theme or multiple themes simultaneously.

Neuroanatomical regions responsible for the genesis of delusions have not been thoroughly understood [22]. A number of studies have suggested functional and/or structural abnormalities in the frontal and temporal lobes and their connectivity. Given the complexity of most delusional systems, involvement of the networks responsible for memory, affect, and conceptualization is suspected [23].

In accordance with Jaspers' diagnostic characteristics, delusions were once considered as a binary condition (i.e., present or absent), leaving a large number of anomalous beliefs undiagnosed. This resulted in reduced diagnostic sensitivity with increased false-negative episodes. For example, patients with long-lasting delusions may have a double bookkeeping system on their delusions, showing a paradoxical combination of an apparent total certainty with and an awareness of the nature of their delusion [24]. Certainty and incorrigibility can be thoughts or feelings on the personal inner mind of normal individuals [24, 25]. It is plausible that delusions finally turn out to be true [13, 26]. Certain groundless confidence (e.g., the subject's worthiness) as well as religious or philosophical beliefs cannot be attested whether real or unreal, possible or impossible [20]. In order to overcome these issues, further characteristics of diagnosing delusions have been found useful. As a consequence, delusions are seen as a continuum from normal to severe, the triad of criteria, each distributing to a degree. The additional characteristics are a self-evident truth with personal significance and not shared by common social or cultural backgrounds [23]; the level of preoccupation; subjective distress; and interference in functioning [26].

Some psychopathology may be similar to those of delusions, but have to be differentiated:

- *Overvalued ideas* are isolated convictions understandable in the context of the person's personality and life experiences [23]. They are considered an intermediary group on the borders of normal beliefs and delusions [20, 27].
- *Obsessional thoughts* are ideas, images, or impulses that enter the person's mind repeatedly in a stereotyped form [19]. They are almost invariably distressing, and the person often tries to resist them. Their insights about the irrational contents are considered to be different from those with delusions [28].
- *Confabulation* is defined as the production of false memories without deliberate intent to lie [29] or false narratives purporting to convey information about oneself or the world [30]. It can be observed in people with a variety of memory impairments that mostly involve the frontal lobes.
- *Delirium* is a transient organic mental syndrome of acute onset. It is characterized by global impairment of cognitive functions, a reduced level of consciousness, abnormalities in attention, increased or decreased psychomotor activity, and a disordered sleep-awake cycle [11].

The review article by Freeman [31] summarized that approximately 10–15 % of nonclinical population had fairly regular delusional ideation. A further 5–6 % had delusions, which were not as severe as those of psychotic disorders, but still with social and emotional difficulties. A further 1–3 % had delusions of which severity is comparable to clinical cases of psychoses. Van Os et al. [32] reviewed that approximately 75–90 % of psychotic experiences were transitory and disappeared over time.

Hallucinations

Hallucinations are defined as perception-like phenomena that occur without external stimuli [3]. Hallucinations can range from "elementary" to "complex." For example, simple auditory hallucinations are the perception of simple sounds. Complex hallucinations include voices, music, or well-formed sounds. Auditory and visual hallucinations are more common; however, hallucinations can occur in any sensory modality [33]. Auditory hallucinations are experienced more frequently in functional psychoses than in organic or substance-induced psychoses. Visual and other hallucinations were relatively often seen in those with organic or physiological dysfunctions, that is, delirium and dementia [33, 34].

Abnormal perceptions, in particular, elementary hallucinations, may derive from the abnormality of the cortical areas responsible for that perceptual modality, for example, elementary visual hallucinations occur with impairment in the visual cortex [35]. In the case of complex hallucinations, areas responsible not only for specific modality in the perception but also for attention, memory, language, and self-monitoring are likely to be involved [36].

Several perceptual phenomena need to be differentiated from "true" hallucinations. These incorrect perceptual phenomena are in principle nonclinical on their own.

- *Pseudohallucinations* are defined when the person is fully aware of the unreality of the experiences [34]. Visual or auditory perception is often involved, for example, visual hallucinations in elder persons with impaired eyesight and musical hallucinations in patients with hearing difficulties.
- *Illusions* are defined as false sensory perception of real external stimuli that may be misinterpreted and perceived in a distorted way [28, 34].
- *Imagery* is as an experience appearing in inner subjective space and lacking the concrete reality of perception, which is usually self-evoked and under control of the will [37].

The prevalence of hallucinations was reported with a wide range (median prevalence 4–13 %) of nonclinical individuals due to variation of the evaluation methods [38]. The first cross-national study across 52 countries on psychotic symptoms in the general population reported an age and gender-adjusted estimate of 5.8 % for hallucinations [15].

Relationships Between Delusions and Hallucinations

Strauss [39] suggested that hallucinations and delusions represent points on dimensions of perceptual and ideational continua function, rather than two separate entities. Patients hearing unpleasant voices tend to be convinced of the presence of persecutors [20]. Several psychotic experiences, such as audible thoughts, control of thinking, and thought broadcasting, have characteristics of both delusions and hallucinations [28]. Cenesthopathy (anomalous somatic sensations) can be classified as either somatic hallucinations or hypochondriac delusions. Some patients have a single form of psychotic symptom, either delusions or hallucinations. Others have both symptoms, whereas one can be predominant to the other. A dominant symptom may transform into the other in the course of the psychotic illness [40].

Delusions and Hallucinations in Epilepsy

At the beginning of the twentieth century, when epilepsy as a whole was excluded from being a mental disorder [2, 12], there was no consistency as to the causative relationship between epilepsy and psychoses. Psychotic symptoms were thought to be rare in people with epilepsy, leading to a concept that epilepsy and psychosis are antagonistic to each other [41]. In the middle of the twentieth century, the invention of EEG and subsequent advancement of clinical epileptology, and treatment with AED resulted in developing more sophisticated classifications of psychoses in epilepsy and further thinking of relations between epilepsy and psychoses. Gibbs [42] showed that patients with psychotic symptoms were likely to have temporal lobe epilepsy. This observation led to the hypothesis that psychoses originated from the temporal lobes. More recent studies in a larger community-based, population-based cohort showed a higher prevalence of psychosis in patients with epilepsy [4, 5], and bidirectional relations between epilepsy and psychoses in their genesis [7–9].

As for the operational diagnostic criteria, organic mental disorders in the ICD-10 [14] or psychoses due to epilepsy in the *DSM-5* [3] are applied. The current diagnostic systems entail that epilepsy-related psychoses emerge as a "secondary" condition to epilepsy (*DSM-5*) or due to epilepsy as the "organic" cause (ICD-10), implying an orthodox dichotomy between "organic" and "functional" psychoses [43, 44]. There seems to be little understanding or acceptance of the bidirectional relation between epilepsy and psychoses.

Studies on psychoses in people with epilepsy have focused on "positive symptoms" and often not evaluated "negative symptoms" [45]. Moreover, few studies examined "positive symptoms" in detail. In the following chapters, we will discuss delusions and hallucinations in people with epilepsy. We will use "psychoses" in the place of delusions or hallucinations at times, due to the limited evidence available of clear psychopathological descriptions.

Ictal Phenomena

Ictal delusions and hallucinations can be observed in two different ways [18, 46]. Psychotic symptoms occur as a seizure phenomenon per se, either as a single, isolated partial seizure, or as a precursor (aura) of subsequent progression to a complex partial seizure, which last for seconds to a few minutes. Alternatively, psychotic symptoms occur during a series of seizures, such as status epilepticus with complex partial seizures or absences [47].

During a single partial seizure, a variety of hallucinations or delusions can happen. Visual hallucinations are most frequently observed; auditory hallucinations are also experienced. Olfactory or somatosensory hallucinations may also occur. Gastaut [48] considered these "epileptic hallucinations" as complex sensory manifestations or perceptions; they occurred in the absence of any corresponding stimuli and constituted the essential and occasionally the sole clinical symptom (sometimes initial) of partial epileptic seizures. Subsequently, similar epileptic hallucinations were captured under monitoring with EEG or neuroimaging, permitting identification of the contributing neuroanatomical or neurophysiological regions and/or functions [35, 49].

Delusions do not occur as frequently as hallucinations ictally [50]; this may be because the duration of a single seizure is too short to generate such complex mental activities. Some delusions that are not systematized (e.g., feelings of persecution or guilt) can present with accompanying paroxysmal anxiety and delusional moods.

These ictal psychotic symptoms are traditionally termed psychic aura or psychic seizures. These phenomena are sometimes classified as simple partial seizures. The person's consciousness during more complicated psychiatric seizures, however, is generally disturbed to some degree; thus, classification as complex partial seizures seems appropriate [51].

A short-run of delusions, hallucinations, and extreme psychomotor excitements may occur during nonconvulsive status epilepticus [52]. The period during and shortly after these seizures is called the epileptic twilight state, characterized by inaccessibility, delusions, visual or auditory hallucinations, ideas of reference, paranoia, thought disorder, illogical responses, and a curious perseverative obsessive insistence [53]. Intense affective symptoms, either panic-like attacks or mood swings, frequently accompany them [47]. Such states may be classed as an intermediate condition between very slightly clouded consciousness and confusions. For example, approximately 20 % of the cases of absence status showed reduced levels of consciousness, which manifested with simple slowing of thought process and expression, but not to a level of distinct mental confusion [54]. The psychotic symptoms experienced under this level of alertness have been regarded as similar to those observed in "clear" consciousness; therefore, they have been distinguished from the symptoms of prolonged post-ictal confusions. Several cases of various psychotic symptoms have been reported during long-term EEG monitoring [55, 56].

Hesdorffer and Hauser [57] described ictal psychosis as an acute psychotic episode that may be an extension of the ictal perceptions or aura. Some caveats in this theory should be pointed out. It is unclear whether the person's disturbance in functioning and/or distress could be due to the seizure per se or the psychiatric symptoms. It is essential for the diagnosis of psychosis that the functional disturbance and distress result from the psychiatric symptoms. These psychotic episodes are usually too short-lived to produce such dysfunctions or complicated mental activities, in particular, the characteristics for delusions (e.g., incorrigibility). It is extremely difficult to evaluate whether the symptoms have characteristics needed for the diagnosis of psychotic symptoms or nonclinical phenomena such as pseudohallucinations [46]. Obviously, these episodes would not meet the requirement of operational diagnostic criteria of psychotic symptoms: 1 day or longer in acute and transient psychotic disorders of the ICD-10 [14], and brief psychotic disorder of the *DSM-5* [3]. Finally, it may not always be possible to recognize the point of the seizure cessation for the person or the witnesses in order to ensure that the experiences are "ictal" rather than "post-ictal". Taken all together, the diagnostic validity and reliability of "ictal psychosis" appear to be limited.

Post-ictal Phenomena

Psychomotor excitements and extreme aggression including self-harm immediately after seizures were described in the late nineteenth to early twentieth centuries [1]. Slater and Roth [58] coined psychotic episodes emerging under clear consciousness, "schizophrenia-like psychosis in epilepsy." Since this concept was widely accepted, marked psychomotor excitements following a seizure were frequently regarded as symptoms occurring during a prolonged period of post-ictal confusion. This trend continued until Toone and his colleagues [17, 59] re-evaluated these symptoms and classed them as post-ictal psychosis (PIP) in 1980s.

PIP was defined as a psychotic episode occurring within 7 days after a decisive seizure or cluster of seizures [59, 60]. The period between the cessation of the seizure and onset of the psychotic episode is called the lucid interval, a unique characteristic of PIP [59]. The lucid interval is observed in approximately 60 % of the episodes [61, 62]. Kanemoto and his colleagues [62, 63] proposed subclassifications of PIP: the nuclear type with a lucid interval and initial hypomanic stage, and the atypical peri-ictal type without these features. There appears to be considerable overlapping between atypical PIP and ictal psychosis during status epilepticus (Fig. 5.1a, b).

As for psychopathological features, visual hallucinations are more common than auditory hallucinations in PIP [64]. Grandiose and religious delusions are frequently observed [64, 65]. These delusions may be associated with hypomanic symptoms, prolonged insomnia, and hyperactivity as a precursor. While most PIP episodes are self-remitting in nature, even relatively short duration of the episodes can accompany astonishingly violent behavior, extreme agitation, or seriously incoherent behavior [65–69]. The level of consciousness during the episode is thought to be intact, because the patient appears orientated and can perform complex tasks. The patient's postepisodic recall about the episode, however, is often absent or fragmental.

PIP episodes mostly occur in patients with partial epilepsies, in particular, TLE or FLE [61, 62]. The presence of either diffuse or bilateral brain disturbance is suggested as a risk factor. Age of onset (mean 30–35 years) is higher than that of IIP (mean 25–30 years) [60]. Family history of affective disorders [60] or functional psychosis [70] is often present. Some patients have a history of psychosis, previous to the initial PIP episode [60, 71, 72].

It is at times difficult to identify the point of cessation of the seizure and beginning of the post-ictal period, even with use of EEG monitoring [73]. In the cases of repeated seizures, the psychotic phenomena may start in between the seizures, making it hard to determine as to whether the phenomena occur during or after the seizures. During a seizure status, the level of consciousness may fluctuate for a prolonged period of time; thus, the onset and cessation may not be clearly identified for each seizure (see Fig. 5.1b). In these instances, the psychotic symptoms can be classified as post-ictal (or peri-ictal) symptoms rather ictal symptoms. This raises two crucial questions as to the diagnosis of ictal and post-ictal psychoses. First, due

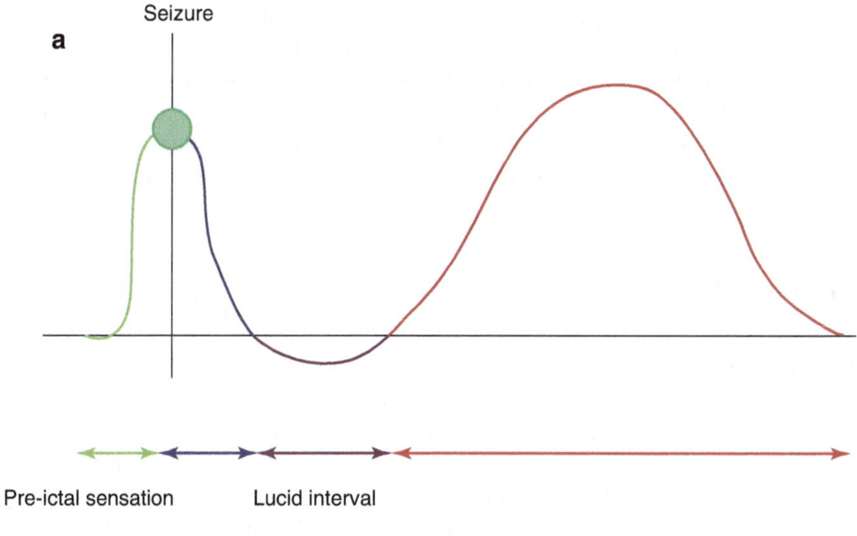

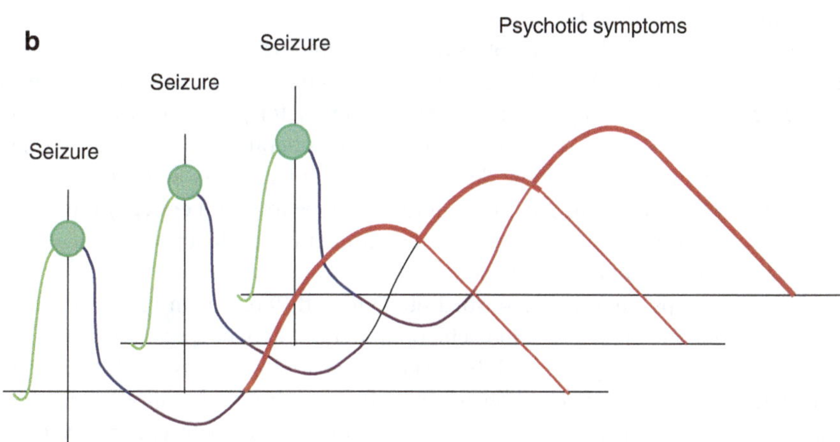

Fig. 5.1 (**a**) A model of post-ictal psychosis. A pre-ictal sensation (*green line*) may occur preceding a seizure. A post-ictal confusion (=delirium, *blue line*) may occur just after the seizure. Thereafter, a short-lasting lucid interval (*purple line*) and post-ictal psychotic symptoms (*red line*) may develop. (**b**) A model of psychotic symptoms during a cluster of seizures. When a cluster of seizures occur, it is difficult to clarify whether psychotic symptoms are pre-ictal, ictal, or post-ictal phenomena. Psychotic symptoms (*bold red line*) may not be clearly differentiated from some pre-ictal sensations, ictal symptoms, post-ictal confusions (deliriums), lucid intervals, and previous/ subsequent psychotic symptoms

to the difficulties in distinguishing the onset of the psychotic symptoms in relation to the seizures, the validity and usefulness of the terms of ictal and post-ictal psychoses may be reduced, and putting both together under "peri-ictal" psychoses may be more appropriate [46]. Second, it is questionable that all the cases of ictal and post-ictal psychoses occur under "clear" consciousness. Some may emerge during a prolonged period of ictal or post-ictal confusions, making these episodes closer to delirium.

Inter-ictal Phenomena

Psychoses can occur without a chronological relationship to seizures. This type of psychoses used to be called "epileptic psychosis" and regarded as the most common form of psychosis in epilepsy. From their large case series, Slater and colleagues [58, 74] coined this "schizophrenia-like psychosis in epilepsy," defining a chronic paranoid state that occurred under clear consciousness in people previously having epilepsy. The onset of the psychosis was not necessarily during or immediately following a seizure. This was later classed "inter-ictal psychosis (IIP)" by Toone [17] in contrast to PIP. Slater's criterion is concise and practical, and has been used for approximately four decades.

Slater and Roth [58] stated that psychotic symptoms seen in IIP were proper to epilepsy, rather than universal phenomena in psychoses in general. Their concept was based on three findings: (i) no genetic tendency for psychoses was found, (ii) some psychopathological features were unique to epileptic psychosis, and (iii) psychosis always occurred after the development of epilepsy. As a consequence, the idea that psychoses may be a mere comorbidity in people with epilepsy diminished until population-based studies revealed the bidirectional relationship between epilepsy and psychosis in the twenty-first century.

British neuropsychiatrists described qualitative differences in psychopathology between "epileptic" psychosis and schizophrenia as "nonepileptic" functional psychosis [58, 75, 76]. They reported that, when compared with those with schizophrenia, patients with IIP tended to show warmer affect and less personality deterioration, and exhibit paranoid delusions with a religious coloring (a relatively common occurrence of mystical delusional experiences) and more visual hallucinations. Subsequent controlled studies with structured evaluation tools [77–82] failed to show distinct qualitative difference in psychopathology between IIP and schizophrenia (Table 5.1). These studies employed more scientific approaches than traditional descriptive studies, although they still had several limitations, including binary evaluations, small sample cohorts, or insufficiently controlled clinical conditions.

Vulnerability factors for IIP have been reported in three categories: (i) epilepsy related, (ii) brain damage related, and (iii) individual related [18, 83]. Epilepsy-related (epileptic) vulnerability factors include age of onset of epilepsy, type and frequency of seizures, lateralization and localization of epileptogenic regions, and use of antiepileptic drugs. Brain damage related (organic) vulnerability factors consist of lateralization and localization of brain lesions and acquired cognitive impair-

Table 5.1 Comparison of delusions and hallucinations between inter-ictal psychosis (IIP) and functional psychosis (schizophrenia) [77–82]

Papers	IIP (n)	FP (n)	Evaluation tools	Findings
Toone et al. 1982 [77]	41	40	PSE	Delusions of persecution, IIP > FP Delusions of reference, IIP > FP (slight tendencies) Catatonic symptoms, IIP < FP (slight tendencies)
Perez et al. 1985 [78]	24	11	PSE	Delusions of grandeur, IIP < FP Visual hallucinations, IIP < FP Other items, IIP = FP
Mendez et al. 1993 [79]	62	62	Conventional psychopathology	Delusions, IIP = FP Hallucinations, IIP = FP
Matsuura et al. 2004 [80]	44 IIP 14 PIP	58	OPCRIT	Positive symptoms, IIP&PIP < FP (thought withdrawal, delusions of passivity, organized delusion, thought insertion)
Tadokoro et al. 2007 [81]	13	59	PANSS	Positive symptoms, IIP = FP
Ito et al. 2010 [82]	76	184	BPRS	Positive symptoms, IIP = FP

IIP inter-ictal psychosis, *PIP* post-ictal psychosis, *FP* functional psychosis, *PSE* Present State Examination, *OPCRIT* Operational Criteria Checklist, *PANSS* Positive and Negative Syndrome Scale, *BPRS* Brief Psychiatric Rating Scale

ment. Individual-related (general) vulnerability factors include sex, family history of psychoses, level of education, and intellectual functioning. These factors may overlap or interact with one another [60, 84].

Since Slater's initial study of schizophrenia-like psychosis, epileptic and organic factors have been well studied and identified [18]. Recent large-scale studies have confirmed the contribution of some of these vulnerability factors to the genesis of IIP, including partial epilepsies and complex partial seizures [60, 79, 84, 85]. These studies did not replicate many factors of previously shown significance, such as the left-sided foci and sinistrality. They also added some factors previously dismissed, such as partial epilepsies with extratemporal lobe foci [60, 86].

In contrast, general vulnerability factors have been ignored or underestimated. Recent studies highlighted the presence of certain general vulnerabilities, for example, low intellectual functioning [60, 87]. While Slater and colleagues [74] reported no genetic tendency for psychoses, recent controlled studies [5, 60, 78, 88, 89] suggested the presence of genetic vulnerability to psychosis (Table 5.2).

The administration of antiepileptic drugs (AED) can be associated with the development or exacerbation of psychotic symptoms [90, 91]. AED-induced psychoses can be a consequence of differing aspects from epilepsy-related, individual-related, and iatrogenic factors. AED is prescribed for controlling the epileptic seizures, and their adversarial response may vary from person to person. A rapid titration of AED, use of extraordinarily high dosage of AED, or unnecessary polypharmacy may be the contributing factors [91]. In accordance with the international

Table 5.2 Studies on family history of psychosis in inter-ictal psychosis (IIP) [5, 60, 78, 88, 89]

Papers	Study design (controlled/ population-based)	Study groups	Findings	Genetic tendency
Flor-Henry (1969) [88]	Controlled	IIP 50, EP 50	Equivalent, no detail	No
Perez et al. (1985) [78]	Controlled	IIP 24, FP 11	IIP (FH+/FH-) 3/21, FP (FH+/FH-) 3/11	Yes
Jensen & Larsen (1979) [89]	Controlled	IIP 20, EP 54	IIP (FH+/FH-) 13/7, EP (FH+/FH-) 21/33	Yes
Adachi et al. (2002) [60]	Controlled	IIP 246, EP 658, FP 612	IIP (FH+/FH-) 13/233, FP (FH+/FH-) 70/542, EP (FH+/FH-) 2/656	Yes
Qin et al. (2005) [5]	Population-based	IIP 519, EP 34494	Relative risk of psychosis (FH+/FH-) 4.03/1	Yes

IIP inter-ictal psychosis, *EP* epilepsy without psychosis, *FP* functional psychosis, *FH* family history of psychosis

diagnostic criteria, psychoses induced by AED are classified into mental and behavioral disorders due to psychoactive substance use (ICD-10) [14] and substance/medication-induced psychotic disorder (*DSM-V*) [3].

Most studies have shown a gap of approximately 14–15 years between the onset of epilepsy and that of IIP [18]. This delayed period is often thought to be required for the development of psychoses as a result of epilepsy-related adversities, for example, repeated seizures, AED administrations, and psychosocial disadvantages. The delay, however, is not observed in all the reported IIP cases; in particular, those with IGE, normal intellectual functioning, or the presence of family history of psychosis [82]. These patients likely develop IIP much sooner after the onset of their epilepsies. This may be because they tend to have greater individual-related vulnerability factors than epilepsy and organic-related factors.

New Concept for the Genesis of IIP

Figure 5.2 shows a new concept for the genesis of IIP [92], applying a vulnerability continuum of general psychopathology [93]. Every person with epilepsy has congenitally a degree of general vulnerability factors as in those without epilepsy. When the congenital general vulnerabilities are significantly high, they develop IIP, regardless of the degree of epilepsy-related and/or organic-related vulnerabilities. When the congenital general vulnerabilities are not high, the development of IIP will increasingly depend on the level of acquired vulnerabilities related to either epilepsy or organic causes, including high seizure frequency, frequent inter-ictal discharges, or use of AED. The latter group seems equivalent to Slater's epileptic psychosis [58].

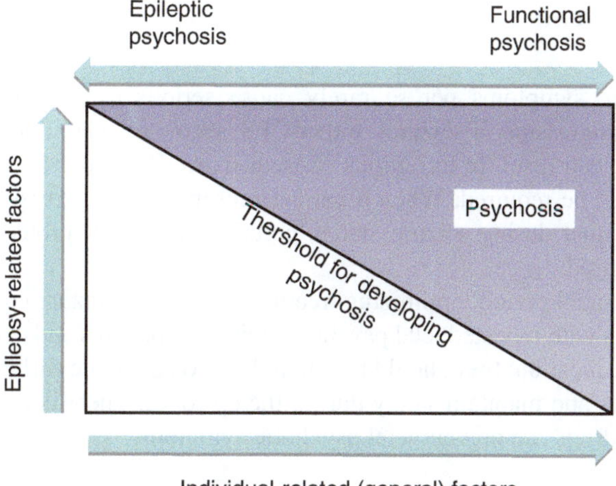

Fig. 5.2 A new concept for the development of inter-ictal psychosis. The model shows that psychosis emerges when the sum of the two sets of psychosis vulnerability factors exceeds the threshold: the individual-related (general and congenital; *vertical axis*), and epilepsy-related (acquired), vulnerability factors (*horizontal axis*). When the individual-related factors are high (toward the *bottom left*), the development of psychosis will increasingly depend on this level, regardless of epilepsy-related factors. Thus, the psychosis once developed, appears similar to functional psychosis (schizophrenia), despite the comorbid presence of epilepsy. In contrast, when the epilepsy-related factors are high (toward the *top right*), but individual-related factors low (toward the *left*), the genesis of psychosis is associated with this level, equivalent to Slater's epileptic psychosis

Treatment

Although our understanding of vulnerability factors for developing psychotic symptoms in epilepsy has been improving, it is as yet not possible to predict who would develop these symptoms in the first instance. The first step for treatment is to detect symptoms and establish diagnosis [94]. Once the type of epilepsy-related psychosis is suspected or confirmed, symptomatic treatment should commence to contain acute symptoms and associated problems. In the cases of recurrent episodes, preventative measures should be implemented inter-ictally. This should include reducing polypharmacy and optimizing AED treatment, while monitoring serum AED levels where possible [91, 95].

Evidence for treatment of psychotic symptoms in epilepsy is limited [96, 97]. Most treatment strategies for psychotic symptoms in epilepsy are empirical. The strategies have hitherto been in line with well-established treatment protocols for schizophrenia and related psychotic illnesses [98, 99].

Treatment targets should depend on the severity of the episodes determined by a combination of risks to self and others by the symptoms and subsequent behavioral changes, and impairment of daily function and quality of life [95, 97].

Ictal Phenomena

Ictal psychotic symptoms per se rarely cause serious dysfunction in patients, whereas the progression of seizures, either CPS, secondary GTC, or nonconvulsive seizure status, can result in hazardous consequences. Particular treatment for psychosis may not be required. When a patient presents with aggressive behavior or self-harm conduct during seizure status, certain sedation or protective seclusion would be required.

In the inter-ictal period, optimizing treatment for better seizure control is essential. In patients with repeated ictal psychotic episodes, patients and carers should be given psychoeducation; they should be taught how to notice the early warning signs of the episodes and maintain safety during the episodes. There is no evidence that psychotropic drugs can prevent ictal psychotic symptoms.

Post-ictal Phenomena

Acute protective measures prioritize the management of risk in the early stages of PIP. The most important point is to notice an unusual state (e.g., elevated mood or peculiar irritability) after a seizure or seizure clusters and to be aware of its potential as a precursor of PIP [100]. Psychotropic agents, either benzodiazepine or antipsychotic drugs, can be used for the purpose of sedation [66, 97, 101]. If the precursor symptoms are treated successfully, the episodes can be contained within the early stage, interrupting the progression to a full-blown episode.

Once PIP develops fully, immediate protective custody is required in many cases when the patient becomes violent or try to commit serious self-harm [66, 69]. The judicious application of local mental health legislation will be necessary [97, 101]. Antipsychotic drugs can be used to control or reduce psychomotor excitements [66]. Sedation and cessation of the process of the present PIP episode should take priority over possible risks of antipsychotic drugs, such as lowering seizure thresholds [97].

In the cases with recurrent PIP, preventative procedures are necessary, including optimizing seizure control by adjusting AEDs or by surgical treatment [62, 70]. Like in ictal psychotic phenomena, patients and carers should have an opportunity of psychoeducation to improve early detection and management of further episodes [97].

Inter-ictal Phenomena

In general, psychotic symptoms are better managed earlier rather than later [102]. In cases of mild symptoms or where the patient does not give consent to be treated with psychotropic drugs, they can be offered psychosocial interventions, or be carefully monitored [95, 103]. Psychotic symptoms with serious distress and/or functional disturbance inevitably need pharmacological treatment in outpatient or inpatient settings [97].

Any mainstream APD can be used for inter-ictal psychotic symptoms; the choice of APD should be due to a balance between pharmacological profiles, efficacy, and adverse effects [97, 98]. Among the readily available APD, there appears to be no significant difference in the psychotropic effects for IIP when the dosage of equivalent antipsychotic strength is used [104–106]. In patients treated with AED, most APD can be safely administered without seizure exacerbation [107]. General rules of APD titration are: to commence at low dose, titrate slowly to a minimum therapeutic dose, and continue at a fixed therapeutic dose for a sufficient period of time [91, 97]. When the patients have particular conditions, such as distinct brain damage and impaired hepatic/renal function, a smaller initiation dose with slower titration is recommended [108].

In addition to pharmacological interventions, psychoeducation, self-help, and reframing may be provided. As well as patients, family and carers often need support. The existing therapeutic relationship helps ensure that epilepsy patients with psychoses are more likely to be cooperative with their treating doctors than are patients with first-episode psychosis who are treatment-naïve [96].

Prognosis

Ictal Phenomena

Ictal hallucinations or delusions per se are short lasting, and rarely result in harmful consequences. Psychotic episodes during nonconvulsive seizure status last a longer period, depending on the duration of the status. Secondary risks may exist due to clouded consciousness (e.g., accidents), or self-harm due to psychotic symptoms (e.g., delusions of guilt and voices commanding killing oneself).

There is no evidence on the long-term prognosis of ictal psychotic symptoms, either during a single seizure or seizure status. It should be linked with the prognosis of their seizures. The long-term prognosis of nonconvulsive seizure status is related to the cause and the type. Most patients with absence status have a single episode, while some have a marked tendency to recur despite AED treatment [55]. Unprovoked CPS status, or CPS status as part of chronic epilepsy, is very likely to recur [53, 109].

Post-ictal Phenomena

PIP episodes are generally benign because of their self-remitting nature. In a seizure monitoring setting [66, 110], PIP episodes tend to resolve within 1 week in an overwhelming majority of patients. In the community and standard inpatient settings

[61], approximately 95 % of PIP episodes resolved within 1 month, with a mean duration of 10.5 days (SD 11.2, median 7 days, and mode 3 days). It should be noted that suicidal attempts are frequent complications of PIP episodes; without interventions, there is an increased risk of mortality.

Approximately half the patients with PIP have only one single episode. In the remaining half, PIP episodes tend to recur. Even extreme cases of quasiregular episodes have been reported after a cluster of complex focal seizures or secondary generalization [59, 66, 67]. Some patients develop into chronic IIP after recurrent PIP episodes [71, 72, 111].

Inter-ictal Phenomena

IIP episodes often take a chronic course. In a longitudinal follow-up study of 320 IIP episodes in 155 patients, the mean duration of the episodes was reported to be 82.7 weeks (median 17 weeks). Approximately 90 % of all IIP episodes lasted for 1 month or longer; 65 % had episodes which lasted for 6 months or longer [102]. The study considered only the periods during which the patients manifested hallucinations and/or delusions. The duration of the episodes is likely to be more prolonged if formal thought disorders, negative symptoms, and/or nonpsychotic symptoms (e.g., depression, anxiety, and irritability) were included.

IIP episodes often recur even after remission of the previous episodes. Onuma et al. [112] reported that during a 10-year follow-up period, almost two-thirds of IIP patients had episodes of relapse after remission or chronic episodes with further worsening. In the course of the illness, patients sometimes exhibit different types of psychoses, which include acute-transient and chronic [102], AED-induced and AED-unrelated [80, 85], and even IIP and PIP [71, 72]. Some IIPs recur after discontinuation of APD treatment [96, 112].

Patients with mental disorders in general have an increased risk of premature death due to either natural or unnatural causes [113]. Patients with epilepsy also have higher risks of early death by sudden unexpected death, status epilepticus, suicide, or accidents [114]. Synergism of the two conditions can lead to an increased risk in mortality.

Conclusions

We have described delusions and hallucinations in people with epilepsy and presented newer concepts on the genesis of these symptoms. Many characteristics are common between ictal (particularly seizure status-related) and post-ictal phenomena. This may indicate the possibility of pathogenesis common to these two subcategories; thus, there may be some practical value to have them unified and classed as peri-ictal phenomena.

We have also reviewed accumulating evidence illustrating characteristics common between “epileptic” psychosis and “functional” psychosis. This highlights the importance of individual-related (general) vulnerability factors in the genesis of delusions and hallucinations in people with epilepsy. There is a potential risk to overestimate epilepsy-related vulnerability factors for epileptic psychosis, based on the historical dichotomy between “organic (epileptic)” and “functional” psychoses.

Acknowledgments The authors are grateful to Ms. Emiri Adachi for help with computer graphing.

References

1. Temkin O. The falling sickness. A history of epilepsy from the Greeks to the beginnings of modern neurology. Baltimore: The Johns Hopkins Press; 1945.
2. Uchimura Y. Seishin-igaku no kihon-mondai. (Basic problems in psychiatry. Structural concepts for understanding mental disorders). Tokyo: Igaku Shoin; 1972 [Japanese].
3. American Psychiatric Association. Diagnostic and statistical manual of mental disorders. 5th ed. Washington DC: American Psychiatric Association; 2013.
4. Cockerell OC, Moriarty J, Trimble M, Sander JWAS, Shorvon SD. Acute psychological disorders in patients with epilepsy: a nation-wide study. Epilepsy Res. 1996;25:119–31.
5. Qin P, Xu H, Laursen TM, Vestergaard M, Moriensen PB. Risk for schizophrenia and schizophrenia-like psychosis among patients with epilepsy: population based cohort study. Br Med J. 2005;331:23–5.
6. Onuma T, Adachi N, Ishida S, Kato M, Uesugi H. Prevalence and annual incidence of paranoid state in epilepsy. Psychiatry Clin Neurosci. 1995;49:S267–8.
7. Cascella N, Schretlen DJ, Sawa A. Schizophrenia and epilepsy: is there a shared susceptibility? Neurosci Res. 2009;63:227–35.
8. Adachi N, Onuma T, Kato M, Ito M, Akanuma N, Hara T, et al. Analogy between psychosis antedating epilepsy and epilepsy antedating psychosis. Epilepsia. 2011;52:1239–44.
9. Chang Y, Chen PC, Tsai IJ, Sung FC, Chin ZN, Kuo HT, et al. Bidirectional relation between schizophrenia and epilepsy: a population-based retrospective cohort study. Epilepsia. 2011;52:2036–42.
10. Berrios GE. Delirium and confusion in the 19th century. A conceptual history. Br J Psychiatry. 1981;139:439–49.
11. Lipowski ZJ. Delirium: acute confusional states. New York: Oxford University Press; 1990.
12. Kraeperin E. Psychiatrie. Ein Lehrbuch fur Studierende und Arzte. Leipzig: Verlag von Johann Ambrosius Barth; 1913. (Trans; Nishimaru S, Nishimaru T. Tokyo: Misuzu Shobo; 1986 [Japanese]).
13. Jaspers K. General psychopathology. Berlin: Springer; 1913. (Trans. Uchimura Y, Nishimaru S, Shimazaki T, Okada K, Tokyo: Iwanami Shoten; 1953 [Japanese]).
14. World Health Organization. The ICD-10 classification of mental and behavioural disorders: clinical descriptions and diagnostic guidelines. Geneva: World Health Organization; 1992.
15. Nuevo R, Chatterji S, Verdes E, Naidoo N, Arango C, Ayuso-Matos JL. The continuum of psychotic symptoms in the general population: a cross-national study. Schizophr Bull. 2012;38:475–85.
16. Crow TJ. Positive and negative schizophrenic symptoms and the role of dopamine. Br J Psychiatry. 1980;137:383–6.
17. Toone B. Psychoses of epilepsy. In: Reynolds EH, Trimble MR, editors. Epilepsy and psychiatry. Edinburgh: Churchill Livingstone; 1981. p. 113–37.

18. Trimble M. The psychoses of epilepsy. New York: Raven; 1991.
19. World Health Organization. Lexicon of psychiatric and mental health term. 2nd ed. Geneva: World Health Organization; 1994.
20. Garety PA, Hemsley DR. Delusions. Investigations into the psychology of delusional reasoning. Oxford: Oxford Univ Press; 1994.
21. Maher B, Ross JS. Delusions. In: Adams HE, Sutker PB, editors. Comprehensive handbook of psychopathology. New York: Plenum; 1984. p. 383–411.
22. Gilleen J, David AS. The cognitive neuropsychiatry of delusions: from psychopathology to neuropsychology and back again. Psychol Med. 2005;35:5–12.
23. Menon V. Large-scale brain networks and psychopathology: a unifying triple network model. Trends Cogn Sci. 2011;15:483–506.
24. Mullen P. The phenomenology of disordered mental function. In: Hill P, Murray R, Thorley A, editors. Essentials of post graduate psychiatry. London: Academic; 1979. p. 25–54.
25. Spitzer M. On defining delusions. Compr Psychiatry. 1990;31:377–97.
26. Oltmanns TF. Approaches to definition and study of delusions. In: Oltmanns TF, Maher BA, editors. Delusional beliefs. New York: John Wiley & Sons; 1988. p. 3–11.
27. Mullen R, Linscott RJ. A comparison of delusions and overvalued ideas. J Nerv Ment Dis. 2010;198:35–8.
28. Hamada H. Seishin-shoukougaku. (Semiologie psychiatrique). Tokyo: Koubundo; 1994 [Japanese].
29. Gilboa A, Moscovitch M. The cognitive neuroscience of confaburation: a review and model. In: Baddeley AD, Kopelman MD, Wilson BA, editors. Handbook of memory disorders. 2nd ed. Chichester: Wiley; 2002. p. 315–42.
30. Berrios GE. Confabulations. In: Berrios GE, Hodges JR, editors. Memory disorders in psychiatric practice. Cambridge: Cambridge University Press; 2000. p. 348–68.
31. Freeman D. Delusions in the nonclinical population. Curr Psychiatry Rep. 2006;8:191–204.
32. van Os J, Linscott RJ, Myin-Germeys I, Delespaul P, Krabbendam L. A systematic review and meta-analysis of the psychosis continuum: evidence for a psychosis proneness-persistence-impairment model of psychotic disorder. Psychol Med. 2009;39:179–95.
33. Blom JD. Hallucinations and other sensory deceptions in psychiatric disorders. In: Jardi R, Cachia A, Thomas P, Pins D, editors. The neuroscience of hallucinations. New York: Springer; 2013. p. 43–57.
34. Assad G. Hallucinations in clinical psychiatry. A guide for mental health professionals. New York: Brunner Mazel; 1990.
35. Jobst BC. Focal seizures with visual hallucinations. In: Panayiotopoulos C, editor. Atlas of epilepsies. London: Springer; 2010. p. 457–62.
36. Benetti S, Pettersson-Yeo W, Mechelli A. Connectivity issues of 'hallucinating' brain. In: Jardi R, Cachia A, Thomas P, Pins D, editors. The neuroscience of hallucinations. New York: Springer; 2013. p. 417–43.
37. Sedman G. A comparative study of pseudo-hallucinations, imagery, and true hallucinations. Br J Psychiatry. 1966;112:9–17.
38. Johns LC, Kompus K, Connell M, Humpston C, Lincoln TM, Longden E, et al. Auditory verbal hallucinations in persons with without a need for care. Schizophr Bull. 2014;40 Suppl 4:255–64.
39. Strauss JS. Hallucinations and delusions as points on continua function. Rating scale evidence. Arch Gen Psychiatry. 1969;21:581–6.
40. Hafner H, der Heiden W. Course and outcome of schizophrenia. In: Hirsh SR, Weinberger D, editors. Schizophrenia. 2nd ed. Malden: Blackwell Science; 2003. p. 101–41.
41. Glaus A. Uber Kombinationen von Schizophrenie und Epilepsie. Zeitschr Ges Neurol Psychiat. 1931;135:450–500.
42. Gibbs F. Ictal and non-ictal psychiatric disorders in temporal lobe epilepsy. J Nerv Ment Dis. 1951;11:522–8.
43. Craddock N, Owen MJ. The Kraepelinian dichotomy – going, going…but still not gone. Br J Psychiatry. 2010;196:92–5.

44. Adachi N, Akanuma N, Ito M, Kato M, Hara T, Oana Y, et al. Authors' reply. Br J Psychiatry. 2010;197:76.
45. Adachi N. Epilepsy and psychosis. Issues on clinical research in epilepsy psychosis. Seishin Shinkeigaku Zasshi. 2006;108:260–5 [Japanese].
46. Kanner AM. Peri-ictal psychiatric phenomena; clinical characteristics and implications of past future psychiatric disorders. In: Ettinger AB, Kanner AM, editors. Psychiatric issues in epilepsy, a practical guide to diagnosis and treatment. 2nd ed. Philadelphia: LWW; 2007. p. 321–45.
47. Benatar M. Cognitive manifestations of status epilepticus. In: Drislane F, editor. Status epilepticus. A clinical perspective. Totowa: Humana Press; 2004. p. 221–44.
48. Gastaut H. Dictionary of epilepsy. Part 1: definitions. Geneva: World Health Organization; 1973.
49. Jobst BC. Focal seizures with auditory hallucinations. In: Panayiotopoulos C, editor. Atlas of epilepsies. London: Springer; 2010. p. 447–50.
50. Kasper BS, Kerling F, Graf W, Stefan H, Pauli E. Ictal delusion of sexual transformation. Epilepsy Behav. 2009;16:356–9.
51. Commission on Classification and Terminology of the International League Against Epilepsy. Proposal for revised clinical and electroencephalographic classification of epileptic seizure. Epilepsia. 1981;22:489–501.
52. Sachdev P. Schizophrenia-like psychosis and epilepsy: the status association. Am J Psychiatry. 1998;155:325–36.
53. Shorvon S. Status epilepticus. Its clinical features and treatment in children and adults. Cambridge: Cambridge University Press; 1994.
54. Thomas P, Sned OC. Absence status epilepticus. In: Engel Jr J, Pedley TA, editors. Epilepsy. A comprehensive textbook. 2nd ed. Philadelphia: Lippincott Wiliams & Wilkins; 2008. p. 693–703.
55. Seeck M, Alberque C, Spinelli L, Michel CM, Jallon P, De Tribolet N, et al. Left temoral rhythmic electrical activity: a correlate for psychosis? A case report. J Neural Transm. 1999;106:787–94.
56. Takeda Y, Inoue Y, Tottori T, Mihara T. Acute psychosis during intracranial EEG monitoring: close relationship between psychotic symptoms and discharges in amygdala. Epilepsia. 2001;42:719–24.
57. Hesdorffer DC, Hauser AH. Epidemiological considerations. In: Ettinger AB, Kanner AM, editors. Psychiatric issues in epilepsy. A practical guide to diagnosis and treatment. 2nd ed. Philadelphia: LWW; 2007. p. 1–16.
58. Slater E, Roth M. Mayer-gross, Slater and Roth clinical psychiatry. 3rd ed. London: Bailliere Tindal; 1969.
59. Logsdail SJ, Toone BK. Postictal psychoses. A clinical and phenomenological description. Br J Psychiatry. 1988;152:246–52.
60. Adachi N, Matsuura M, Hara T, Oana Y, Okubo Y, Kato M, Onuma T. Psychoses and epilepsy: are interictal and postictal psychoses distinct clinical entities? Epilepsia. 2002;43:1574–82.
61. Adachi N, Ito M, Kanemoto K, Akanuma N, Okazaki M, Ishida S, et al. Duration of postictal psychotic episodes. Epilepsia. 2007;48:1531–7.
62. Kanemoto K. Postictal psychoses, established facts and new clinical questions. In: Trimble M, Schmitz B, editors. The neuropsychiatry of epilepsy. 2nd ed. Cambridge: Cambridge University Press; 2011. p. 67–79.
63. Oshima T, Tadokoro Y, Kanemoto K. A prospective study of postictal psychoses with emphasis on the periictal type. Epilepsia. 2006;47:2131–4.
64. Kanemoto K. Postictal psychoses, revisited. In: Trimble M, Schmitz B, editors. The neuropsychiatry of epilepsy. Cambridge: Cambridge University Press; 2002. p. 117–31.
65. Devinsky O. Postictal psychosis: common, dangerous, and treatable. Epilepsy Curr. 2008;8:31–4.
66. Kanner AM, Stagno S, Kotagal P, Morris HH. Postictal psychiatric events during prolonged video-electroencephalographic monitoring studies. Arch Neurol. 1996;53:258–63.

67. Kanemoto K, Kawasaki J, Kawai I. Postictal psychosis: a comparison with acute interictal and chronic psychoses. Epilepsia. 1996;37:551–6.
68. Kanemoto K, Kawasaki J, Mori E. Violence and epilepsy: a close relation between violence and postictal psychosis. Epilepsia. 1999;40:107–9.
69. Fukuchi T, Kanemoto K, Kato M, Ishida S, Yuasa S, Kawasaki J, et al. Death in epilepsy with special attention to suicide cases. Epilepsy Res. 2002;51:233–6.
70. Alper K, Devinsky O, Westbrook L, Luciano D, Pacia S, Perrine K, Vazquez B. Premorbid psychiatric risk factors for postictal psychosis. J Neuropsychiatry Clin Neurosci. 2001;13:492–9.
71. Tarulli A, Devinsky O, Alper K. Progression of postictal and interictal psychosis. Epilepsia. 2001;42:1468–71.
72. Adachi N, Kato M, Sekimoto M, Ichikawa I, Akanuma N, Uesugi H, et al. Recurrent postictal psychoses after remission of interictal psychosis: Further evidence of bimodal psychosis. Epilepsia. 2003;44:1218–22.
73. Shorvon S, Trinka E. Nonconvulsive status epileptics and postictal state. Epilepsy Behav. 2010;19:172–5.
74. Slater E, Beard AW, Glithero E. The schizophrenia-like psychoses of epilepsy. Br J Psychiatry. 1963;109:95–150.
75. Hill D. Psychiatric disorders of epilepsy. Med Press. 1953;229:473–5.
76. Pond DA. Psychiatric aspects of epilepsy. J Indian Med Prof. 1957;3:1421–51.
77. Toone B, Garralda ME, Ron MA. The psychoses of epilepsy and the functional psychoses: a clinical and phenomenological comparison. Br J Psychiatry. 1982;141:256–61.
78. Perez M, Trimble MR, Murray NMF, Reider I. Epileptic psychosis: an evaluation of PSE profiles. Br J Psychiatry. 1985;146:155–63.
79. Mendez MF, Grau R, Doss RC, Taylor JL. Schizophrenia in epilepsy: seizure and psychosis variables. Neurology. 1993;43:1073–7.
80. Matsuura M, Adachi N, Oana Y, Okubo Y, Kato M, Nakano T, et al. A polydiagnostic and dimensional comparison of psychopathology of epileptic psychoses and schizophrenia spectrum disorders. Schizophr Res. 2004;69:189–201.
81. Tadokoro Y, Oshima T, Kanemoto K. Interictal psychosis in comparison with schizophrenia. A prospective study. Epilepsia. 2007;48:2345–51.
82. Ito M, Adachi N, Adachi T, Kato M, Onuma T, Matsubara R, et al. Evaluation of psychiatric symptoms in epilepsy psychosis using BPRS. Epilepsia. 2010;51 Suppl 4:29.
83. Adachi N, Akanuma N, Ito M, Kato M, Hara T, Oana Y, et al. Epileptic, organic, and genetic vulnerabilities for timing of the development of onset of interictal psychosis. Br J Psychiatry. 2010;196:212–6.
84. Adachi N, Matsuura M, Okubo Y, Oana Y, Takei N, Kato M, et al. Predictive variables of interictal psychosis in epilepsy. Neurology. 2000;55:1310–4.
85. Kanemoto K, Tsuji T, Kawasaki J. Reexamination of interictal psychoses based on DSM IV psychosis classification and international epilepsy classification. Epilepsia. 2001;42:98–103.
86. Adachi N, Onuma T, Hara T, Matsuura M, Okubo Y, Kato M, et al. Frequency and age-related variables in interictal psychoses in localization-related epilepsies. Epilepsy Res. 2002;48:25–31.
87. Mellers J, Toone BK, Lishman WA. A neuropsychological comparison of schizophrenia and schizophrenia-like psychosis of epilepsy. Psychol Med. 2000;30:325–35.
88. Flor-Henry P. Psychosis and temporal lobe epilepsy: a controlled investigation. Epilepsia. 1969;10:363–95.
89. Jensen I, Larsen JK. Mental aspects of temporal lobe epilepsy. Follow-up of 74 patients after resection of a temporal lobe. J Neurol Neurosurg Psychiatry. 1979;42:256–65.
90. Matsuura M. Epileptic psychoses and anticonvulsant drug treatment. J Neurol Neurosurg Psychiatry. 1999;67:231–3.
91. Mula M, Monaco F. Antiepileptic drugs and psychopathology of epilepsy: an update. Epileptic Disord. 2009;11:1–9.

92. Adachi N. Epilepsy as a risk factor for schizophrenia. Presented in the 13th Pacific Rim College of Psychiatrists Scientific Meeting. Tokyo, 2008.
93. Ingram RE, Price JM. The role of vulnerability in understanding psychopathology. In: Ingram RE, Price JM, editors. Vulnerability to psychopathology. Risk across the lifespan. New York: Guilford press; 2001. p. 3–19.
94. Koutroumanidis M, Adachi N, Howard R. History, physical and mental examination, and assessment. In: Panayiotopoulos CP, editor. Atlas of epilepsies. London: Springer; 2010. p. 671–80.
95. Onuma T. Therapeutic approach to epileptic patients with psychiatric symptoms. Jpn J Psychiatry Treat. 1987;2:553–60 [Japanese].
96. Adachi N. Treatment of mental disorders in epilepsy patients. Jpn J Psychiatry Treat. 2005;20(Suppl):370–3 [Japanese].
97. Adachi N, Kanemoto K, de Toffel B, Akanuma N, Oshima T, Mohan A, et al. Basic treatment principles for psychotic disorders in patients with epilepsy. Epilepsia. 2013;54 Suppl 1:19–33.
98. Kerr M, Mensah S, Besag F, de Toffol B, Ettinger A, Kanemoto K, et al. International consensus clinical practice statements for the treatment of neuropsychiatric conditions associated with epilepsy. Epilepsia. 2011;52:2133–8.
99. American Psychiatric Association. Practice guideline for the treatment of patients with schizophrenia. Am J Psychiatry. 1998;154 Suppl 4:1–63.
100. Krauss G, Theodore WH. Treatment strategies in the postictal state. Epilepsy Behav. 2010;19:188–90.
101. Lancman ME, Craven WJ, Asconapé JJ, Penry JK. Clinical management of recurrent postictal psychosis. J Epilepsy. 1994;7:47–51.
102. Adachi N, Akanuma N, Ito M, Okazaki M, Kato M, Onuma T. Interictal psychotic episodes in epilepsy: duration and associated clinical factors. Epilepsia. 2012;53:1088–94.
103. Francey SM, Nelson B, Thompson A, Parker AG, Kerr M, Macneil C, et al. Who need antipsychotic medication in the earliest stage of psychosis? A reconsideration of benefits, risks, neurobiology and ethics in the era of early intervention. Schizophr Res. 2010;119:1–10.
104. Crossley NA, Constante M, McGuire P, Power P. Efficacy of atypical v. typical antipsychotics in the treatment of early psychosis: meta-analysis. Br J Psychiatry. 2010;196:434–9.
105. Girgis RR, Phillips MR, Li X, Li K, Jiang H, Wu C, et al. Clozapine v. chlorpromazine in treatment-naïve, first-episode schizophrenia: 9-year outcomes of a randomized clinical trial. Br J Psychiatry. 2011;199:281–8.
106. Hara K, Adachi N, Okazaki M, Ito M, Akanuma N, Kato M, et al. Duration of interictal psychotic episodes by antipsychotic drug treatments. Epilepsy Behav. 2013;27:342–5.
107. Okazaki M, Adachi N, Akanuma N, Hara K, Ito M, Kato M, Onuma T. Do antipsychotic drugs increase seizure frequency in epilepsy patients? Eur Psychoneuropharmachol. 2014;24:1738–44.
108. Gardner DM, Murphy AL, O'Donnel H, Centorrino F, Baldessarini RJ. International consensus study of antipsychotic dosing. Am J Psychiatry. 2010;167:686–93.
109. Cockerell OC, Walker MC, Sander JWAS, Shorvon SD. Complex partial status epilepticus: a recurrent problem. J Neurol Neurosurge Psychiatry. 1994;57:835–7.
110. Devinsky O, Abramson H, Alper K, FitzGerald LS, Perrine K, Calderon J, Luciano D. Postictal psychosis: a case control series of 20 patients and 150 controls. Epilepsy Res. 1995;20:247–53.
111. Kanner AM, Ostrovskaya A. Long-term significance of postictal psychotic episodes II. Are they predictive of interictal psychotic episodes? Epilepsy Behav. 2008;12:154–6.
112. Onuma T, Adachi N, Hisano T, Uesugi S. 10-year follow-up study of epilepsy with psychosis. Jpn J Psychiat Neurol. 1991;45:360–1.
113. Harris EC, Barraclough B. Excess mortality of mental disorder. Br J Psychiatry. 1999;173:11–53.
114. Hitiris N, Mohanraj R, Norrie J, Brodie MJ. Mortality in epilepsy. Epilepsy Behav. 2007;10:363–76.

Chapter 6
Obsessiveness and Viscosity

Bruce Hermann

Abstract There has been a long and controversial history concerning the relationship between epilepsy, and specific epilepsy syndromes, and the presence and characteristics of diverse personality and behavioral changes. Here we focus on several distinct traits that have been included in this area of research including obsessiveness, viscosity, hypergraphia, and verbosity. Aspects of this interesting history are reviewed, the development and elaboration of theories concerning these personality and behavioral traits and epilepsy are discussed, and segments of the empirical research that has been conducted in the field are examined. The presence, rate, and correlates of these target behaviors (e.g., hypergraphia, viscosity) vary as a function of important details of the research methodology (e.g., mode of assessment, operational definition of behavior). The clinical significance and underlying neurobiology of these characteristics remain to be determined.

Keywords Temporal Lobe Epilepsy • Behavioral Change • Hypergraphia • Circumstantiality • Bear-Fedio Inventory • Viscosity • Epilepsy • Personality

Introduction

The topic of this chapter is a gateway to an interesting, complex, and contentious literature—one with an interesting history. One aspect of the discussion of alterations in personality and behavior, and behavior change in epilepsy, temporal lobe epilepsy (TLE) in particular, arguably dates to the work of Gibbs and colleagues in the late 1940s and early 1950s [1] (Fig. 6.1), work that in retrospect initiated the so-called period of psychomotor peculiarity in epilepsy-behavioral research [2]. Two developments led to re-popularization of the controversial concept of the "epileptic personality" that was attributed to TLE. First, there developed a better appreciation of the role of the limbic system in emotion and behavior, and second, it was recognized that a

B. Hermann, PhD
Department of Neurology, University of Wisconsin School of Medicine and Public Health, Madison, WI 53705, USA
e-mail: hermann@neurology.wisc.edu

M. Mula (ed.), *Neuropsychiatric Symptoms of Epilepsy*, Neuropsychiatric Symptoms of Neurological Disease, DOI 10.1007/978-3-319-22159-5_6

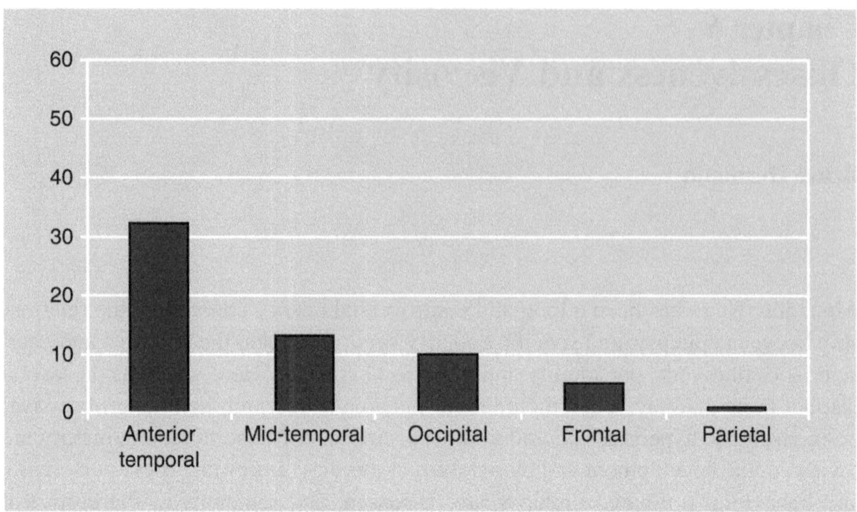

Fig. 6.1 Severe personality disorder and EEG focus [1]. "To use a figure of speech, the Sylvian fissure is one of the chief boundaries between neurology and psychiatry" [1]

sizeable proportion of partial seizures had their origin in the temporal lobes and limbic system. Case studies published over the years also stimulated interest in unusual personality and behavioral traits/changes associated with epilepsy and TLE specifically, which included sudden religious conversions, increased philosophical interest, and humorlessness. Waxman and Geschwind [3, 4] eventually formally proposed a specific inter-ictal behavioral syndrome consisting of alterations in sexual behavior, increased religiosity, and a tendency toward extensive writing (hypergraphia).

This theme of thinking and research was further developed by Bear and Fedio [5], who proposed that progressive changes in limbic system structure occurred secondary to a temporal-limbic epileptiform focus which produced new functional connections between neocortical and limbic structures—termed *sensory-limbic hyperconnection*, resulting in enhanced affective associations to previously neutral stimuli, events, or concepts—subsequently resulting in progressive changes in 18 proposed changes in personality, behavior, and affect. It was argued that as these behavioral changes were neither maladaptive nor psychopathologic in the traditional sense, new and different assessment techniques were needed to demonstrate their existence. Questionnaires to assess these characteristics were devised by Bear and Fedio including a patient self-report form (*Personal Inventory*) and a companion proxy-based measure (*Personal Behavior Survey*). In their influential initial paper, and related to the theme of this chapter, Bear and Fedio [5] reported that circumstantiality, obsessiveness, and viscosity were among the most discriminating traits identifying TLE from controls.

This was and remains a very highly cited paper (591 citations as of March 2015) and it initiated a long and very intense debate surrounding the question of personality change in epilepsy. Some 20+ years later, Devinsky and Najjar [6] critically reviewed 17 papers specifically using the inventories developed by Bear and Fedio and concluded: (1) TLE and other epilepsy groups exhibited increased (abnormal) scores versus healthy controls and/or neurobehavioral controls; (2) differences between patients with TLE versus other epilepsies, such as primary generalized epilepsies, were inconsistent; (3) epilepsy patients were poorly distinguished from patients with psychiatric disorders; (4) laterality differences in relation to the presentation of these personality and behavioral changes in TLE were not strongly marked; (5) factors that could affect personality were not systematically studied; (6) a behavioral syndrome distinctive or specific for TLE was not defined; and (7) the behavioral inventories developed by Bear and Fedio focused interest in behavior and epilepsy.

Additional research at the time included the development of additional assessment techniques to assess the behaviors of interest including semi-structured interview techniques (Behavior Rating Scales for Epilepsy [7]), other similar questionnaires (Neurobehavioral Inventory [8]), questionnaire measures of specific behaviors such as viscosity [9], and direct behavioral investigations of the traits of interest which will be reviewed in more detail.

Definition of Terms

In the original Bear and Fedio publication, the proposed behavioral changes were presented as having been based on specific clinical observations reflected in published case studies and reports. Obsessionalism was based in observations of ritualism, orderliness, and compulsive attention to detail. Viscosity was based in observations of stickiness and a tendency to repetition. Related traits were circumstantiality (characterized by loquacious, pedantic, overly detailed and peripheral speech) and hypergraphia (characterized by keeping extensive diaries, detailed notes, and writing autobiography or novel).

All of these terms and behaviors of course have additional meanings and some traits have been of longer-standing interest in epilepsy. For example, in a more conventional characterization, circumstantiality can be defined as a communication disorder in which the focus of conversation drifts, but often comes back to the point. Unnecessary details and irrelevant remarks cause a delay in getting to the point. This is less severe than tangential speech where the speaker wanders and drifts but usually never returns to the original topic. Pertinent symptoms may include slowed thinking and speaking at length about trivial details, and eliciting information can be difficult as circumstantiality makes it hard for the person to stay on topic. In most instances, the relevant details are eventually achieved. For example, if one asks “At what age did your mother die?”, the speaker may respond by talking at length about his mother, accidents, and how too many people die in accidents, and then eventually state the age at which his mother died (due to an accident) [10]. This particular trait had been of interest and early views, such as expressed by Kraepelin [11], suggested a link to epilepsy:

> Here we observe a unique sign, the circumstantiality of the epileptic patient. The patient begins each answer with many details that initially don't seem to be related to the question. He adds so many unnecessary details that he does not seem to move forward. He does not lose his train of thought, though, and eventually gets to the point, albeit circuitously.

As noted, over time, the link between circumstantially and epilepsy began to focus on an association with specific epilepsy syndromes, included as part of a broader set of personality characteristics linked to epilepsy and temporal lobe epilepsy in particular, attributed to nonspecific psychiatric complications of the epilepsies, and posited to perhaps reflect a more generally disordered language system.

Hypergraphia and Viscosity: Written and Oral Reflections of Circumstantiality or Obsessiveness?

Overlapping and related traits such as hypergraphia [3, 12–15] and verbosity/viscosity [14] were topics of direct investigation in their own right. Hypergraphia was defined and operationalized to include: (a) writing styles that were *unusual* (e.g., mirror images, codes, different colored inks, ritualized script), (b) writing that was *excessive* (e.g., length, frequency, duration of writing), and (c) preoccupation with selected *themes* (e.g., philosophical, moral, ethical). Others added additional features such as "writing goes beyond social, occupational, or educational requirements" and "associated with a pressure to express self and ideas, perception of having unique thoughts and ideas."

Operational definitions made it possible to interrogate these traits in ways that were arguably more precise than assessment via questionnaires. For example, assessing hypergraphia specifically, and in an operational fashion, Sachdev and Waxman [12] used a standard stimulus question ("Describe to the best of your ability, your present state of health, understanding of the disease, and the changes in your life resulting from it"). Letters were then mailed to 63 patients and dependent measures of interest included the response rate, length of written response, and qualitative features of the syndrome. The response rate was 53 % for TLE and 21 % for non-TLE, and the median length of responses for TLE was 403 words versus other epilepsies with a median length of response of 100 words. Qualitative features of the responses suggested that two patients exhibited the behavioral syndrome.

In one of our own attempts to examine hypergraphia [12], a standard written stimulus question was posed to patients who were undergoing inpatient EEG monitoring:

> We are very interested in learning about how epilepsy affects our patients' lives. Please begin writing below and tell us, in as much detail as you think important, how epilepsy has affected you and the course of your life, both for the better as well as for the worse. Use as many additional sheets as necessary. Everything you write will be held strictly confidential.

Two dependent measures were derived from the writing samples: (1) the total number of words contained in the response; and (2) the presence or absence of references to the meaning or significance of their seizures—philosophical, ethical or religious themes, and unusual writing styles (e.g., calligraphy, use of unusual symbols or drawings). These assessments were conducted by an independent rater blinded to all characteristics of each responder. This was done in a fashion identical to that used previously by the present investigators.

The sample consisted of 50 epilepsy patients and 6 % of the responses were hypergraphic with the predictors of response length being the MMPI Depression scale ($p < .05$) (decreased length with increased depression), the MMPI Mania scale ($p < .05$) (increased length of response with increased Ma scale score), and the presence of adverse life events ($p = .04$) (increased response length with elevated mania scale and increased life events).

In addition to this direct measure of writing behavior, the subjects were clinically evaluated regarding their writing behavior using an interview-based Research Diagnostic Criteria-like procedure. Using this procedure, 30 % of the sample was classified as hypergraphic. While the proportion of patients classified as hypergraphic differed between the two methods, there was a significant correlation between the number of words written and a clinical-interview-based rating of hypergraphia. Predictors of interview determined hypergraphia included primary generalized epilepsy ($r = 0$–35), a previous psychiatric history ($r = 0.45$), increased MMPI Hypomania ($r = 0.34$) and Schizophrenia ($r = 0.27$) scales, an increased number of life events ($r = 0.38$), and being female ($r = 0.25$).

Thus, operational definitions help to focus attention on the behavior of interest, provide estimates of the frequency of occurrence and the predictors of the behavior. The operational definitions have varied across studies of hypergraphia, there are demonstrated differences in the same subject pool when assessed by direct behavior versus interview, and clear is the fact that these behaviors occur in a modest subset of epilepsy patients in general and TLE in particular. Many of the classic features are not observed (i.e., different inks, mirror writing), suggesting that such behaviors are even more uncommon, and predictors of these abnormal behaviors include markers of psychopathology.

Similar objective approaches examined *verbosity or viscosity*. Examining verbosity, Hoeppner et al. [15] characterized the actual speech of patients with various types of epilepsy and various foci, and compared it with the speech of control individuals. They also investigated the influence of several variables on speech including intelligence, memory, and age of onset and duration of epilepsy.

All subjects were shown the “cookie thief card” from the Boston Diagnostic Aphasia Examination and all responses were tape-recorded and then transcribed verbatim. Transcriptions were blindly reviewed, and examined were topical shifts, trivial details, length of response and dysfluencies (i.e., part-word repetitions, word-repetitions, revisions, incomplete phrases, broken words, prolonged sounds). The results showed that only 4 of 29 (14 %) epilepsy participants were verbose. All had complex partial seizures with left hemisphere EEG foci, not quite half of all epilepsy participants with left-sided complex partial seizures. They tended to be older than other epilepsy participants, with longer seizure and medication histories. They tended to introduce extra-list intrusions into recall, but were not otherwise distinguishable from nonverbose epilepsy participants with complex partial seizures in other aspects of memory or intelligence. Finally, their verbosity was marked by references to nonessential details, including subjective, peculiar, illusory, and one extrapictorial elaboration.

Rao et al. [9] examined viscosity and social cohesion in TLE. As they pointed out that viscosity had different meanings:

> This trait has had two meanings in the epilepsy literature: stickiness of thought processes or enhanced interpersonal adhesiveness; also referred to as increased social cohesion. Such patients are often described as talking repetitively and circumstantially, sticking to restricted topics, and having difficulty in breaking off conversations. Increased social cohesion is characterised by a tendency to form clinging relationships with family members and close friends.

They developed self-report and rater scales for both viscosity, defined strictly as repetitive and circumstantial speech, and social cohesiveness. They embedded these two scales within a longer test, which provided additional scales for paranoid tendencies and a defensive response style. They examined a total subject pool consisting of 118 participants that included patients with left, right, or bilateral TLE as well as patients with absence or generalized epilepsy, a psychiatric control group consisting of panic disorder patients, and normal controls.

All subjects completed a 32-item true-false questionnaire that yielded four summary scales: viscosity, social cohesion, paranoia, and five items from the lie scale of the MMPI. Similar traits were also rated by a close relative (spouse, parent, sibling) or friend with a 24-item true-false questionnaire assessing the same traits.

There were no group differences in social cohesion, but viscosity, as measured by self-report and rater scales, was observed more often in patients with left-sided or bilateral temporal lobe seizure foci. The authors speculated that viscosity is caused by a critical deficit in the TLE patient's ability to perceive social cues in conversation including posture, facial expressions, and eye contact in addition to linguistic communication.

As they explained:

> During normal conversation, participants assume mutual responsibility for assuring that what is said has been heard and understood before the conversation proceeds. TLE patients with viscosity may fail to perceive that the listener has understood what was said, resulting in speech repetition or disjointed conversational switches. In addition, mental slowing, which is common in epilepsy patients partly due to seizure medications, may contribute to the perception of viscosity by observers.

Conclusion

When *operationally defined and behaviorally assessed*, "traits" such as circumstantiality, hypergraphia, and verbosity occur in a small subset of epilepsy patients; therefore, these behaviors are the exception rather than the rule. Varying methods of analysis (direct behavioral observations vs. rating scales) of the same behavior will result in different frequencies. An imprecise understanding of what underlies the expression of these unusual behavioral phenotypes remains, as does the relationships across traits and their underlying anatomy. The relationship of these atypical behaviors to disorders of social interaction and related anatomical substrate as well as fundamental abnormalities in the underlying language system appear to be potentially promising paths to pursue.

Acknowledgments Thanks to Guenter Kraemer, MD, for providing the quote by Kraepelin and Susanne Seeger, MD, for translation.

References

1. Gibbs FA. Ictal and non-ictal psychiatric disorders in temporal lobe epilepsy. J Nerv Ment Dis. 1951;113(6):522–8.
2. Guerrant J, Anderson WW, Fischer A, Weinstein MR, Jaros M, Deskins A. Personality in epilepsy. Springfield: Charles C Thomas Publisher; 1962.
3. Waxman SG, Geschwind N. Hypergraphia in temporal lobe epilepsy. Neurology. 1974;24(7):629–36.
4. Waxman SG, Geschwind N. The interictal behavior syndrome of temporal lobe epilepsy. Arch Gen Psychiatry. 1975;32(12):1580–6.
5. Bear DM, Fedio P. Quantitative analysis of interictal behavior in temporal lobe epilepsy. Arch Neurol. 1977;34(8):454–67.
6. Devinsky O, Najjar S. Evidence against the existence of a temporal lobe epilepsy personality syndrome. Neurology. 1999;53(5 Suppl 2):S13–25.
7. Mungas D. Interictal behavior abnormality in temporal lobe epilepsy. A specific syndrome or nonspecific psychopathology? Arch Gen Psychiatry. 1982;39(1):108–11.
8. Blumer D. Personality in epilepsy. Semin Neurol. 1991;11(2):155–66.
9. Rao SM, Devinsky O, Grafman J, Stein M, Usman M, Uhde TW, et al. Viscosity and social cohesion in temporal lobe epilepsy. J Neurol Neurosurg Psychiatry. 1992;55(2):149–52.
10. Green B. Problem-based psychiatry. 2nd ed. United Kingdom: Radcliffe Publishing Ltd; 2009.
11. Kraepelin E. Psychiatrie. Ein kurzes Lehrbuch für Studirende und Aerzte. Dritte, vielfach umgearbeitete Auflage. Leipzig: Abel Verlag; 1899.
12. Sachdev HS, Waxman SG. Frequency of hypergraphia in temporal lobe epilepsy: an index of interictal behaviour syndrome. J Neurol Neurosurg Psychiatry. 1981;44(4):358–60.
13. Hermann BP, Whitman S, Arntson P. Hypergraphia in epilepsy: is there a specificity to temporal lobe epilepsy? J Neurol Neurosurg Psychiatry. 1983;46(9):848–53.
14. Hermann BP, Whitman S, Wyler AR, Richey ET, Dell J. The neurological, psychosocial and demographic correlates of hypergraphia in patients with epilepsy. J Neurol Neurosurg Psychiatry. 1988;51(2):203–8.
15. Hoeppner JB, Garron DC, Wilson RS, Koch-Weser MP. Epilepsy and verbosity. Epilepsia. 1987;28(1):35–40.

Chapter 7
Aggressive Behavior

Hesham Yousry Elnazer and Niruj Agrawal

Abstract Epilepsy was considered to be commonly associated with aggression historically. It has also been emphasized in medicolegal settings. However, the link between epilepsy and directed aggression is now noted to be less clear-cut even though brief and non-directed aggression can occur not so uncommonly. Aggression in epilepsy could be linked to a number of factors including seizures or the underlying electrophysiological activity of the brain, neuropsychiatric comorbidities, anti-epileptic drugs or underlying brain damage which may cause aggression and epilepsy both. Common clinical presentations of aggressive behaviors in epilepsy and their pathogenesis are discussed. A clinical approach to assess and manage these problems is described and related evidence is discussed.

Keywords Epilepsy • Aggression • Agitation • Automatism • Intermittent Explosive Disorder

Introduction

Epilepsy is one of the oldest known illnesses. Seizures were believed to be associated with evil procession causing violent movements and aggressive behaviors. Throughout history, the disorder was thought to be of a spiritual nature. The world's oldest description of an epileptic seizure goes back to Mesopotamia around 2000 BC. A person was described as being under the influence of a moon god with violent movements and disruptive behaviour and subsequently underwent exorcism. Epileptic seizures are listed in the Code of Hammurabi (c. 1790 BC) as reason for

H.Y. Elnazer, MBBch, MRCPsych • N. Agrawal, MBBS, MD, MSc, Dip CBT, FRCPsych (✉)
Department of Neuropsychiatry, St. George's Hospital, Blackshaw Road, London SW17 0QT, UK
e-mail: doctor_hesham@yahoo.com; niruj.agrawal@swlstg-tr.nhs.uk

M. Mula (ed.), *Neuropsychiatric Symptoms of Epilepsy*, Neuropsychiatric Symptoms of Neurological Disease, DOI 10.1007/978-3-319-22159-5_7

which a purchased slave may be returned for a refund [1]. The Edwin Smith Papyrus (c. 1700 BC) describes cases of individuals with epileptic convulsions [2].

The Babylonian tablet 1067 BC (currently at the British Museum in London) describes different seizure types, similar to what we recognize today. It also emphasizes the supernatural nature of epilepsy, with each seizure type associated with the name of a spirit or god—usually evil alluding to development of bad/aggressive behaviors. The text gives signs and symptoms, different types, and details treatment and likely outcomes [2]. Punarvasu 900 BC Atreya described epilepsy as loss of consciousness; this definition was carried forward into the Ayurvedic text of Charaka Samhita (400 BC) [3].

The idea that epilepsy is a supernatural or spiritual disorder persisted with widespread beliefs that it was due to possession by the devil. This notion gained popularity through the common observation—at the time—of violent movements, behavioral changes, and aggression. Epilepsy was also viewed as a result of a person perpetrating evil doings, or as a consequence of cycles of the moon or mystic magical phenomenon.

Hippocrates (c. 400 BC) was first to regard epilepsy and its associated motor and behavioral changes as a physical disorder due to natural causes. This was contradictory to the wide belief understanding of epilepsy as a spiritual phenomenon. Galen of Pergamon (AD 130–200) described three types of fits, and deduced that epilepsy was a brain disorder related to an accumulation of thick humors. Galen postulated that the moon governs the periods of epileptic cases [4].

It was not before the nineteenth and twentieth centuries that scientific explanations replaced and dominated the previous concepts. Nevertheless, the belief that epilepsy is linked to violent behavior acquired popularity in the late nineteenth century when the criminologist Cesare Lombroso promoted the association of epilepsy with aggressive, sociopathic tendencies on the basis of degenerative theory, which was prevalent at that time [4]. The notion of a close association between epilepsy and violence persisted long after the Degenerative theory became widely refuted. Up until the early 1980s, aggressive and self-destructive impulses were linked to people with epilepsy in a popular psychiatric textbook [5, 6]. This view gradually lost general acceptance in the 1990s following several studies which showed that aggressive phenomena, including destructive acts, can arise during epileptic seizures, but are extremely rare [7, 8].

Epidemiology

Epilepsy is a common condition with a prevalence of 8.2/1000 [9]. Risk factors for aggression in epilepsy include organic cerebral disease, low socioeconomic status, and poor upbringing [10]. Some data suggests higher vulnerability for patients with intractable epilepsy to develop aggressive disorder following epilepsy surgery including hippocampectomy or temporal lobectomy. The hippocampus and related area have been implicated in seizure-induced behavioral and cognitive disorders and also aggression [11].

A multicenter study measured aggression in 503 patients from nine centers using the Aggression Questionnaire. This study concluded that aggressive behaviors in patients with epilepsy were different from that in the normal population. After adjustment for age and sex, when appropriate, the results showed that the presence of compromised intellectual functioning, psychiatric disturbances, and disability status, number of medications, geographic distribution, education, chronologic age, and disease duration all significantly affected aggressiveness [12].

A retrospective study at a residential epilepsy center found the prevalence of aggression to be 27.2 % in 1 year compared to age and sex matched controls. The overall frequency was estimated at between 121 and 207 incidents per 100 persons per year. A few incidents (0.7 %) were related to an acute psychosis but they were more likely to result in significant injury. Offenders were younger than non-aggressive residents. Gender, age of onset of epilepsy, history of psychosis, mobility, abnormality on MRI scan, learning disability, and seizure frequency were not associated with aggressive conduct [13].

An earlier review suggested a two- to four-times greater prevalence of epilepsy in prisoners than controls although it maintained that the prevalence is similar to the prevalence in other socioeconomic populations from which the prisoners came. The review refuted that violence was more common among epileptic patients than non-epileptics or in patients with temporal lobe epilepsy compared to other subtypes of epilepsy. Ictal violence is rare, and usually in the form of resistive violence due to confusion as the result of physical restraint at the end of a seizure. Violence early in a seizure is extremely rare, stereotyped, and never supported by consecutive series of purposeful movements [14].

The chronological relationship between seizures and violent behaviors in patients with epilepsy is significant. A study on patients with post-ictal psychosis (PIP) showed that well-directed violent attacks occurred during 22.8 % of the post-ictal psychosis episodes, 4.8 % of the inter-ictal psychosis episodes, and 0.7 % of the post-ictal confusions. Proneness to violence (and also suicidal attempts) stood out in the post-ictal psychotic episodes. Purposeful, organized violence as a direct manifestation of seizures or ictal automatism is highly exceptional. Violent acts could occur in post-ictal confusion as an expression of unconscious, vigorous resistance against efforts of surrounding people to prevent the affected patient from sustaining accidental injury. On the other hand, some post-ictal psychotic episodes can be risky, especially if a violent act has been reported in preceding episodes. Violent acts by patients with epilepsy should be treated differently according to the various pathophysiological backgrounds from which the violence arises [15].

Post-ictal behavioral changes (PBCs) include psychosis, aggression, and mood change, and are commonly observed in patients with epilepsy. Recognition and description of the clinical manifestations of PBCs is important in patients' management. Additionally, various quantified objective scales available in clinical psychiatry could be used to assess PBCs. There are few reports in which objective rating scales have been used to assess neuropsychiatric symptoms in patients with epilepsy. In contrast, there have been a small number of studies on inter-ictal psychosis and depression in which either the Brief Psychiatric Rating Scale or the Hamilton

Depression Scale was used. These can be useful for the assessment of PBCs but may not be routinely required [15].

Clinical Description/Presentation

Epilepsy is often complicated by behavioral symptoms including aggression or various psychiatric disorders. Behaviour symptoms associated with epilepsy may be pre-ictal, ictal, post ictal or inter ictal [16]. Seizures-related behavioral changes, including aggressive behaviors, have been interpreted as the emergence of "archeical" or innate motor patterns [17].

One third of patients with epileptic seizures—especially secondarily generalized seizures—develop pre-ictal prodromal symptoms hours to days before the seizures. These can include mood changes or depression, irritability, restlessness or motor hyperactivity, and poor frustration tolerance; all of which can lead to aggressive or emotional outbursts. These symptoms are often relieved by the occurrence of the seizure although might persist for few days afterwards. It has been suggested that these prodromal symptoms may represent biophysiological processes involved in initiation of abnormal emotions and seizures or a subclinical seizure activity [16].

Ictal behavioral symptoms occur in nearly in 25 % of auras (especially when long), following a cluster of complex partial and secondary generalized seizures of temporal lobe epilepsy (TLE) or non-convulsive status epilepticus [18]. These can include depression (which ranges from mild sadness to profound hopelessness, despair feelings of anhedonia, guilt, and suicidal ideation) [16], fear, distress, nervousness, anger, irritability, panic attacks, phobias [19, 20], forced thinking, obsession [12, 13], and aggression [21]. Ictal aggression is unorganized and accidental. Directed aggression towards people is observed as resistive aggression as a result of physical restraint in the context of ictal confusion [22].

Ictal behavioral symptoms tend to be stereotyped, paroxysmal, of brief duration, and unprovoked by environmental stimuli. These are sometimes associated with other characteristics of temporal discharges such as bizarre behavior, mutism and amnesia, depersonalization and déjà vu, as well as automatism and altered consciousness [23].

Post-ictal behavioral symptoms occur after seizures, particularly with TLE and last hours to days. The symptoms include anxiety, dysphoria, depression, psychosis, suicidal ideas, and transient aggression [24–26]. Aggression is frequently reported in post-ictal confusional states or post-ictal psychoses. Post-ictal psychosis might ensue between 12 h and up to 7 days following the seizure episode, with symptoms lasting from few hours to few days or rarely for up to 4 weeks. Post-ictal psychosis may be associated with irritability and aggression along with affective and psychotic symptoms [25].

Inter-ictal behavioral symptoms are often mild and spontaneously reversible [27]. Complex partial seizures (CPS) of temporal lobe origin may be accompanied by inter-ictal emotional disturbances [28] such as sadness or dysphoria, anxiety, irritability, and aggression [29].

Personality changes have been reported in association with epilepsy (as epileptic personality), schizophreniform psychosis, impulse control disorder (including aggression), somatoform disorder (conversion, somatization), dissociative amnesia, and fugue and psychogenic non-epileptic seizures [27]. Inter-ictal aggressive behavior is among the frequent psychiatric comorbidities with epilepsy, with prevalence varying between 4.8 and 50 % (not taking into account the specific epileptic sub-syndromes) compared to aggression in general population comparing for socioeconomic profile, public and family circumstances, and ethnic social vulnerabilities [21].

Aggression in patients with epilepsy can also manifest as episodic and independent from observable seizures and may not be classifiable as ictal post-ictal or inter-ictal. This could either be due to AEDs, psychiatric comorbidities, or associated with underlying neurological conditions (episodic dyscontrol) [23].

Investigations and Diagnosis

The mainstay of diagnosis of aggressive behavior is a detailed history rather than any particular investigation. Obtaining detailed and complete neuropsychiatric history and pre-existing aggressive behaviors or other behavioral disturbances is crucial. Vulnerability factors to aggression in epilepsy should be investigated.

Early detection of neuropsychiatric comorbidities including history of head trauma, brain surgeries, or hemorrhage can increase the risk of behavioral changes in epilepsy and aggression. Pre-existing or subsequently developed depression, anxiety, or psychotic disorders increases the risk of developing aggressive behaviors.

In contrast to EEG, brain imaging may not be a part of the essential practice in the diagnosis and management of epilepsy. Nevertheless, utilizing neuroimaging to detect early or old brain changes can be helpful to determine the vulnerability of the patient to develop behavioral changes and aggression. EEG may show increase of slow-waves in individuals with aggressive behavior [17].

Brain imaging studies have reported that patients with epilepsy and severe aggression (intermittent explosive disorder) had a significantly higher incidence of encephalitic brain disease and left-handedness, more bilateral EEG abnormality, and less frequent hippocampal sclerosis than controls. A sub-group in the aggressive patients showed severe amygdala atrophy. In a further analysis using voxel-based morphometry, reductions of gray matter density over large areas of the left extratemporal neocortex, maximal in the left frontal neocortex, were observed [30].

Aggression associated with epilepsy can be discriminated from a non-ictally related aggression by its directionality. That is, ictal aggression is not planned and focused. However, ictal aggression might ensue if post-ictal delirium is forcibly contained [31, 32]. Suggested criteria to diagnose specific violent behaviors of epilepsy include: a. the diagnosis of epilepsy should be established by a neurologist with special competence in epilepsy; b. the presence of epileptic automatisms should be documented by the case history and closed-circuit TV-EEG; c. aggression during epileptic automatisms should be documented on closed-circuit TV-EEG; d. the aggressive act should be characteristic of the patient's habitual seizures; and e. a clinical judgment should be made by the neurologist as to the possibility that the violent act was part of a seizure [14].

Pathogenesis

The relationship between epilepsy and psychiatric presentations suggests involvement of similar—if not the same—neuroanatomical structures, pathogenic mechanisms, and neurotransmitters. Recurrent epileptiform discharges, kindling, and related neurobiological abnormalities will result in prolonged aura, hypometabolism of other brain areas, disrupted neuronal plasticity, epilepsy intractability cognitive deficits, and behavioral phenomena [32–35]. It has been suggested that post-ictal psychiatric manifestations are a direct manifestation of epileptic discharges in the brain, although it might be a consequence of the inhibitory mechanisms involved in the termination of seizures [23–25].

The repeated focal or generalized ictal and inter-ictal epileptiform results in an abnormal recurrent synaptic bombardment of distant projection areas. This may induce plastic changes sensory-limbic hyper-connection and impair the naturally occurring homeostatic which maintain the inter-ictal state and therefore disturbing the normal neuronal and psychological functions [32, 35, 36].

Disturbances of the limbic system, frontal-limbic-subcortical circuits, frontostriatal systems, limbic-brainstem connections or amygdala, amygdala-hypothalamic connection, amygdala-locus coeruleus connection are postulated to be among the potential causes of behavioral disorders in patients with epilepsy and are likely to be linked with aggression in epilepsy as well [32, 34, 37].

Available literature is consistent with the explanation that epilepsy-like neuronal hyperexcitability is a biological substrate of disturbed emotional behavior [38]. The hippocampus and the amygdala are common foci from which CPS originate. The amygdala is involved in normal and abnormal emotional behaviors and serves an important role in fear, anxiety, and emotional memory. The amygdala is also involved in complex social behaviors such as aggression and impulse control. In CPS, the emotional behavior system can become supersensitized, resulting in an epilepsy-like state of neuronal hyperexcitability that produces emotional disturbances and abnormal behavior. This facilitates an adaptive, rapid, subcortical processing of the emotional salience of objects and events in the surrounding environment. Abnormal behavior can result from the over activity of this mechanism. In the extreme, the over activity produces seizures [38].

At a sub-seizure level, cellular and molecular mechanisms may underlie the abnormal emotional processes that contribute to emotional dysfunction, namely, inappropriate aggression and lack of impulse control [38]. Afferent input to the amygdala activates both excitatory and inhibitory amino acid receptors [39–42] and thus, alteration of excitatory and inhibitory transmission may change the functional output of the amygdala. Neurobiological processes that depend on the amygdala occur with changes in excitability of neurons within the amygdala.

Mechanisms of synaptic plasticity, including long-term potentiation [43, 44] and long-term depression [45], have been shown to occur at specific synapses in the amygdala. Plastic changes in neurotransmission also occur following epilepsy [46, 47] and following fear-conditioning [42, 48].

Following induced epilepsy, several physiological alterations have been demonstrated. A comprehensive study investigating lasting changes in amygdala neuronal excitability used a sharp electrode and whole-cell recordings from brain slices containing the baso-lateral nucleus of the amygdala (BLA) [47], has shown that glutamate and GABA receptors are altered after eliciting fully induced (stage 5) seizures [49]. Neurons in the BLA become hyper-excited following kindling [38].

Aggressive behaviors are relatively rare during epileptic fits [50]. A case study of a patient with intractable CPS, had depth electrodes implanted in the amygdala to map the focus of epileptic activity prior to surgery. This study showed that delivering a short stimulus via the implanted electrodes evoked a seizure that included angry facial grimaces with baring of the teeth (a primate "threat display") and a sudden and unexpected violent attack. Although the reported violent behaviors were directed toward an inanimate object (the wall), the suddenness of the aggressive outburst explained why others had been harmed during similar stereotyped outbursts in prior seizures [51]. The study highlights the overlap between aggressive behavior and seizure activity, even though the violent outbursts are phenomenologically different from violence in people without epilepsy [38].

Other brain areas involved in generating epileptic discharges and behavioral symptoms include: limbic system, temporal lobe, orbitofrontal regions, anterior insula, anterior cingulate gyrus, and basal ganglia [52–54]. The most important brain structures implicated in the mediation of aggressive behavior are the amygdala and associated-limbic structures, the frontal lobes, periaqueductal gray, and the hypothalamus. The amygdala is thought to play a crucial role in the mediation of fear-induced aggression [55].

Antiepileptics and Aggression

Some antiepileptic drugs (AEDs) have demonstrated mood improvement and a therapeutic potential for patients with epilepsy. However, other AEDs have been reported to have a negative behavioral effect in patients with epilepsy [56, 57].

The negative behavioral disturbances may result from the direct action of the drug via alteration of ion channels and neurotransmitter system functions and modulation of the electrochemical systems [57–59]. AEDs negative effects may indirectly result from the effect of the drug on the epilepsy itself leading to what is known as forced normalization phenomenon. This occurs when successful seizure control with AED is associated with negative impact of worsening of behavior with concomitant improvement in seizure control.

Many AEDs exert their effect via potentiating GABA inhibitory transmission. Some studies report phenobarbital to have the greatest behavioral toxic potential with dose-related impairment in attention and reaction time, performance intelligence quotient, and short-term memory, and inducing a hyperkinetic syndrome in children [60]. Gradual conversion to a non-barbiturate AED in epileptic patients with depressed, irritable, or aggressive manifestations may avoid the need for prescribing a psychotropic medication [27].

Valproate causes sedation and less often cognitive impairment, irritability, depression, hyperactivity, and aggressive behavior [61]. Gabapentin can cause irritability and agitation and minimal negative cognitive and behavioral side effects in patients with epilepsy [62]. Vigabatrin was reported to be associated with increased occurrence of depression and psychosis, agitation, and irritability. Hyperkinesia and agitation were commonly reported in children receiving vigabatrin [62].

Antigultamatergic AEDs may cause anxiety, insomnia, and agitation. Lamotrigine was reported to cause insomnia, irritability, hyperactivity, and stereotypic or aggressive behavior. Also, felbamate has stimulant properties, which can cause anxiety, irritability, or insomnia [56, 57, 63, 64].

Some AEDs act on serotonin receptors. In patients with existing behavioral difficulties, carbamazepine may cause irritability, impaired attention, and behavioral problems. Carbamazepine-epoxide (active metabolite) is partly responsible for the mild cognitive and psychomotor effects attributed to carbamazepine. Mild degrees of confusion, nervousness, agitation, irritability, abnormal thinking, and fatigue have been reported with zonisamide therapy. High rates of psychosis and depression have been reported for zonisamide and topiramate (highlighting their action as carbonic anhydrase-inhibitors) [65].

The mechanism of action psychotropic effects for some AEDs is not known. Reports suggest a Phenytoin's dose-related decline in concentration, memory, visuomotor functions, and mental speed, generating anxiety, aggression, fatigue, and depression [65]. In contrast to these reports a double-blind crossover study on impulse and premeditated aggression in in-mates reported that during the phenytoin treatment, the frequency of impulsive aggressive behaviors were significantly diminished compared with that in the placebo control condition. The anti-aggressive effect of phenytoin was concluded to be selective for impulsive aggression as it was without effect on aggression in the premeditated group. Similar results were reported in a non-inmate population showing that carbamazepine and valproate are also as efficacious as phenytoin in reducing impulsive aggressive acts. These anticonvulsants have been used in psychiatric patients with impulsive aggressive symptoms [66, 67]. The selective properties of phenytoin on impulsive aggression suggest that biological mechanisms of excitability distinguish impulsive and premeditated aggression [38].

Phenytoin and levetiracetam may cause anxiety, impair mood, and cognitive functions, and consequently increased risk of suicide. Ethosuximide is used to treat absence seizures. It may cause confusion, sleep disturbances as insomnia, aggressive behavior, depression, and rarely psychosis [68].

It has been reported that ~ nearly 5–10 % of adults taking levetiracetam manifest with irritability, hostility, nervousness, emotional lability, anxiety, depression, and other behavioral and cognitive disorders [69, 70]. In a study of 288 consecutive patients with epilepsy on levetiracetam (90 % polytherapy, mean dose = 2689 mg), 43 patients on other AEDs as a control group and 135 relatives, to determine whether levetiracetam caused a positive or negative behaviors. Levetiracetam was rated as very effective by 40 % of the patients. In contrast to only 9 % of the controls, a considerable number of patients reported a behavioral change while taking levetiracetam (12 % very negative, 25 % negative, 16 % positive, 6 % very positive). Negative ratings included—predominantly—aggression, loss of self-control, restlessness, and sleep problems. Positive ratings were related to increased energy, vigilance, and activation. Increases in psychomotor speed, concentration, and remote memory indicated subjectively experienced positive effects on cognition. The proxy reports indicated reliable self-reports. Levetiracetam exerts a dose-independent stimulating effect that can be positive or negative. Aggression is a prominent feature. Lack of efficacy, mental retardation, and presumably also pre-intake disposition (organic psychosyndrome, impulsivity) may be helpful in predicting whether additional activation under levetiracetam will be positive or negative [71]. However, more recently, aggression associated with levetiracetam in epilepsy has been shown to correlate to clinical and subclinical depression [72].

There is RCT evidence showing worsening of aggressive behavior in children with adjunctive treatment with levetiracetam as compared to placebo [73]. Similar evidence exists for levetiracetam mono-therapy in late onset post-stroke seizures leading on to aggressive behavior in 8.55 % at 3000 mg which lead to termination of the treatment [74]. In an open label treatment multicenter observational study in a cohort of 285 pediatric patients with a mean age of 9.9 years, diagnosed with refractory generalized and focal epilepsy who received levetiracetam as an add-on, somnolence (23.9 %), general behavioral changes (15.4 %), aggression (10.5 %), and sleep disturbances (3.2 %) were reported [75]. In a multicenter, open label, study assessing cognition and behavior in 103 patients aged 4–16 years with partial-onset seizures levetiracetam was associated with treatment-emergent adverse events including aggression [7.8 %] and irritability [7.8 %]. Of these patients, 4.9 % discontinued levetiracetam because of treatment-emergent adverse events [76].

In a study of perampanel as an adjunct treatment of patients with partial seizures in three phase trials, overall, depression and aggression were reported more frequently in patients taking perampanel, particularly at higher doses, than in patients taking placebo. Reported side effects necessitated the withdrawal of perampanel in 99 patients (9.5 %) and placebo in 21 patients (4.8 %) [77].

Epilepsy, Psychiatric Comorbidities, and Aggression

Epilepsy is commonly complicated with psychiatric disorders. Among these, depression is the most, with prevalence of 20–55 %, some references report up to 80 % [78, 79]. Aggression may be a consequence of a pre-existing psychiatric disorder or a psychiatric disorder that developed subsequent to epilepsy [23]. A wide range of psychiatric comorbidities in epilepsy can present with aggressive behavior.

Commonly depression and anxiety can be associated with increased irritability which could result in verbal or physical aggression [23, 80]. Issue of correlation of depression with aggression in epilepsy was studied using Beck Depression Inventory II (BDI-II), Centre for Epidemiologic Studies Depression Scale (CES-D), and Buss-Perry Aggression Questionnaire (BAQ) in patients with epilepsy and depression compared to patients with idiopathic depression [81]. The results showed the BAQ and BDI scores were closely related within a group of patients with epilepsy and depression, while BAQ and BDI scores were not correlated with each other within a group of patients with idiopathic depression. This suggests that depression in people with epilepsy is more likely to lead to aggression than idiopathic depression. There is some emerging evidence that suggests that depression may modulate drug-induced aggression particularly with levetiracetam in epilepsy [72].

Aggression in epilepsy can be due to a comorbid antisocial personality disorder [23]. High risk of aggressive behavior in epilepsy has been found to be frequently related to left TLE, intractable epilepsy, low intelligence quotient in particular verbal intelligence, early onset of seizures, dominant-hemisphere electroencephalographic (EEG) focus, and antisocial personality disorders [23].

Epilepsy and aggression can often present together as a consequence of other neurological or psychiatric conditions such as traumatic brain injury, vascular disorders, limbic encephalitis, alcohol or drug dependence, or due to learning disability. In such situations epilepsy may not be causally linked to aggression and may be merely an incidental comorbidity [80].

Medicolegal Aspects

The link between epilepsy and aggression against humans has been disproportionally emphasized in the medicolegal settings. Available evidence lacks the precise description of seizures as well as the chronological relationship of violence and seizures [82]. However, a few studies have attempted to study the link between epileptic seizures and aggressive behavior.

Well-directed attacks on surroundings are unlikely to occur with ictal automatism. More organized aggressive response may be possible during post-ictal confusion. Sudden serious emotional upset while in clear consciousness is commonly produced by psychic aura, and could serve as a potential source of aggressive behavior, especially if the amygdala is involved and the episode lasts for an extended period [30, 83–85]. If the violent act is post-ictal and sudden-onset, it is more likely to occur after a cluster of seizures and is usually related with alcohol abuse.

A study of groups matched age and age of onset of epilepsy, examined 30 patients with post-ictal confusion, 30 patients with post-ictal psychosis, and 33 patients with inter-ictal psychosis. All patients had complex partial seizures and EEG temporal foci. The study monitored aggressive behaviors towards humans following spontaneous complex focal seizures and were directly observed and documented by the medical staff within 1 month of admission. Well-directed and well-documented attacks against humans were counted as incidents of violent behavior, which was defined as irrational behavior that resulted in a severe injury, such as bone fracture, or a life-threatening situation, such as strangulation. Aggressive behavior such as cursing and menacing gestures, without physical attacks were not included. Episodes of resistive violence, in which attempts to restrain patients followed a violent reaction, were counted separately. Well-directed violent attacks occurred during 22.8 % of the post-ictal psychosis episodes, 4.8 % of the IIP episodes, and 0.7 % of the episodes of post-ictal confusion. Compared with the other two situations, proneness to violence stood out in the post-ictal psychosis episodes. Resistive violence was observed only during episodes of post-ictal confusion (3.0 %) [86].

In patients with frequent, hyperkinetic seizures of frontal origin, well-targeted, highly organized violent acts have not been reported. On the other hand, violent acts could occur in post-ictal confusion as an expression of unconscious, vigorous resistance to efforts of surrounding people to prevent the affected individual from roaming or fumbling about. If caretakers can avoid direct physical contact and only watch as the situation may allow, it will require at most half an hour before the unorganized behavior ceases and the individual becomes settled.

Some post-ictal psychosis episodes can be highly alarming, especially if a violent act has been committed in preceding episodes. Even without any apparent physical intervention, unpredictable outrage can be targeted toward people incidentally in the area. Post-ictal psychosis episodes are biologically based and closely linked to seizures; thus, successful seizure control also controls violent acts. In contrast, in IIP episodes, aggression based on frank psychotic experience is typically not directed toward those who are incidentally in the area, but rather toward an imaginary culprit suggested by a hallucinatory voice or delusional idea [86].

Intermittent explosive disorder (also known as episodic dyscontrol syndrome) was described as a condition with associated cranial neurophysiological abnormality although the validity of the concept has been disputed. It presents as sudden episodes of spontaneously released violence, often in the setting of minimal provocation, which tend to be short-lived. They may be provoked by small amounts of alcohol, and after the events, patients may feel remorse. Generally, the condition is associated with non-specific abnormalities that are also seen in epilepsy, with evidence of minimal neurologic damage, soft neurologic signs, and abnormal EEG studies, although there is no evidence that these episodes have the same pathophysiology as epileptic seizures [87].

Management of Aggression in Epilepsy

Aggressive behavior and related behavioral difficulties in patients with epilepsy can often be missed. Screening for behavioral changes and psychiatric comorbidities such as depression is crucial for early identification and adequate management. Chronological prospective needs to be adopted when considering whether behavioral changes are premorbid, related to the illness, psychiatric comorbidities, or a consequence of treatment. Early recognition and treatment can help patients and carers to cope better and in turn a better quality of life [88].

Optimizing seizure control is important when managing any epilepsy-related aggression, but particularly in cases of ictal, post-ictal, and inter-ictal aggression symptoms [27] and aggression. In addition, psychological and behavioral measures, such as anger management, relaxation training, and if necessary, individual psychotherapy particularly cognitive behavioral therapy (CBT), can help [27]. If optimization of AEDs, seizure control, and behavioral and psychological measures are not sufficient, psychopharmacological measures can be used.

There are no RCTs to guide treatment of aggression in people with epilepsy. Generally the pharmacological approach followed would be similar to management of aggression in other neurological settings including traumatic brain injury. Atypical antipsychotic medications such as risperidone or quetiapine can be used in smaller doses and if there is lack of tolerance or lack of response then other atypical antipsychotics such as olanzapine or aripiprazole can be used. If aggression is linked to depression then use of SSRIs is indicated. In patients where aggression is linked to emotional lability or impulsivity then the use of mood stabilizers or choice of AEDs with mood stabilizing properties such as carbamazepine and valproate can be helpful.

When aggression is believed to be due to AED, reducing or discontinuing that AED and replacing it with a suitable alternative is indicated. After a thorough assessment, if a salient psychiatric symptom or aggression persists and the AED cannot be changed, both behavioral and pharmacology intervention should be added. Caution must be used while choosing a psychotropic medication to avoid drugs with known significant effect on the seizure threshold. The adverse effects and drug interactions should be carefully considered [89].

Untreated comorbid psychiatric disorders can lead to aggressive behaviors. The relationship between psychiatric disorders and epilepsy has therapeutic implications which should be directed towards a comprehensive biopsychosocial approaches. Continuous re-evaluation of the management plan and the anticonvulsant treatment is important. Pre-ictal and ictal depression does not usually require any specific psychopharmacological or psychological treatment [27]. In more severe cases of personality disorders with epilepsy where aggression is evident, lithium, antipsychotics, carbamazepine, and valproic acid should be considered [90].

When treating comorbid depression with epilepsy, priority should be given to AEDs that might improve mood along with antidepressant and attention enhancing efficacy, and reduce anxiety and suicidal tendencies. Some AEDs with antiglutamatergic and serotonergic properties may confer antidepressant, mood stabilizing effects [56]. AEDs with serotonergic properties will improve mood and reduce the anxiety risk, because they exert effects similar to antidepressants (i.e., selective serotonin reuptake inhibitors or SSRIs), whereas AEDs that lack serotonergic mechanisms would not be effective in improving mood, reduction of anxiety and suicidality. Sedating drugs have anxiolytic, antimanic, and sleep-promoting benefits [27].

Both antiepileptic and antidepressants drugs are metabolized by the hepatic microsomal cytochrome P450 oxidases (3A4, 1A2, 2C19, 2C9, and, possibly, 2B6)

[91] and also influence the 2D6 cytochrome. Antidepressants and AEDs can influence these enzymes by inducing or inhibiting them. The levels of AED that act as a substrate for the cytochrome may be decreased if an inducing antidepressant drug is added, with decreasing of seizure threshold while enzyme inhibitor may decrease the metabolism of AEDs, thus increasing toxicity from the AED. Serotonin syndrome is a rare disorder that may result from drug interactions between AEDs of serotonergic properties and SSRIs. It is caused by excessive serotonergic stimulation; symptoms include restlessness, myoclonus, hyperthermia, convulsions, and possibly death [92].

Careful follow-up of the serum levels of antiepileptic and antidepressants may be required while treating comorbid depression with epilepsy. The AEDs most commonly reported for interactions with antidepressants are the cytochrome-inducing drugs and the inhibitory agent valproate [93, 94]. Significant levels of these AEDs have been observed when used in combination with fluoxetine and thus fluoxetine should not be used in combination with carbamazepine, phenytoin, or phenobarbital, or, at the least, serum monitoring is required.

Slow titration in antidepressant dosages is recommended while treating comorbid depression and epilepsy as fast titration can cause an increase in seizure frequency with antidepressants. Other methods of treatment should be considered for severe, treatment-resistant, or psychotic depression and independent of effect on seizure frequency which include: neuroleptics [95], electro convulsive therapy (ECT) [96], and vagus nerve stimulation [97].

Buspirone at low dosages has been found to be useful for ameliorating aggression. It does not appear to interact with anticonvulsants. However, in animal models, buspirone has been shown to be pro-convulsant [98]. In addition, one case report cites a patient who sustained a seizure after an overdose of buspirone [99].

Beta-blockers (propranolol) may be useful for modulating overstimulation and to treat aggression in patients with epilepsy [100]. The beta-blockers decrease hyperarousal, restlessness, and tension. They decrease anxiety and cause little cognitive compromise. Nadolol works peripherally, whereas propranolol is more lipophilic and exerts more CNS effects. Both medications, especially propranolol, may require titration to obtain an effective dosage. However, propranolol has been noted to be associated with seizure activity in over dosage. In some animal models, however, it appears to increase the seizure threshold [101]. In addition, depression is a rare side effect of propranolol [100]. Benzodiazepines and barbiturates should not be used as anxiolytics in people with epilepsy because of the danger of dependence and the potential for withdrawal seizures [27].

In a small study of deep brain stimulation (DBS) of the posterior hypothalamus (pHyp) in the treatment of drug-refractory and severe painful syndromes of the face, disruptive and aggressive behavior was associated with epilepsy and below-average intelligence. Six (75 %) of eight patients presenting with aggressive behavior and mental retardation benefited from pHyp stimulation; six patients were part of the authors' series and two were reported in the literature [80]. However, DBS is not clinically indicated at this stage in treating aggression in epilepsy based on the current level of evidence.

References

1. Saraceno B, Avanzini G, Lee P, editors. Atlas: epilepsy care in the world. World Health Organization; 2005. Retrieved 20 Dec 2013. http://www.who.int/mental_health/neurology/epilepsy_atlas_r1.pdf
2. Magiorkinis E, Kalliopi S, Diamantis A. Hallmarks in the history of epilepsy: epilepsy in antiquity. Epilepsy Behav. 2010;17(1):103–8.
3. Epilepsy: an historical overview. World Health Organization; 2001. Retrieved 27 Dec 2013. htpp://www.who.int/mediacentre/factsheets/fs168/en/
4. Lombroso-Ferrero G. Criminal man according to the classification of Cesare Lombroso. Montclair: Patterson Smith; 1972.
5. Kolb LC, Brodie HKH. Modern clinical psychiatry. 10th ed. Philadelphia: WB Saunders; 1982.
6. Pincus J. Violence and epilepsy. N Engl J Med. 1981;305:696–8.
7. Delgado-Escueta AV, Mattson RH, King L, Goldensohn ES, Spiegel H, Madsen J, et al. Special report: the nature of aggression during epileptic seizures. N Engl J Med. 1981;305:711–6.
8. Treiman DM. Psychobiology of ictal aggression. In: Smith D, Treiman DM, Trimble M, editors. Neurobehavioral problems in epilepsy. New York: Raven; 1991. p. 341–56.
9. Hauser WA. Incidence and prevalence. In: Engel J, Pedley TA, editors. Epilepsy: a comprehensive textbook. Philadelphia: Lippincott-Raven; 1997. p. 47–57.
10. Hermann BP, Whitman S. Behavioural and personality correlates of epilepsy: a review methodological critique, and conceptual model. Psychol Bull. 1984;95:451–92.
11. Engel Jr J. Update on surgical treatment of the epilepsies. Summary of the second international palm desert conference on the surgical treatment of the epilepsies (1992). Neurology. 1993;43(8):1612–7.
12. Piazzini A, Bravi F, Edefonti V, Turner K, Vignoli A, Ferraroni M, Canevini MP. Aggressive behavior and epilepsy: a multicenter study. Epilepsia. 2012;53(10):e174–9.
13. Bogdanovic MD, Mead SH, Duncan JS. Aggressive behaviour at a residential epilepsy centre. Seizure. 2000;9(1):58–64.
14. Treiman DM. Epilepsy and violence: medical and legal issues. Epilepsia. 1986;27 Suppl 2:S77–104.
15. Ito M. Neuropsychiatric evaluations of postictal behavioral changes. Epilepsy Behav. 2010;19(2):134–7.
16. Blanchet P, Frommer GP. Mood change preceding epileptic seizures. J Nerv Ment Dis. 1986;174(8):471–6.
17. Bronsard G, Bartolomei F. Rhythms, rhythmicity and aggression. J Physiol Paris. 2013;107(4):327–34.
18. Manchanda R, Freeland A, Schaefer B, McLachlan RS, Blume WT. Auras, seizure focus, and psychiatric disorders. Neuropsychiatry Neuropsychol Behav Neurol. 2000;13(1):13–9.
19. Biraben A, Taussig D, Thomas P, Even C, Vignal J, Scarabin J, Chauvel P. Fear as the main feature of epileptic seizures. J Neurol Neurosurg Psychiatry. 2001;70(2):186–91.
20. Alemayehu S, Bergey GK, Barry E, Krumholz A, Wolf A, Fleming CP, Frear Jr EJ. Panic attacks as ictal manifestations of parietal lobe seizures. Epilepsia. 1995;36(8):824–30.
21. Kanemoto K, Kawasaki J, Mori E. Violence and epilepsy: a close relation between violence and postictal psychosis. Epilepsia. 1999;40(1):107–9.
22. Treiman DM. Violence and the epilepsy defense. Neurol Clin. 1999;17(2):245–55.
23. Kanner AM. Recognition of the various expressions of anxiety, psychosis and aggression in epilepsy. Epilepsia. 2004;45 Suppl 2:22–7.
24. Kanner AM, Stagno S, Kotagal P. Postictal psychiatric events during prolonged video-electroencephalographic monitoring studies. Arch Neurol. 1996;53(3):258–63.
25. So NK, Savard G, Andermann F, Olivier A, Quesney LF. Acute postictal psychosis: a stereo EEG study. Epilepsia. 1990;31(2):188–93.

26. Kanner AM, Trimble M, Schmitz B. Postictal affective episodes. Epilepsy Behav. 2010;19(2):156–8.
27. Hamed SA. Psychiatric symptomatologies and disorders related to epilepsy and antiepileptic medications. Expert Opin Drug Saf. 2011;10(6):913–34.
28. Devinsky O. Interictal behavioral changes in epilepsy. In: Devinsky O, Theodore WH, editors. Epilepsy and behavior. New York: Wiley–Liss; 1991. p. 1–21.
29. Bear DM, Fedio P. Quantitative analysis of interictal behavior in temporal lobe epilepsy. Arch Neurol. 1977;34:454–67.
30. Wieser HG, Hailemariam S, Regard M. Unilateral limbic epileptic status activity: stereo-EEG, behavioral, and cognitive data. Epilepsia. 1985;26:19–29.
31. van Elst LT, Woermann FG, Lemieux L, Thompson PJ, Trimble MR. Affective aggression in patients with temporal lobe epilepsy, a quantitative MRI study of the amygdala. Brain. 2000;123(Pt 2):234–43.
32. Engel J, Wilson C, Lopez-Rodriguez F. Limbic connectivity: anatomical substrates of behavioural disturbances in epilepsy. In: Trimble M, Schmitz B, editors. The neuropsychiatry of epilepsy. Cambridge: Cambridge University Press; 2002. p. 18–37.
33. Mula M, Marotta AE, Monaco F. Epilepsy and bipolar disorders. Expert Rev Neurother. 2010;10(1):13–23.
34. Drevets WC. Functional neuroimaging studies of depression: the anatomy of melancholia. Annu Rev Med. 1998;49:341–61.
35. Hamed SA. Neuronal plasticity: implications in epilepsy progression and management. Drug Dev Res. 2007;68(8):498–511.
36. Engel J, Shewmon DA. Impact of the kindling phenomenon on clinical epileptology. In: Morrell F, editor. Kindling and synaptic plasticity: the legacy of Graham Goddard. Cambridge: Birkhauser; 1991. p. 195–210.
37. Steriade M. Corticothalamic resonance, states of vigilance and mentation. Neuroscience. 2000;101(2):243–76.
38. Keele NB. The role of serotonin in impulsive and aggressive behaviors associated with epilepsy-like neuronal hyperexcitability in the amygdala. Epilepsy Behav. 2005;7(3):325–35.
39. Mahanty NK, Sah P. Excitatory synaptic inputs to pyramidal neurons of the lateral amygdala. Eur J Neurosci. 1999;11:1217–22.
40. Rainnie DG, Asprodini EK, Shinnick-Gallagher P. Excitatory transmission in the basolateral amygdala. J Neurophysiol. 1991;66:986–98.
41. Rainnie DG, Asprodini EK, Shinnick-Gallagher P. Inhibitory transmission in the basolateral amygdala. J Neurophysiol. 1991;66:999–1009.
42. McKernan MG, Shinnick-Gallagher P. Fear conditioning induces a lasting potentiation of synaptic currents in vitro. Nature. 1997;390:607–11.
43. Huang CC, Hsu KS, Gean PW. Isoproterenol potentiates synaptic transmission primarily by enhancing presynaptic calcium influx via P- and/or Q-type calcium channels in the rat amygdala. J Neurosci. 1996;16:1026–33.
44. Gean P-W, Chang F-C, Huang C-C, Lin J-H, Long-Joy W, et al. Longterm enhancement of EPSP and NMDA receptor-mediated synaptic transmission in the amygdala. Brain Res Bull. 1993;31:7–11.
45. Wang SJ, Gean PW. Long-term depression of excitatory synaptic transmission in the rat amygdala. J Neurosci. 1999;19:10656–63.
46. Asprodini EK, Rainnie DG, Shinnick-Gallagher P. Epileptogenesis reduces the sensitivity of presynaptic gamma-aminobutyric acid B receptors on glutamatergic afferents in the amygdala. J Pharmacol Exp Ther. 1992;262:1011–21.
47. Shinnick-Gallagher P, Keele NB, Neugebauer V. Long-lasting changes in the pharmacology and electrophysiology of amino acid receptors in amygdala kindled neurons. In: Corcoran M, Moshe S, editors. Kindling 5. New York: Plenum; 1997.
48. Rogan MT, Staubli UV, LeDoux JE. Fear conditioning induces associative long-term potentiation in the amygdala. Nature. 1997;390:604–7.

49. Racine RJ. Modification of seizure activity by electrical stimulation. II. Motor seizure. Electroencephalogr Clin Neurophysiol. 1972;32:281–94.
50. Fenwick P. Aggression and epilepsy. In: Devinsky O, Theodore WH, editors. Epilepsy and behavior. New York: Wiley–Liss; 1991. p. 85–96.
51. Mark VH, Ervin FR. Violence and the brain. New York: Harper & Row; 1970.
52. Broicher S, Kuchukhidze G, Grunwald T, Krämer G, Kurthen M, Trinka E, Joiket H. Association between structural abnormalities and fMRI response in the amygdala in patients with temporal lobe epilepsy. Seizure. 2010;19(7):426–31.
53. Helmstaedter C. Behavioral aspects of frontal lobe epilepsy. Epilepsy Behav. 2001;2(5):384–95.
54. Elst LT, Groffmann M, Ebert D, Schulze-Bonhage A. Amygdala volume loss in patients with dysphoric disorder of epilepsy. Epilepsy Behav. 2009;16(1):105–12.
55. Eron LD, Gruder CL. Some topics closely related to the study of abnormal behavior: aggression and fantasy. In: Reiss S et al., editors. Abnormality: experimental and clinical approaches. New York: Macmillan; 1977. p. 579–638.
56. Ketter TA, Post RM, Theodore WH. Positive and negative psychiatric effects of antiepileptic drugs in patients with seizure disorders. Neurology. 1999;53 Suppl 2:S53–67.
57. Nadkarni S, Devinsky O. Psychotropic effects of antiepileptic drugs. Epilepsy Curr. 2005;5(5):176–81.
58. Koneski JA, Casella EB. Attention deficit and hyperactivity disorder in people with epilepsy: diagnosis and implications to the treatment. Arq Neuropsiquiatr. 2010;68(1):107–14.
59. Kuzniecky R, Ho S, Pan J. Modulation of cerebral GABA By topiramate, lamotrigine, and gabapentin in healthy adults. Neurology. 2002;58(3):368–72.
60. Yanai J, Fares F, Gavish M, Greenfeld Z, Katz Y, Marcovici G, et al. Neural and behavioral alterations after early exposure to phenobarbital. Neurotoxicology. 1989;10(3):543–54.
61. Meador KJ, Loring DW, Hulihan JF, Kamin M, CAPSS-027 Study Group, Karim R. Differential cognitive and behavioural effects of topiramate and valproate. Neurology. 2003;40(9):1279–85.
62. Harden CL, Lazar LM, Pick LH, Nikolov B, Goldstein MA, Carson D, et al. A beneficial effect on mood in partial epilepsy patients treated with gabapentin. Epilepsia. 1999;40(8):1129–34.
63. McConnell H, Snyder PJ, Duffy JD, Weilburg J, Valeriano J, Brillman J, et al. Neuropsychiatric side effects related to felbamate. J Neuropsychiatry Clin Neurosci. 1996;8(3):341–6.
64. Fakhoury TA, Miller JM, Hammer AE, Vuong A. Effects of lamotrigine on mood in older adults with epilepsy and co-morbid depressive symptoms: an open-label, multicentre, prospective study. Drugs Aging. 2008;25(11):955–62.
65. Cavanna AE, Ali F, Rickards HE, McCorry D. Behavioral and cognitive effects of anti-epileptic drugs. Discov Med. 2010;9(45):138–44.
66. Gardner DL, Cowdry RW. Positive effects of carbamazepine on behavioral dyscontrol in borderline personality disorder. Am J Psychiatry. 1986;143:519–22.
67. Kavoussi RJ, Coccaro EF. Divalproex sodium for impulsive aggressive behavior in patients with personality disorder behavior in patients with personality disorder. J Clin Psychiatry. 1998;59:676–80.
68. Wolf P, Trimble MR. Biological antagonism and epileptic psychosis. Br J Psychiatry. 1985;146:272–6.
69. Cramer JA, De Rue K, Devinsky O, Edrich P, Trimble MR. A systematic review of the behavioral effects of levetiracetam in adults with epilepsy, cognitive disorders, or an anxiety disorder during clinical trials. Epilepsy Behav. 2003;4(2):124–32.
70. Mecarelli O, Vicenzini E, Pulitano P, Vanacore N, Romolo FS, Di Piero V, et al. Clinical, cognitive and neurophysiologic correlates of short-term treatment with carbamazepine, oxcarbazepine and levetiracetam in healthy volunteer. Ann Pharmacother. 2004;38(11):1816–22.
71. Helmstaedter C, Fritz NE, Kockelmann E, Kosanetzky N, Elger CE. Positive and negative psychotropic effects of levetiracetam. Epilepsy Behav. 2008;13(3):535–41.

72. Mula M, Agrawal N, Mustafa Z, Mohanalingham K, Cock HR, Lozsadi DA, von Oertzen TJ. Self-reported aggressiveness during treatment with levetiracetam correlates with depression. Epilepsy Behav. 2015;45:64–7.
73. de la Loge C, Hunter SJ, Schiemann J, Yang H. Assessment of behavioral and emotional functioning using standardized instruments in children and adolescents with partial-onset seizures treated with adjunctive levetiracetam in a randomized, placebo-controlled trial. Epilepsy Behav. 2010;18(3):291–8.
74. Belcastro V, Costa C, Galletti F, Autuori A, Pierguidi L, Pisani F, et al. Levetiracetam in newly diagnosed late-onset post-stroke seizures: a prospective observational study. Epilepsy Res. 2008;82(2–3):223–6.
75. Opp J, Tuxhorn I, May T, Klugerc G, Wiemer-Krueld A, Kurlemanne G, et al. Levetiracetam in children with refractory epilepsy: a multicenter open label study in Germany. Seizure. 2005;14(7):476–84.
76. Schiemann-Delgado J, Yang H, Loge Cde L, Stalvey TJ, Jones J, Legoff D, Mintz M. A long-term open-label extension study assessing cognition and behavior, tolerability, safety, and efficacy of adjunctive levetiracetam in children aged 4 to 16 years with partial-onset seizures. J Child Neurol. 2012;27(1):80–9.
77. Rugg-Gunn F. Adverse effects and safety profile of perampanel: a review of pooled data. Epilepsia. 2014;55 Suppl 1:13–5. doi:10.1111/epi.12504.
78. Ettinger A, Reed M, Cramer J. Depression and comorbidity in community-based patients with epilepsy or asthma. Neurology. 2004;63(6):1008–14.
79. Mensah SA, Beavis JM, Thapar AK. The presence and clinical implications of depression in a community population of adults with epilepsy. Epilepsy Behav. 2006;8(1):213–9.
80. Riggio S. Traumatic brain injury and its neurobehavioral sequelae. Psychiatr Clin North Am. 2010;33(4):807–19.
81. Beyenburg S, Mitchell AJ, Schmidt D, Elger CE, Reuber M. Anxiety in patients with epilepsy: systematic review and suggestions for clinical management. Epilepsy Behav. 2005;7(2):161–71.
82. Brower MC, Price BH. Epilepsy and violence: when is the brain to blame? Epilepsy Behav. 2000;1:145–9.
83. Kanemoto K. Periictal Capgras syndrome following clustered ictal fear. Epilepsia. 1997;38:847–50.
84. Hermann BP, Chhabria S. Interictal psychopathology in patients with ictal fear: examples of sensory-limbic hyperconnection? Arch Neurol. 1980;37:667–8.
85. Takeda Y, Inoue Y, Tottori T, Mihara T. Acute psychosis during intracranial EEG monitoring: close relationship between psychotic symptoms and discharges in amygdala. Epilepsia. 2001;42:719–24.
86. Kanemoto K, Tadokoro Y, Oshima T. Violence and postictal psychosis: a comparison of postictal psychosis, interictal psychosis, and postictal confusion. Epilepsy Behav. 2010;19(2):162–6.
87. Monroe R. Episodic behaviour disorder. Boston: Harvard University Press; 1970.
88. Mrabet H, Mrabet A, Zouari B, Ghachem R. Health-related quality of life of people with epilepsy compared with a general reference population: a Tunisian study. Epilepsia. 2004;45(7):838–43.
89. Leppik IE, Gram L, Deaton R, Sommerville KW. Safety of tiagabine: summary of 53 trials. Epilepsy Res. 1999;33(2–3):235–46.
90. Trimble M. Treatment issues for personality disorders in epilepsy. Epilepsia. 2013;54 Suppl 1:41–5.
91. Harvey AT, Preskorn SH. Cytochrome P450 enzymes: interpretation of their interactions with selective serotonin reuptake inhibitors (part 1). J Clin Psychopharmacol. 1996;16(4):273–85.
92. Dursun SM, Mathew VM, Reveley MA. Toxic serotonin syndrome after fluoxetine plus carbamazepine. Lancet. 1993;342(8868):442–3.

93. Grimsley SR, Jann MW, Carter JG, D'Mello AP, D'Souza MJ. Increased carbamazepine plasma concentrations after fluoxetine coadministration. Clin Pharmacol Ther. 1991;50(1):10–5.
94. Lucena MI, Blanco E, Corrales MA, Berthier ML. Interaction of fluoxetine and valproic acid. Am J Psychiatry. 1998;155(4):575.
95. McConnell H, Duncan D. Treatment of psychiatric comorbidity in epilepsy. In: McConnell H, Snyder PJ, editors. Psychiatric comorbidity in epilepsy: basic mechanisms, diagnosis, and treatment. Washington, DC: American Psychiatric Press; 1998. p. 245–61.
96. Baghai TC, Moller HJ. Electroconvulsive therapy and its different indications. Dialogues Clin Neurosci. 2008;10(1):105–17.
97. Elger G, Hoppe C, Falkai P, Rush AJ, Elgera CE. Vagus nerve stimulation is associated with mood improvements in epilepsy patients. Epilepsy Res. 2000;42(2–3):203–10.
98. Ninan TN, Cole JO, Yonkers KA. Nonbenzodiazepine anxiolytics. In: Schatzberg AF, Nemeroff CB, editors. Textbook of psychopharmacology. 2nd ed. Washington, DC: American Psychiatric Press; 1998. p. 287–300.
99. Catalano G, Catalano MC, Hanley PF. Seizures associated with buspirone overdose: case report and literature review. Clin Neuropharmacol. 1998;21(6):347–50.
100. Yudofsky SC, Silver JM, Hales RE. Treatment of agitation and aggression. In: Yudofsky SC, Hales RE, editors. The American psychiatric press textbook of neuropsychiatry. Washington, DC: American Psychiatric Press; 1997. p. 881–900.
101. Raju SS, Gopalakrishna HN, Venkatadri N. Effect of propranolol and nifedipine on maximal electroshock-induced seizures in mice: individual and in combination. Pharmacol Res. 1998;38(6):449–52.

Chapter 8
Epilepsy and Sleep: Close Connections and Reciprocal Influences

Paolo Tinuper, Francesca Bisulli, and Federica Provini

Abstract Epilepsy and epileptic seizures affect every aspect of a patient's cognitive, social, and emotional well-being. Also sleep disorders have an adverse impact on daily living for both patients and their caregivers . This chapter is devoted to the relationship between epilepsy and sleep and its disorders. The effects of epilepsy on sleep architecture and the quality of sleep are reviewed discussing how sleep may affect epilepsy and the role of antiepileptic therapy on sleep structure. Evidence on the relation between epilepsy and sleep disorders is summarized with a brief discussion highlighting the differences between these disturbances. This chapter ends with an outline of the evaluation and treatment of epileptic patients with a sleep disorder.

Keywords Sleep • Epilepsy • Arousal Disorders • Nocturnal Frontal Lobe Seizures

The Influence of Epilepsy on Sleep Architecture and the Quality of Sleep

Epilepsy and epileptic seizures affect every aspect of a patient's cognitive, social, and emotional well-being. Also sleep disorders have an adverse impact on daily living for both patients and their caregivers [1, 2].

Epilepsy may have an important effect on sleep and the sleep–wake cycle affecting the quality, quantity, and architecture of sleep. Epileptic seizures may provoke an alteration in total sleep time, sleep latency, and spontaneous awakenings. Moreover, epileptiform discharges themselves may affect sleep by disrupting normal sleep architecture. The effects of epilepsy on sleep vary depending on the different epileptic syndromes and seizure type. The amount of REM sleep is decreased by 50 % in

P. Tinuper, MD (✉) • F. Bisulli, MD, PhD • F. Provini, MD, PhD
IRCCS Institute of Neurological Sciences, Via Altura 3, Bologna 40139, Italy

Department of Biomedical and Neuromotor Sciences, University of Bologna, Bellaria Hospital, Via Altura 3, Bologna 40139, Italy
e-mail: paolo.tinuper@unibo.it; francesca.bisulli@unibo.it; federica.provini@unibo.it

M. Mula (ed.), *Neuropsychiatric Symptoms of Epilepsy*, Neuropsychiatric Symptoms of Neurological Disease, DOI 10.1007/978-3-319-22159-5_8

patients with primary generalized tonic–clonic seizures, while it may be as low as 41 % in those suffering from secondarily generalized seizures [3]. Young children with infantile spasms and hypsarrhythmia and children with Lennox–Gastaut syndrome also have decreased REM sleep [4], whereas patients with childhood absence epilepsy and epilepsy with myoclonic absences did not show such disturbances [5]. The total non-REM sleep duration was higher (46.7 %) in patients with juvenile myoclonic epilepsy than in age-matched controls (23 %). Sleep disruption is less common in focal epilepsies and only in patients with multiple nocturnal seizures is the proportion of REM sleep significantly lowered. Interestingly, the pattern of sleep is largely unimpaired in benign focal epilepsy, a disorder with no apparent impairment of mentation or symptoms of daytime dysfunction, despite nocturnal seizures [6, 7].

The negative effect of epilepsy on the quality of sleep is particularly evident in children, who have more sleep problems than siblings or healthy controls. In addition, children with active seizure disorders have more complaints than epileptic children who are seizure-free. Age is also a factor, with younger children having more sleep problems than older children [8]. A correlation between nighttime awakening and daytime problems in learning and behavior in children with epilepsy has also been described [3].

An increase in daytime sleepiness-related symptoms in patients with epilepsy is a matter of debate. The few studies applying validated tools to investigate sleepiness failed to demonstrate a difference with respect to healthy controls [9]. Patients with Nocturnal Frontal Lobe Epilepsy, a particular epileptic condition with seizures occurring almost only during sleep [10], occasionally many times per night, may report non-restorative sleep and they often feel tired during the day [11–13]. However, daytime sleepiness is not significantly higher in patients with SHE than in controls [14].

The Influence of Sleep on Epileptic Activity

The influence of sleep stages on paroxysmal activity and seizures is well known. Epileptic inter-ictal discharges may be influenced by the state of arousal and seizures, particularly in some epileptic conditions, precipitated by sleep or occur primarily according to a recognizable circadian rhythm [15]. Drowsiness and NREM sleep EEG activity facilitate the propagation and synchronization of epileptiform discharges. In the presence of diminished, but still preserved, muscle tone, these discharges facilitate the clinical manifestation of seizures [2, 16].

The opposite occurs in REM sleep, when postural tone is inhibited and EEG activity desynchronized. For these reasons, inter-ictal discharges of focal epilepsies tend to propagate during NREM sleep whereas they become topographically restricted during REM episodes. On the other hand, the thalamocortical volleys that physiologically evoke the K-complexes and spindles in NREM stages facilitate the occurrence of generalized discharges in idiopathic generalized epilepsies (IGE). Seizures in IGE with Grand Mal (GTC) seizures on awakening appear exclusively or predominantly after awakening or while relaxing [17]. In these patients routine awake EEG could be normal, whereas EEG after sleep deprivation and during early sleep stages or soon after awakening may disclose generalized spike-and-wave discharges. The myoclonic jerks characteristic of juvenile myoclonic epilepsy (JME), another type of IGE, usually occur after awakening and are often precipitated by sleep deprivation [18]. Sleep is an important activating state of seizures in Benign Epilepsy of Childhood with Centrotemporal Spikes (BECT) [19], a form of idiopathic (with age-related onset) focal epilepsy. Drowsiness is a strong trigger of the typical EEG paroxysmal abnormalities on the centrotemporal areas and spikes appear only during sleep in about one third of patients.

Focal seizures in lesional or cryptogenetic partial epilepsy may have a random occurrence. However, seizures in some patients may adopt a more regular circadian rhythm during the illness, irrespective of the clinical form, and tend to concentrate preferentially during sleep.

Infantile spasms also occur more frequently in the period preceding or just following sleep, whereas they rarely occur during non-REM sleep and never during REM. Generalized tonic seizures associated with Lennox–Gastaut syndrome occur more frequently in clusters upon awakening.

Patients with sleep disorders may exhibit an increase in seizure frequency and more difficulty with seizure control secondary to sleep fragmentation. Patients with obstructive sleep apnea syndrome or restless legs syndrome may have poor seizure control. Patients with altered sleep patterns may also experience increased seizures. Central nervous system abnormalities that alter or interrupt circadian pathways may also affect sleep and seizure control.

Epilepsy and Sleep Disorders

Sleep disorders or sleep-related physiological events frequently coexist in patients with epilepsy and may mimic epileptic seizures. Prompt recognition of phenomena mimicking epilepsy is vital to prevent patients undergoing unnecessary and costly investigations, and clinicians instigating potentially harmful therapeutic regimens. Furthermore, it is important to recognize these cases because treatment of the sleep disorder may contribute to seizure control by decreasing sleep disruption [6, 20].

Sleep-Related Breathing Disorders

Obstructive Sleep Apnea (OSA)

Obstructive sleep apnea (*OSA*) is characterized by snoring associated with repetitive episodes of upper airway obstruction or cessation of breathing during sleep, associated with blood oxygen saturation reduction and consequent arousals and sleep disruption [21]. Awakenings with feelings of suffocation, fear due to sleep apnea, and intense distress are common; they may be mistaken for a nightmare, sleep terror, seizure or panic attack, but obstructive apneas occur repeatedly during the night, compared to the typical single occurrence per night for nocturnal panic (awaking from sleep in a state of panic, that is an abrupt and discrete period of intense fear or discomfort, accompanied by tachycardia, sweating, shortness of breath, chest pressure, etc.) [22]. When chronic, this pattern leads to sleep deprivation and excessive daytime sleepiness [21, 23]. OSA can be confirmed with polysomnography. The severity of OSA has been defined by use of apnea/hypopnea index (AHI) criteria alone.

Patients complain of daytime sleepiness and fatigue. Behavioral problems, hyperactivity, and neurocognitive deficits are much more common in children with sleep apnea compared to normal controls.

The prevalence of OSA is estimated at 10 % in unselected adult patients with epilepsy and 30 % of patients with medically refractory epilepsy [24–28].

Sleep-Related Groaning (Catathrenia)

Sleep-related groaning (*catathrenia*) is an expiratory groaning noise occurring almost every night, mainly during REM sleep and in the second half of the night [29–31]. The noise occurs without any respiratory distress or concomitant motor phenomena; patients are unaware of their groaning, and upon awakening in the morning do not recall anything particular about the night and feel restored. Affected patients have no overt neurological or respiratory diseases and during the groaning arterial oxygen saturation remains normal. Its predominant or exclusive occurrence during REM sleep, its duration (groaning usually lasts few seconds, often repeated in clusters) and the absence of any concomitant motor phenomena distinguish this nocturnal sound from moaning occurring during epileptic seizures. Patients usually decline any treatment because they are unconcerned about the problem.

Narcolepsy

Narcolepsy is a chronic neurologic disorder occurring in approximately one in 2000 persons and peaks in the second decade of life. There is no significant gender difference. Symptoms include excessive daytime sleepiness with or without cataplexy (a bilateral loss of muscle tone, triggered by strong emotion such as laughter or crying with consciousness usually unaffected), hypnagogic hallucinations, sleep paralysis, and fragmented nighttime sleep [20]. Narcolepsy characterized by excessive daytime sleepiness and cataplexy is actually classified as Narcolepsy type 1. It has now been firmly established that narcolepsy type 1 is caused by a deficiency of hypothalamic hypocretin (orexin) signaling. Narcolepsy characterized by excessive daytime sleepiness without cataplexy, although some atypical sensations of weakness triggered by unusual emotions such as stress and anger may be reported, is classified as Narcolepsy type 2 [21]. As sleepiness may be the only symptom in children, the diagnosis of narcolepsy may be more difficult in this age group [32–34]. Narcolepsy is likely an under recognized disorder in pediatric practice; 30 % of adults report symptom onset before 15 years, perhaps 16 % before 10 years of age, and possibly 4 % before the age of 5 [35, 36].

The symptoms of narcolepsy are frequently misdiagnosed as neurologic, psychiatric, or behavioral [37–39]. Diagnostic confusion arises because a lack of responsiveness due to excessive sleepiness is mistaken for epileptic absences, and cataplexy is confused with a variety of seizure types. In young children recognition of excessive sleepiness can be confounded by the occurrence of daytime naps in normal children. However, these should normally cease by the age of 3–4 years after which the reappearance of repeated napping is significant. The variety in the degree and distribution of loss of tone in cataplexy can be mistaken for different types of focal and generalized epileptic seizures. A lack of responsiveness associated with tiredness can be confused with facial myoclonia associated with absences.

The identification of triggers for cataplexy (usually strong emotions such as laughter or crying) is important in differentiating these paroxysmal events. Home-video recording of events can be more useful than attempting to capture events in unfamiliar environments such as hospitals because a degree of familiarity with surroundings and a relatively relaxed state is often required for cataplexy to occur. The relative frequency of attacks, their relation to emotional experience and preservation of consciousness are useful guides to genuine cataplexy. Polysomnography with a multiple sleep latency test (MSLT) may provide clear evidence of narcolepsy. Narcolepsy with cataplexy is strongly associated with hypocretin deficiency and human leukocyte antigen (HLA) DQB1*06:02 and the reduced or absent cerebrospinal fluid hypocretin may aid diagnosis [40].

The current treatment recommendations for narcolepsy include education (with the family and the other individuals with whom the child interacts), sleep hygiene (appropriate sleep scheduling and daily naps), and pharmacological interventions. Modafinil was reported to be effective for treating sleepiness, venlafaxine for cataplexy, and sodium oxybate for all symptoms, also in children [33].

Parasomnias

Parasomnias are considered benign phenomena, especially in children, and do not usually have a serious impact on sleep quality and quantity. They include disorders of arousal (arising from NREM sleep), parasomnias usually associated with REM sleep, and other parasomnias [21].

Disorders of Arousal

Disorders of arousal are common pediatric sleep disorders that tend to cease with development [41]. The three basic types of arousal disorders recognized in the International Classification of Sleep Disorders-ICSD-3 are confusional arousals, sleep terrors, and sleepwalking.

Confusional arousals, affecting up to 20 % of children, are characterized by mental confusion and disorientation, relative unresponsiveness to environmental stimuli and difficulty awakening the subject [42] (Fig. 8.1). They are sometimes associated with incontinence. These events present a difficult diagnostic problem since they can resemble post-ictal confusion typical in a patient with seizures. *Sleep terrors*, affecting 1–7 % of children, are "arousals from slow-wave sleep accompanied by a cry or piercing scream and autonomic nervous system and behavioral manifestations of intense fear" generally lasting 1–5 min [21] (Fig. 8.2). Although appearing alert, the child typically does not respond when spoken to, and more forceful attempts to intervene may meet with resistance and increased agitation.

Sleepwalking, peaking by age 8–12 years [41], is defined as "a series of complex behaviors (such as changes in bodily position, turning and resting on one's hand, playing with the sheets, sitting up in bed, resting on knees, etc.) that are usually initiated during arousals from slow-wave sleep and culminate in walking around with an altered state of consciousness and impaired judgment" [21].

During disorders of arousal, although individuals are asleep, they may appear awake (eyes open), but they may not recognize their parents or bed partner and resist attempts to be comforted or soothed, with attempts to wake the patient often

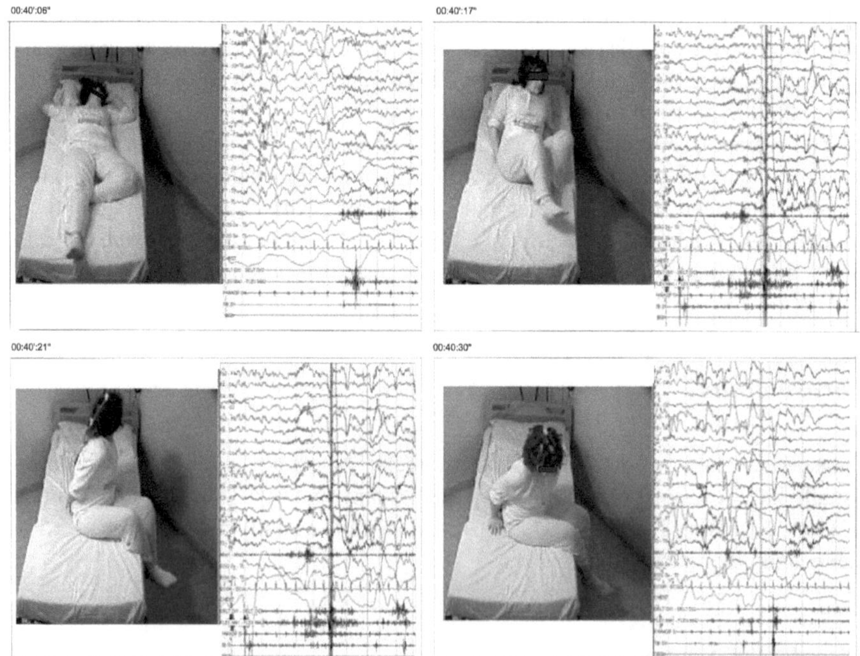

Fig. 8.1 Confusional arousal in a young girl. The patient sits on the bed and turns her head left and right pronouncing unintelligible words, unresponsive to environmental stimuli. Polysomnographic tracing during the event documents a delta-theta activity associated with increased muscle tone and change in respiratory and heart rates

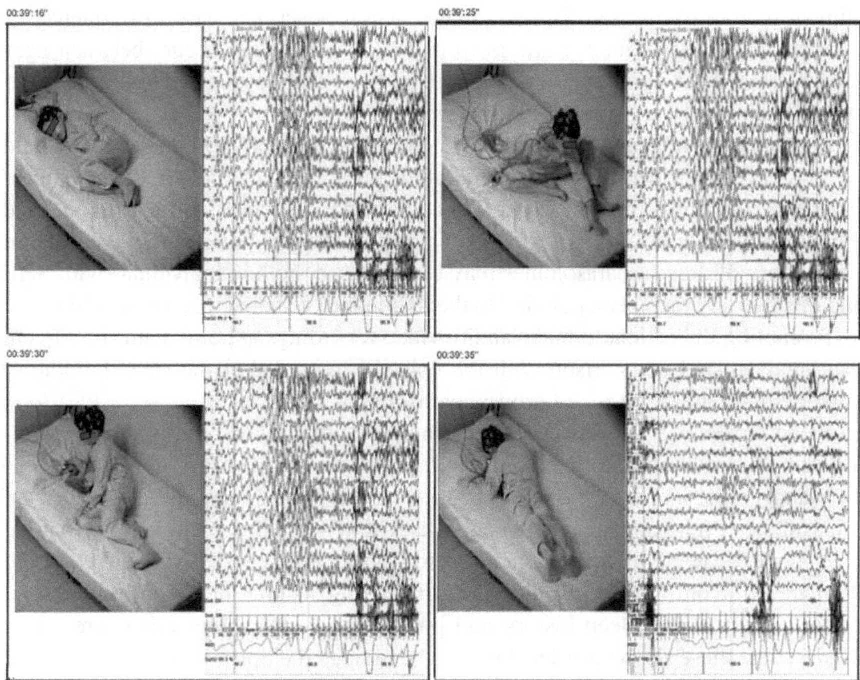

Fig. 8.2 Sleep terror in a 7-year-old boy. The patient sits on his bed, opens his eyes, touches the objects around him with his left hand looking around frightened, and then rapidly goes back to sleep. Polysomnographic tracing during the event documents a rhythmic delta activity associated with increased muscle tone and marked increase of heart rate

prolonging the event. Typical parasomnias resolve spontaneously with the patient rapidly returning to sleep, with no recollection of the event in the morning.

Disorders of arousal tend to occur in the first part of the night, when NREM stages 3 and 4 predominate, and may be triggered by a variety of factors including sleep deprivation, a disruption to the sleep environment or sleep schedule, stress, febrile illness, medications, alcohol, emotional stress in susceptible individuals or sleep-disordered breathing [43]. Polysomnography during the events reveals a rhythmic delta activity pattern associated with a marked increase in muscle tone, and changes in respiratory and heart rates.

Arousal parasomnias may mimic epileptic seizures, namely Nocturnal Frontal Lobe Seizures (NFLS), and the differential diagnosis can be challenging but can usually be accomplished by attention to the description of the events, their frequency, clustering, and timing in relationship to sleep onset [44]. Features that suggest an NREM parasomnias rather than NFLS are a low rate of same-night recurrence of the episodes, long duration, appearance within the first few hours of sleep (seizures may occur throughout the night), and the characteristic motor pattern (parasomnias are not stereotypical, and complex and repetitive behavior with abnormal movements, such as dystonic and dyskinetic postures, are absent) [45]. Moreover, the clinical picture of arousal disorders (early age at onset, decrease in frequency or disappearance after puberty) differs from NFLE which first occurs between ages 10–20 years, often persists into adulthood, and could be responsive to low doses of antiepileptic drugs, especially carbamazepine (Fig. 8.3).

Many parasomnias can be diagnosed on the basis of history-taking. Patients should be considered for video-EEG monitoring if events are stereotypic or repetitive, occur frequently (minimum one event per week), have not responded to medications, and the history is suggestive of potentially epileptic events [46]. Interestingly, prevalence of a history of arousal parasomnias may be increased, both in individuals with SHE and other family members, pointing to the likelihood of shared mechanisms [47].

Prompting the patient to make audio–video recordings at home with subsequent data analysis and comparison with the episodes recorded at the sleep laboratory may facilitate the diagnosis of arousal parasomnia.

Sleep terrors are also distinguished from nocturnal panic attacks by being followed by a quick return to sleep without recall of the event [22].

Management includes reassuring parents or bed partners that these episodes are a harmless developmental phenomenon, and they should not awaken the patient who should be gently redirected back to bed without awakening. Every effort should be made to avoid any predisposing and triggering factors identified by a careful general medical and sleep history and polysomnography. Medications are rarely used to treat these sleep disorders but may be indicated if episodes are very frequent or when the patient or others in the home are in danger of the behavior. In these cases imipramine or clonazepam at bedtime are beneficial in some patients.

REM Parasomnias

The most common and best-studied REM sleep parasomnia is the *REM sleep behavior disorder* (RBD). RBD is characterized by episodes of motor agitation of varying intensity arising during REM sleep, because the absence of the physiological muscle atonia of REM sleep permits the "acting out" of dreams [48]. The dreams are usually vivid, accompanied by vigorous, often violent sleep behaviors enacting attack or defense reactions; patients and bed partners are frequently injured, leading to bruising, lacerations, and fractures—the violence of the sleep-related behavior often being discordant with the waking personality. During the episodes autonomic activation is usually absent or mild. RBD patients tend to have from one to multiple events per night; the duration of the behavior is brief, and on awakening from an episode there is a rapid return to alertness and orientation with the patient's report of dream mentation appropriate to the observed behavior.

The events are more frequent in the middle of the night or early in the morning. RBD is more common in people older than 50 years of age and males [49, 50] antidepressants (tricyclic antidepressants, particularly the serotonin-specific reuptake inhibitors, SSRIs) [51] or associated with their withdrawal (alcohol, barbiturates or meprobamate) [52, 53]. The chronic form represents usually a prodromal sign of neurodegenerative diseases, particularly the synucleinopathies such as multiple sys-

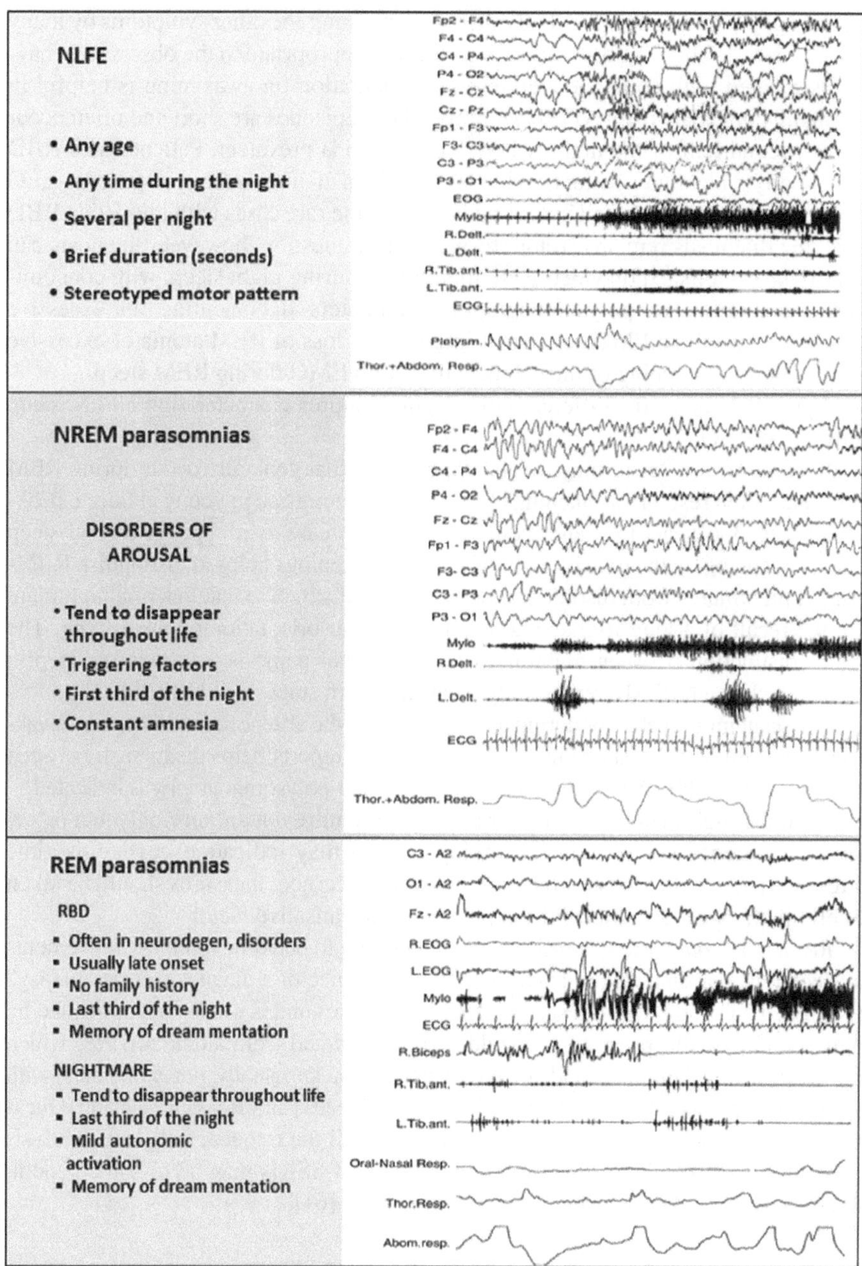

Fig. 8.3 Typical features distinguishing nocturnal paroxysmal episodes. In each field only the distinctive clinical features of the phenomenon are listed

tem atrophy (MSA) and Lewy body disease, preceding the other symptoms by many years [54–57]. The memory of dream mentation appropriate to the observed behavior associated with complete alertness and orientation on awakening is helpful in distinguishing RBD from NFLS. Moreover RBD episodes are short and often occur in the second half of the night, where REM sleep is prevalent. Patients with RBD are usually older than patients with NFLS. Even if inter-ictal epileptiform EEG abnormalities were detected in routine EEG of some rare cases with idiopathic RBD [58], the diagnosis remains straightforward. If in question, however, diagnosis can readily be established by video-EEG monitoring during night sleep, with concomitant examination of polysomnographic parameters documenting an excessive amount of sustained EMG activity or intermittent loss of REM atonia or excessive phasic muscle twitching of the submental or limb EMG during REM sleep.

Figure 8.3 shows the different polygraphic features characterizing NFLS, sleep terror, and RBD.

Nightmares are "disturbing mental experiences that generally occur during REM sleep and often result in awakening" [21]. They are common in young children, peaking at ages 3–6 years [59] and their frequency decreases with age. A careful sleep history focusing on the time of night of fearful awakenings helps to distinguish REM-related nightmares from disorders of arousals: the distinctive features of a nightmare are the recall of a long frightening dream, and clear orientation on awakening. The major distinction between nightmares and nocturnal panic is the stage of sleep: a panic attack is a NREM event usually occurring from stages 2–3 NREM [22].

The scant motor behavior during the episodes and the absence of confusion on awakening, as well as the availability of detailed dream reports helps distinguish between nightmares from NFLS [45]. In doubtful cases, video-polysomnography is indicated.

Sporadic nightmares are not worrisome, and require reassurance only, but recurrent nightmares or those with disturbing content may indicate excessive daytime stress [60]. Once the basis for the nightmares is discerned, measures should be taken to eliminate or reduce the child's exposure to the causative factor.

Recurrent isolated sleep paralysis is "an inability to perform voluntary movements at sleep onset or on awaking from sleep in the absence of a diagnosis of narcolepsy" [21]. Each episode lasts from seconds to a few minutes and is usually accompanied by intense anxiety. Sleep paralysis should be differentiated from atonic seizures which occur during wakefulness and nocturnal panic attacks usually not associated with paralysis (patients typically sit up and/or get out of bed) [22]. Reassurance and education are the most useful treatment in isolated cases. If the frequency of sleep paralysis is bothersome to patients, there is a suggestion that SSRIs may be of some benefit, likely because of their REM-suppressing properties [61].

Other Parasomnias

Sleep enuresis is "characterized by recurrent involuntary voiding during sleep." In primary sleep enuresis, recurrent involuntary voiding occurs at least twice weekly during sleep after the age of 5 years in a patient who has never been consistently dry during sleep for six consecutive months [21]. The prevalence of primary nocturnal enuresis is approximately 15–20 % of 5-year-olds and is more common in boys than girls at all ages [21]. Epileptic seizures are excluded because in these cases enuresis is the only symptom and occurs without any motor phenomenon.

Primary nocturnal enuresis is a heterogeneous condition for which various causative factors have been identified so the treatment could be a combination of non-invasive tools and only particular cases and motivated patients should receive a specific pharmacologic treatment [62].

Isolated Symptoms and Normal Variants

Sleep talking is defined as talking during sleep "with varying degrees of comprehensibility" [21]. It can arise from both slow-wave sleep and REM sleep. Although considered the most frequent parasomnia, sleep talking is usually without consequences and is rarely a reason for consultation.

Sleep-Related Movement Disorders

Sleep-related movement disorders are primarily characterized by relatively simple, usually stereotyped, movements that disturb sleep or its onset. They include disorders (a) and isolated symptoms and normal variants (b).

Disorders

Restless legs syndrome (*RLS*). RLS is a sensorimotor disorder characterized by uncomfortable sensations usually involving only the legs that worsen in the evening and with long periods of inactivity (e.g., a long car ride or movie) [21, 63]. Sensations are often described as creepy-crawly or tingling feelings, temporarily alleviated by movement. Patients, especially young children, may have difficulty describing the symptoms. Children may get into trouble at school or at home because they have difficulty sitting still. In younger children Walters et al. [64] demonstrated an association with hyperactivity. In patients with epilepsy RLS may be confused with their underlying seizure disorder. Primary restless legs syndrome occurs frequently in families, indicating significant genetic or shared environmental factors for the disease. Renal failure, iron deficiency, diabetes, and pregnancy are the most common diseases and condition associated to the restlessness.

Periodic limb movement disorder (*PLMD*) commonly co-occurs with RLS but may also appear independently. Periodic limb movements in sleep (PLMS) are brief repetitive movements or jerks, lasting 0.5 to 5 seconds and occurring every 5–90 s in a sequence of 4 or more movements, especially during sleep stages 1 and 2. PLMD is diagnosed when PLMS occur more than 5 per hour of sleep in children and >15/h in adults causing significant sleep disturbance or daytime impairment [21]. Dopamine agonist therapy is the mainstay of RLS treatment in adults.

Sleep bruxism, or teeth-grinding, is "an oral activity characterized by grinding or clenching teeth during sleep, usually associated with sleep arousals" which, when long-lasting, can cause significant tooth wear [21]. Sleep bruxism occurs most commonly in children aged 3–12 years, without any sex prevalence, and then decreases throughout life; in many cases, patients are unaware of the jaw movements [65]. Bruxism occurs in all stages of sleep but is most common during NREM, especially stage 1–2 of sleep, in the absence of associated abnormal EEG activity.

Rhythmic jaw movements could be a semiological feature of epileptic seizures such as temporal lobe attacks, but in these cases the movements represent a more diffuse oro-alimentary behavior, and are often preceded by an arising gastric aura accompanied by other motor automatisms not limited to the face [66].

There is no specific treatment for sleep bruxism: each subject has to be individually evaluated and treated. The three management alternatives are dental, pharmacological, and psychobehavioral therapy [67].

Nocturnal facio-mandibular myoclonus is characterized by nocturnal myoclonic jerks involving the masseter, orbicularis oculi, and oris muscles [68]. These abnormal movements can trigger nocturnal awakenings due to painful tongue biting and bleeding sometimes leading to the misdiagnosis of tongue biting due to an epileptic seizure. A detailed description of the episodes, collected from a bed partner or other observer helps establish the correct diagnosis. Its relationship with sleep bruxism is still a matter of debate.

Sleep-related rhythmic movement disorders (*RMD*) are "repetitive, stereotyped, and rhythmic motor behaviors (not tremors) occurring predominantly during drowsiness or sleep and involving large muscle groups" [21]. They comprise head-banging (Fig. 8.4), head-rolling, and body-rocking. The rhythmic behaviors are generally benign and self-limiting in normal children: they are common in infancy dropping to 5 % by the age of 5 years [69]. Episodes are not restricted to sleep–wake transition, occur more frequently in wake, stages NREM 1 and 2, but also in REM and slow-wave sleep [70, 71]. Movements typically occur at a frequency of 0.5–2 times per second and events last 5–15 min. Children are usually non-responsive during the episodes and do not recall the events on awakening [71]. Although sleep-related epilepsy is a diagnostic consideration, the characteristic movements make epilepsy far less likely: unlike epilepsy, patients can usually arrest waking movements on request. The behaviors only rarely result in a significant complaint (interference with normal sleep or daytime function, or self-inflicted bodily injury requiring medical treatment). Pharmacological treatment is therefore rarely necessary. In severe cases, RMD episodes respond favorably to clonazepam at low doses [72].

Benign sleep myoclonus of infancy (BSMI) is a non-epileptic paroxysmal disorder characterized by repetitive myoclonic jerks during NREM sleep in the early life of healthy newborns [73–75]. BSMI is characterized by rhythmic or arrhythmic, generalized or sometimes segmental jerks, involving one limb or one side of the body, which typically appear during NREM sleep. They frequently occur in clusters, lasting 20–30 min, and terminate with awakening.

According to ICSD-3, the following criteria are necessary for diagnosis: repetitive myoclonic jerks involving the whole body, trunk, or limbs; onset in early

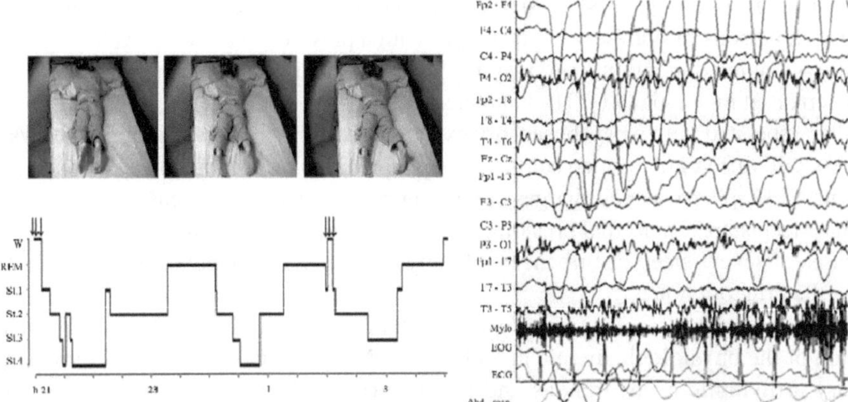

Fig. 8.4 Sleep-related rhythmic movement disorders (head-banging) in a 10-year-old boy. The patient presents repetitive, stereotyped, and rhythmic head movements characterized by forcibly banging his head back and down into the pillow. Polygraphic tracing (*right* of the figure) shows the typical artifact due to movements. The episodes appear during the sleep–wake transition and during infra-sleep wakefulness as shown in the excerpt of the hypnogram (*bottom* of the figure). *Mylo* Mylohyoideus muscle, *EOG* electroculogram, *Abd. resp* abdominal respiration

infancy, typically from birth to 6 months of age; the movements occur only during sleep and stop abruptly and consistently with arousal. In addition, the movements can be precipitated by rocking during sleep [76]. The syndrome is usually sporadic; only a few familial cases have been reported in the literature [77]. No medication is required.

Propriospinal myoclonus (PSM) at sleep onset is a distinctive form of spinal myoclonus characterized by violent muscle jerks arising from the axial muscles (in the neck or trunk), which extends up and down to the rostral and caudal muscles along the propriospinal pathways intrinsic to the cord [78]. In many cases PSM shows a striking relationship with vigilance level as it typically occurs during postural and mental rest, particularly when patients try to fall asleep giving rise to a severe and persistent insomnia [79]. The time of occurrence of the jerks (confined to the wake-sleep transition or to intra-sleep arousals), their frequent recurrence, and suppression of the motor phenomena by mental and sensory stimuli distinguish PSM from epileptic phenomena. Clonazepam (0.5–2 mg) can reduce muscle jerks and make sleep more restful. Opiates are also effective but carry the risk of dependence [79].

Isolated Symptoms and Normal Variants

Sleep starts, also known as *hypnagogic* or *hypnic jerks*, are bilateral, sudden, brief, non-periodic jerks, mainly affecting the legs or arms, just before sleep onset. The jerks are associated with a subjective feeling of falling, or a sensory flash or a hypnagogic dream [21]. Sleep starts are a common and normal phenomenon occurring in persons of both sexes and all ages with a prevalence of 70 %. Although usually a single contraction, they may be so severe as to be a true sleep disorder like sleep onset insomnia [21]. The characteristics of sporadic, isolated, brief jerks, usually associated with a psychosensory experience and mainly present during drowsiness will differentiate sleep starts from epileptic clonias that are always associated with EEG spike-wave discharges of varying complexity. In most cases, reassurance that sleep start is a normal phenomenon is sufficient. If drugs are necessary to treat cases of severe sleep disturbance and daily drowsiness, benzodiazepine appears to be the drug of choice.

Excessive fragmentary myoclonus (*EFM*) consists in an abnormal intensification of the physiologic hypnic myoclonia. EFM is characterized by brief involuntary arrhythmic asynchronous and asymmetric brief twitches involving various body areas. They occur throughout the night, including relaxed wakefulness and all sleep stages [42]. Patients are usually unaware of the twitch-like movements, which may be present during wakefulness or sleep. In many cases, EFM is diagnosed strictly as an incidental finding on polysomnographic recording, that demonstrates recurrent and persistent very brief (75–150 ms) EMG potentials in various muscles occurring asynchronously and asymmetrically in a sustained manner without clustering; more than 5 potentials per minute are sustained for at least 20 min of non-REM sleep stages.

If severe, EFM may disturb sleep onset and sleep continuity [80]. EFM is readily distinguished from epileptic seizures by its atypical motor patterns (minor movements of the fingers and toes or twitching of the corners of the mouth) and prolonged persistence throughout the night across all sleep stages. Pharmacological treatment is rarely required.

Sleep-Related Medical and Neurological Disorders

Sleep-Related Gastro-Esophageal Reflux Disease (GER)

Sleep-related gastro-esophageal reflux disease (*GER*) is caused by symptoms and/or signs related to the reflux of gastric acid or intestinal bile contents onto the esophageal mucosa. The most common and essentially pathognomonic symptoms of GER are heartburn and regurgitation [81]. Chronic acid reflux is often associated with frequent arousals during sleep. According to ICSD-3 diagnostic criteria "the patient complains of recurrent awakenings from sleep with shortness of breath or heartburn or a sour bitter taste in the mouth upon awakening from sleep or sleep-related coughing or choking or awakening from sleep with heartburn." Polysomnography and esophageal pH monitoring demonstrate gastro-esophageal reflux during sleep with associated arousal.

Evaluation and Treatment of Patients with Epilepsy and Sleep Disorder

The proper identification and treatment of common sleep disorders is an essential part of the overall evaluation and management of patients with epilepsy. A sleep history is the essential tool to evaluate sleep problems and involves a thorough review of the patients' 24-h routine, focusing on bedtime habits, nighttime behavior, nap and daytime behavior. Nighttime behavior after sleep onset such as parasomnias and symptoms of OSA (snoring, gasping, breathing pauses, and restless sleep) should also be assessed. A sleep diary can be helpful in delineating the exact sleep pattern.

Insufficient sleep syndrome remains a major problem for adolescents. Adolescents have some degree of delayed sleep phase syndrome, which leads to early morning sleepiness and insufficient sleep. School start times, extracurricular activities, and peer pressure contribute to a chronic state of sleep deprivation, placing most adolescent patients at risk for activation of their seizure disorder. Regular sleep habits must be recommended by physicians and enforced by parents.

Patients with epilepsy frequently complain of daytime sleepiness, usually considered an unavoidable adverse effect of antiepileptic therapy. Nevertheless, in patients with persistent hypersomnia, particularly if on AED monotherapy or with low serum drug concentrations and well-controlled seizures, primary sleep disorders should be suspected [82]. Study of these patients by video-EEG polysomnography or home video may be indicated [83]. Evaluation of sleep with polysomnography should be performed with extended EEG montages in patients with epilepsy to correlate arousal with seizures and inter-ictal activity. Monitoring for sleep-related breathing disorders, restless legs syndrome, or parasomnias should also be performed. Therapy should be directed at resolving any sleep disorder observed, as improved seizure control might result. Anticonvulsant monotherapy should be attempted whenever possible to minimize the side effects of sedation. Less sedating anticonvulsants should be used as primary anticonvulsant therapy avoiding barbiturates, benzodiazepines, and topiramate.

How Treatment of Sleep Disorders Affects Seizures

The treatment of an underlying sleep disorder and improvement of sleep hygiene benefits not only daytime sleepiness but also seizure control. An example is the beneficial effect on seizure frequency of C-PAP treatment in patients with OSA [84, 85], without changes in the drug regimen. Resolution of chronic sleep deprivation, improvement in cerebral hypoxemia, and reduction in arousals from sleep have been postulated to be the reason whereby treatment of a sleep disorder improves seizure control, even if the exact mechanism is unknown [86].

The majority of sleep disorders do not need pharmacological treatment. Behavioral therapy and regular and regularization of sleep habits may reduce the problem in most cases [2].

On the other hand, sleep problems in young children may present with hyperactivity or behavioral problems rather than excessive somnolence. Recognition of the paradoxical response of hyperactivity as the result of excessive daytime sleepiness is central to evaluation of these pediatric patients [2].

Insomnia has been reported in patients with epilepsy and may be caused by different situations. In particular, patients with epilepsy may become disabled, which will lead to "behaviorally" induced circadian rhythm problems because they may choose their own sleep hours if inactive. Nighttime fears may affect patients with epilepsy as well, especially if they have nocturnal seizures. In addition, caregivers may feel anxious about leaving the patient alone in the room [87].

How Treatment of Seizures Affects Sleep

Not only seizures but also antiepileptic drugs (AEDs) may contribute to sleep disorders and adversely affect sleep. For example, in a patient predisposed to OSA, barbiturates and benzodiazepines may worsen the frequency of apneas and hypopneas by reducing the muscle tone of the upper airways and increasing the arousal threshold. Similarly AEDs that are associated with weight gain (i.e., VPA) may worsen OSA. Avoiding these agents in patients with untreated OSA may be advisable, especially if alternative AEDs are available.

Clinicians may base their AED choice not only on the epilepsy syndrome but also on its effects on coexisting sleep disorders and complaints [2]. Somnolence and diurnal sedation are the most common side effects of AEDs especially in patients on polytherapy [86, 88]. Whether it is epilepsy itself or AEDs which cause abnormal sleep architecture is difficult to determine. This adverse effect on sleep is especially relevant to the AED effect on cognitive functions. It is likely that cognitive effects of AEDs on memory and concentration are related to drug effects on the central nervous system mediating arousal rather than the specific effect on cognitive functions. Ideally the AED chosen to treat epilepsy should have the least effect on sleep. This may not be always possible.

AEDs have been shown to have a variety of effects on sleep and daytime vigilance. However, the literature is confounded by significant methodological variations across studies, including composition of the study population, dose, timing and duration of treatment, and failure to control for seizures and concomitant AEDs. Much of the available literature on the older AEDs comes from animal studies, but with the use of newer anticonvulsants in other neurologic and psychiatric conditions, new data are becoming available on patients exposed to AEDs for the first time.

It has been shown that anticonvulsants can improve seizure control by stabilizing sleep [15, 89]. Although it is certainly possible that part of the improved sleep seen with the use of anticonvulsants may be the result of seizure suppression, it seems clear that AEDs also affect sleep independently of their antiepileptic effect. They may also cause state-dependent seizures to become dispersed randomly during the sleep/wake cycle [90].

Effect of AEDs on Sleep Architecture

The effects of some specific AEDs on sleep architecture are discussed below. In general, many of the traditional AEDs can reduce sleep latency and sleep fragmentation, delay REM onset or decrease the percentage of time spent in REM sleep [2, 89].

Phenytoin With chronic phenytoin use most investigators have found a shortened sleep latency, an increase in stages 1 and 2, a small decrease in REM sleep, and increased arousals [91, 92].

Carbamazepine Carbamazepine, the most extensively studied AED, has shown to cause decreased sleep latency, increased total sleep time, decreased fragmentation, and improved sleep continuity [91–94].

Valproate No notable alteration of sleep have been found with valproate which appears to promote a more normal distribution of REM sleep during the night, and can also stabilize the sleep cycle [91, 95].

Ethosuximide The few studies available show an increase in stage 1 of NREM sleep with a concomitant decrease in stage 3, an increased number of awakenings, and an increase in the percentage of REM [91, 92].

Phenobarbital Phenobarbital in chronic treatment shortened sleep latency and led to a reduction in body movements and arousals, increased total sleep time with a higher sleep efficiency [92, 96]. It also caused a reduction in REM sleep and its abrupt withdrawal can cause a rebound of REM parasomnias. Usually phenobarbital may produce excessive daytime sleepiness but in children paradoxical effects on sleep behavior with hyperactivity are noted.

Primidone The effects on sleep of primidone are similar to those of phenobarbital.

Benzodiazepines Most benzodiazepines have been described to cause a decrease in sleep latency and the number of arousals. This is accompanied by an increase in the percentage of stage 2 sleep, with a decrease in the amount of stages 3 and 4 NREM sleep. REM sleep latency is increased, with longer acting benzodiazepines causing a greater suppression of REM sleep [97].

Lamotrigine Compared with the older AEDs, LTG seems to have less effect on disruption of sleep. The only significant effects of LTG treatment included an increase in stage 2 (light sleep) and a decrease in SWS (deep sleep). Although it did not reach statistical significance, treatment with LTG was associated with a slight reduction in arousals and stage shifts and an increase in the number of REM periods without affecting sleep efficiency, suggesting a tendency for sleep to be less disrupted [86]. Other authors reported different effects of LTG on sleep with an increase in the percentage of REM sleep, and a decrease in the fragmentation of REM sleep usually present in epileptic patients. Overall, sleep was also more stable, with a decreased number of phase shifts [98]. There was no correlation between the increase in REM sleep and the decrease in spikes, leading investigators to believe that the sleep stabilizing effect of lamotrigine acts independently of its antiepileptic effect. Another controversial point regarding LTG effects on sleep is insomnia of sufficient severity to require discontinuation or dose reduction. This adverse effect was reported in 6.4 % of patients treated with LTG in a recent series of 109 subjects [99]. Difficulty initiating and maintaining sleep developed shortly after LTG was introduced, increased with dose escalation, and resolved quickly with discontinuation or dose reduction. Symptoms developed at a mean daily dose of 286 mg (100–500). Based on these data, we believe that LTG may be less disruptive to sleep than the older AEDs. Because sleep fragmentation reduces the seizure threshold in some individuals, these changes may contribute to the anticonvulsant effects of the drug.

Gabapentin In general, patients on GBP show a subjective improvement in sleep [97]. An increase in the percentage of REM sleep, and a prolonged duration of REM periods and a decreased number of awakenings have been observed in epileptic patients treated with GBP [100].

Vigabatrin Vigabatrin as add-on therapy showed no difference in sleep latency, total sleep time, or number of awakenings without improvement in daytime sleepiness [101].

Effect of VNS on Sleep

Vagus nerve stimulation (VNS), a nonpharmacological therapy for epilepsy involving intermittent stimulation of the left vagus nerve peripherally, may decrease daytime sleepiness in epilepsy patients documented by MSLTs performed 3 months after VNS treatment was initiated (mean sleep latency from 6.4 to 9.8 min) [102]. However, VNS may also contribute to decreases in respiratory airflow and effort during sleep and exacerbate OSA via central and peripheral mechanisms [2, 103].

Acknowledgments We thank the IRCCS Sleep Laboratory. We thank Mrs. Elena Zoni for graphic production and Anne Collins for editing the manuscript.

References

1. Carney PR, Berry RB, Geyer JD. Clinical sleep disorders. 1st ed. Philadelphia: Lippincott Williams Wilkins; 2005.
2. Tinuper P, Bisulli F, Provini F, Geyer JD, Carney PR. Treating epilepsy in the presence of sleep disorders. In: Pediatric epilepsy. New York: McGraw Hill Medical; 2012. p. 343–61.

3. Rosen I, Blennow G, Risberg AM, Ingvar DH. Quantitative evaluation of nocturnal sleep in epileptic children. In: Sterman MB, Shouse MN, Passouant P, editors. Sleep and epilepsy. New York: Academic; 1982. p. 397–409.
4. Horita H, Khumagai K, Mackawa K. Overnight polygraphic study of Lennox—Gastaut syndrome. Brain Dev. 1987;9:627–35.
5. Tassinari CA, Rubboli G, Volpi L, Billard C, Bureau M. Electrical status epilepsticus during slow sleep (ESES or CSWS) including acquired apileptic aphasia (Landau-Klefner syndrome): chapter 18. In: Roger J, Bureau M, Dravet C, Genton P, Tassinari CA, Wolf P, editors. Epileptic syndromes in infancy, childhood and adolescence. 4th ed. London: John Libbey; 2005. p. 295–314.
6. Clemens B, Olah R. Sleep studies in benign epilepsy of childhood with rolandic spikes. Epilepsia. 1987;28:20–3.
7. Shouse MN, Martins da Silva A, Sammaritano M. Circadian rhythm, sleep and epilepsy. J Clin Neurophysiol. 1996;13:32–50.
8. Cortessi F, Gionnotti F, Ottaviano S. Sleep problems and behavior in childhood idiopathic epilepsy. Epilepsia. 1999;40:1557–65.
9. Manni R, Tartara A. Evaluation of sleepiness in epilepsy. Clin Neurophysiol. 2000;111 Suppl 2:S111–4.
10. Provini F, Plazzi G, Tinuper P, Vandi S, Lugaresi E, Montagna P. Nocturnal frontal lobe epilepsy. A clinical and polygraphic overview of 100 consecutive cases. Brain. 1999;122(Pt 6):1017–31.
11. Oldani A, Zucconi M, Castronovo C, Ferini-Strambi L. Nocturnal frontal lobe epilepsy misdiagnosed as sleep apnea syndrome. Acta Neurol Scand. 1998;98:67–71.
12. Zucconi M, Oldani A, Smirne S, Ferini-Strambi L. The macrostructure and microstructure of sleep in patients with autosomal dominant nocturnal frontal lobe epilepsy. J Clin Neurophysiol. 2000;17:77–86.
13. Nobili L, Francione S, Mai R, Tassi L, Cardinale F, Castagna L, et al. Nocturnal frontal lobe epilepsy: intracerebral recordings of paroxysmal motor attacks with increasing complexity. Sleep. 2003;26:883–6.
14. Vignatelli L, Bisulli F, Naldi I, Ferioli S, Pittau F, Provini F, et al. Excessive daytime sleepiness and subjective sleep quality in patients with nocturnal frontal lobe epilepsy: a case-control study. Epilepsia. 2006;47 Suppl 5:73–7.
15. Shouse MN, Martins da Silva A. Chronobiology. In: Engel J, Pedley TA, editors. Epilepsy: a comprehensive textbook. Philadelphia: Lippincott-Raven; 1997. p. 1917–27.
16. Bazil CW, Walczak TS. Effect of sleep and sleep stage on epileptic and non epileptic seizures. Epilepsia. 1997;38:56–62.
17. Janz D. The grand mal epilepsies and the sleeping-waking cycle. Epilepsia. 1962;3:69–109.
18. Janz D. Epilepsy with impulsive petit mal (juvenile myoclonic epilepsy). Acta Neurol Scand. 1985;72:449–59.
19. Loiseau P, Beaussart M. The seizures of benign childhood epilepsy with rolandic paroxysmal discharges. Epilepsia. 1973;14:381–9.
20. Gastraut H, Roger J, Soulayrol R, Tassinari CA, Régis H, Dravet C, Bernard R, Pinsard N, Saint-Jean M, et al. Childhood epileptic encephalopathy with diffuse slow spike–waves (otherwise known as "petit mal variant") or Lennox syndrome. Epilepsia. 1966;7:139–79.
21. American Academy of Sleep Medicine. International classification of sleep disorders. 3rd ed. Darien: American Academy of Sleep Medicine; 2014.
22. Craske MG, Tsao JCI. Assessment and treatment of nocturnal panic attacks. Sleep Med Rev. 2005;9:173–84.
23. Guilleminault C, Billiard M, Montplaisir J, Demerit WC. Altered states of consciousness in disorders of daytime sleepiness. J Neurol Sci. 1976;26:377–93.
24. Manni R, Terzaghi M. Comorbidity between epilepsy and sleep disorders. Epilepsy Res. 2010;90(9):171–7.
25. Chiorek AM, Abou-Khalil B, Malow BA. Obstructive sleep apnea is associated with seizure occurrence in older adults with epilepsy. Neurology. 2007;69:1823–7.

26. Manni R, Terzaghi M, Arbasino C, et al. Obstructive sleep apnea in a clinical series of adult epilepsy patients: frequency and features of the comorbidity. Epilepsia. 2003;44:836–40.
27. Hollinger P, Khatami R, Gugger M, et al. Epilepsy and obstructive sleep apnea. Eur Neurol. 2006;55:74–9.
28. Malow BA, Weatherwax KJ, Chervin RD, Hoban TF, Marzec ML, Martin C, Binns LA. Identification and treatment of obstructive sleep apnea in adults and children with epilepsy: a prospective pilot study. Sleep Med. 2003;4:509–15.
29. Vetrugno R, Provini F, Plazzi G, Vignatelli L, Lugaresi E, Montagna P. Catathrenia (nocturnal groaning): a new type of parasomnia. Neurology. 2001;56:681–3.
30. DeRoeck J, Van Hoof E, Cluydts R. Sleep-related expiratory groaning: a case report. Sleep Res. 1983;12:237.
31. Pevernagie D, Boon P, Mariman A, Verhaeghen D, Pauwels R. Vocalization during episodes of prolonged expiration: a parasomnia related to REM sleep. Sleep Med. 2001;2:19–30.
32. Ohayon MM, Ferini-Strambi L, Plazzi G, Smirne S, Castronovo V. How age influences the expression of narcolepsy. J Psychosom Res. 2005;59:399–405.
33. Aran A, Einen M, Lin L, Plazzi G, Nishino S, Mignot E. Clinical and therapeutic aspects of childhood narcolepsy-cataplexy: a retrospective study of 51 children. Sleep. 2010;33:1457–64.
34. Pizza F, Franceschini C, Peltola H, Vandi S, Finotti E, Ingravallo F, et al. Clinical and polysomnographic course of childhood narcolepsy with cataplexy. Brain. 2013;136:3787–95.
35. Challamel MJ, Mazzola ME, Nevismalova S, et al. Narcolepsy in children. Sleep. 1994;17:S17–20.
36. Luca G, Haba-Rubio J, Dauvilliers Y, Lammers GJ, Overeem S, Donjacour CE, et al. European Narcolepsy Network. European Narcolepsy Network. Clinical, polysomnographic and genome-wide association analyses of narcolepsy with cataplexy: a European Narcolepsy Network study. J Sleep Res. 2013;22:482–95.
37. Zeman A, Douglas N, Aylward R. Narcolepsy mistaken for epilepsy. BMJ. 2001;322:216–8.
38. Macleod S, Ferrie C, Zuberi SM. Symptoms of narcolepsy in children misinterpreted as epilepsy. Epileptic Disord. 2005;7:13–7.
39. Stores G. The protean manifestations of childhood narcolepsy and their misinterpretation. Dev Med Child Neurol. 2006;48:307–10.
40. Mignot E, Chen W, Black J. On the value of measuring CSF hypocretin 1 in diagnosing narcolepsy. Sleep. 2003;26:646–9.
41. Ohayon MM, Guilleminault C, Priest RG. Night terrors, sleepwalking, and confusional arousals in the general population: their frequency and relationship to other sleep and mental disorders. J Clin Psychiatry. 1999;60:268–76.
42. Broughton R, Tolentino MA. Fragmentary pathological myoclonus in NREM sleep. Electroencephalogr Clin Neurophysiol. 1984;57:303–9.
43. Guilleminault C, Palombini L, Pelayo R, Chervin RD. Sleepwalking and sleep terrors in prepubertal children: what triggers them? Pediatrics. 2003;111:17–25.
44. Derry CP, Harvey AS, Walker MC, Duncan JS, Berkovic SF. NREM arousal parasomnias and their distinction from nocturnal frontal lobe epilepsy: a video EEG analysis. Sleep. 2009;32(12):1637–44.
45. Tinuper P, Provini F, Bisulli F, Vignatelli L, Plazzi G, Vetrugno R, et al. Movement disorders in sleep: guidelines for differentiating epileptic from non-epileptic motor phenomena arising from sleep. Sleep Med Rev. 2007;11:255–67.
46. Kushida CA, Littner MR, Morgenthaler T, Alessi CA, Bailey D, Coleman Jr J, et al. Practice parameters for the indications for polysomnography and related procedures: an update for 2005. Sleep. 2005;28:499–521.
47. Bisulli F, Vignatelli L, Naldi I, Licchetta L, Provini F, Plazzi G, et al. Increased frequency of arousal parasomnias in families with nocturnal frontal lobe epilepsy: a common mechanism? Epilepsia. 2010;51(9):1852–60.
48. Schenck CH, Bundlie SR, Ettinger MG, Mahowald MW. Chronic behavioral disorders of REM sleep: a new category of parasomnia. Sleep. 1986;9:293–308.

49. Olson EJ, Boeve BF, Silber MH. Rapid eye movement sleep behaviour disorder: demographic, clinical and laboratory findings in 93 cases. Brain. 2000;123:33139.
50. Boeve BF. REM sleep behavior disorder: Updated review of the core features, the REM sleep behavior disorder-neurodegenerative disease association, evolving concepts, controversies, and future directions. Ann N Y Acad Sci. 2010;1184:15–54.
51. Mahowald MW, Schenck CH. Insights from studying human sleep disorders. Nature. 2005;43:1279–85.
52. Silber MH. REM sleep behaviour disorder associated with barbiturate withdrawal. Sleep Res. 1996;25:371.
53. Plazzi G, Montagna P, Meletti S, Lugaresi E. Polysomnographic study of sleeplessness and oneiricisms in the alcohol withdrawal syndrome. Sleep Med. 2002;3:279–82.
54. Schenck CH, Bundie SR, Mahovald MW. Delayed emergence of a parkinsonian disorder in 38% of 29 older males initially diagnosed with idiopathic rapid eye movement sleep behaviour disorder. Neurology. 1996;46:388–93.
55. Plazzi G, Corsini R, Provini F, Pierangeli G, Martinelli P, Montagna P, et al. REM sleep behaviour disorders in multiple system atrophy. Neurology. 1997;48:1094–7.
56. Vetrugno R, Provini F, Cortelli P, Plazzi G, Lotti EM, Pierangeli G, et al. Sleep disorders in multiple system atrophy: a correlative video-polysomnographic study. Sleep Med. 2004;5:21–30.
57. Postuma RB, Iranzo A, Hogl B, Arnulf I, Ferini-Strambi L, Manni R, et al. Risk factors for neurodegeneration in idiopathic rapid eye movement sleep behavior disorder: a multicenter study. Ann Neurol. 2015;77(5):830–9.
58. Manni R, Terzaghi M, Zambrelli E, Pacchetti C. Interictal, potentially misleading, epileptiform EEG abnormalities in REM sleep behavior disorder. Sleep. 2006;29:934–7.
59. Leung AK, Robson WL. Nightmares. J Natl Med Assoc. 1993;85:233–5.
60. Levin R, Fireman G. Nightmare prevalence, nightmare distress, and self-reported psychological disturbance. Sleep. 2002;25:205–12.
61. Koran LM, Raghavan S. Fluoxetine for isolated sleep paralysis. Psychosomatics. 1993;34:184–7.
62. Lottmann HB, Alova I. Primary monosymptomaic nocturnal enuresis in children and adolescents. Int J Clin Pract Suppl. 2007;155:8–16.
63. Allen RP, Picchietti DL, Garcia-Borreguero D, Ondo WG, Walters AS, Winkelman JW, et al. International Restless Legs Syndrome Study Group. Restless legs syndrome/Willis-Ekbom disease diagnostic criteria: updated International Restless Legs Syndrome Study Group (IRLSSG) consensus criteria – history, rationale, description, and significance. Sleep Med. 2014;15(8):860–73.
64. Walters A, Picchietti DL, Ehrenberg B. Restless leg syndrome in childhood and adolescence. Pediatr Neurol. 1994;11:241–5.
65. Kato T, Thie N, Montplaisir J, Lavigne G. Bruxism and orofacial movements during sleep. Dent Clin North Am. 2001;45:657–84.
66. Meletti S, Cantalupo G, Volpi L, Rubboli G, Magaudda A, Tassinari CA. Rhythmic teeth grinding induced by temporal lobe seizures. Neurology. 2004;62:2306–9.
67. Bader G, Lavigne G. Sleep bruxism; an overview of an oromandibular sleep movement disorder. Sleep Med Rev. 2000;4:27–43.
68. Vetrugno R, Provini F, Plazzi G, Lombardi C, Liguori R, Lugaresi E, Montagna P. Familial nocturnal facio-mandibular myoclonus mimicking sleep bruxism. Neurology. 2002;58:644–7.
69. Chisholm T, Morehouse RL. Adult headbanging: sleep studies and treatment. Sleep. 1996;19:343–6.
70. Manni R, Terzaghi M. Rhythmic movements during sleep: a physiological and pathological profile. Neurol Sci. 2005;26:s181–5.
71. Mayer G, Wilde-Frenz J, Kurella B. Sleep related rhythmic movement disorder revisited. J Sleep Res. 2007;16:110–6.
72. Manni R, Tartara A. Clonazepam treatment of rhythmic movement disorders. Sleep. 1997;20:812.

73. Resnick TJ, Moshe SL, Perotta L, Chambers HJ. Benign neonatal sleep myoclonus: relation to sleep state. Arch Neurol. 1986;43:266–8.
74. Coulter DL, Allen RJ. Benign neonatal sleep myoclonus. Arch Neurol. 1982;39:191–2.
75. Di Capua M, Fusco L, Ricci S, Vigevano F. Benign neonatal sleep myoclonus: clinical features and video-polygraphic recordings. Mov Disord. 1993;8:191–4.
76. Alfonso I, Papazian O, Aicardi J, Jeffries HE. A simple maneuver to provoke benign neonatal sleep myoclonus. Pediatrics. 1995;96:1161–3.
77. Cohen R, Shuper A, Straussberg R. Familial benign neonatal sleep myoclonus. Pediatr Neurol. 1996;5:334–7.
78. Brown P, Thompson PD, Rothwell JC, Day BL, Marsden CD. Axial myoclonus of propriospinal origin. Brain. 1991;114:197–214.
79. Montagna P, Provini F, Plazzi G, Liguori R, Lugaresi E. Propriospinal myoclonus upon relaxation and drowsiness. A cause of severe insomnia. Mov Disord. 1997;12:66–72.
80. Vetrugno R, Plazzi G, Provini F, Liguori R, Lugaresi E, Montagna P. Excessive fragmentary hypnic myoclonus: clinical and neurophysiologic findings. Sleep Med. 2002;3:73–6.
81. Richter JE. Extraesophageal presentations of gastroesophageal reflux disease. Semin Gastrointest Dis. 1997;8:75–89.
82. Foldary-Schaefer N. Sleep complaints and epilepsy: the role of seizures, antiepileptic drugs and sleep disorders. J Clin Neurophysiol. 2002;19:514–21.
83. Bazil CW, Castro LHM, Walczak TS. Reduction of rapid eye movement sleep by diurnal and nocturnal seizures in temporal lobe epilepsy. Arch Neurol. 2000;57:363–8.
84. Carney PR, Kohrman MH. Relation between epilepsy and sleep during infancy and childhood. In: Bazil CW, Malow BA, Sammaritano MR, editors. Sleep and epilepsy: the clinical spectrum. Amsterdam: Elsevier Science BV; 2002. p. 359–72.
85. Koh S, Ward SL, Lin M, Chen LS. Sleep apnea treatment improves seizure control in children with neurodevelopmental disorders. Pediatr Neurol. 2000;22:36–9.
86. Foldvary N, Perry M, Lee J, Dinner D, Morris HH. The effects of lamotrigine on sleep in patients with epilepsy. Epilepsia. 2001;42(12):1569–73.
87. Rodriguez AJ. Pediatric sleep and epilepsy. Curr Neurol Neurosci Rep. 2007;7:342–7.
88. Giannotti F, Cortesi F, Bruni O. Sleep habitus in children with idiopathic epilepsy. Sleep Res. 1994;23:361 [abstract].
89. Touchon J, Baldy-Moulinier M, Billiard M, Besset A, Cadilhac J. Sleep organization and epilepsy. In: Degen R, Rodin EA, editors. Epilepsy, sleep and sleep deprivation. Amsterdam: Elsevier; 1991. p. 73–81.
90. Kellaway P, Frost JD, Mizrabi EM. Ethosuximide effect on thalamic oscillation mechanisms, spindles and generalized 3-Hz spike-and wave bursts [abstract]. Ann Neurol. 1991;30:293.
91. Declerck AC, Wauquier A. Influence of antiepileptic drugs on sleep patterns. In: Degen R, Rodin EA, editors. Epilepsy, sleep and sleep deprivation. 2nd ed. Amsterdam: Elsevier; 1991. p. 153–62.
92. Wolf P, Röder–Wanner UU, Brede M. Influence of therapeutic phenobarbital and phenytoin medication on the polygraphic sleep of patients with epilepsy. Epilepsia. 1984;25:467–75.
93. Manni R, Galimberti CA, Zucca C, Parietti L, Tartara A. Sleep patterns in patients with late onset partial epilepsy receiving chronic carbamazepine therapy. Epilepsy Res. 1990;7(1):72–6.
94. Obermayer WH, Benca RM. Effects of drugs on sleep. Neurol Clin. 1996;14:827–40.
95. Findji J, Catani P. The effects of valproic acid on sleep parameters in epileptic children: clinical note. In: Sterman MB, Shouse MN, Passouant P, editors. Sleep and epilepsy. New York: Academic; 1982. p. 395–6.
96. Barzaghi N, Gatti G, Manni R, Galimberti CA, Zucca C, Tartara A, Perucca E. Time-dependent pharmacodynamic effects of phenobarbital in humans. Ther Drug Monit. 1990;11:661–6.
97. Ehrenberg B. Importance of sleep restoration in co-morbid disease: effect of anticonvulsants. Neurology. 2000;54 suppl 1:S33–7.

98. Placidi F, Diomedi M, Scalise A, Marciani MG, Romigi A, Gigli GL. Effect of anticonvulsants on nocturnal sleep in epilepsy. Neurology. 2000;54 suppl 1:S25–32.
99. Adler M. Lamotrigine associated with insomnia. Epilepsia. 1999;40(3):322–5.
100. Placidi F, Diomedi M, Scalise A, Silvestri G, Marciani MD, Gigli GL. Effect of long-term treatment with gabapentin on nocturnal sleep in epilepsy. Epilepsia. 1997;38 suppl 8:179–80.
101. Bonanni E, Massetani R, Galli R, Gneri C, Petri M, Iudice A, Murri L. A quantitative study of daytime sleepiness induced by carbamazepine and add-on vigabatrin in epileptic patients. Acta Neurol Scand. 1997;95:193–6.
102. Malow BA, Edwards J, Marzec M, Sagher O, Fromes G. Effects of vagus nerve stimulation on respiration during sleep: a pilot study. Neurology. 2000;55:1450–4.
103. Malow BA, Edwards J, Marzec M, Sagher O, Ross D, Fromes G. Vagus nerve stimulation reduces daytime sleepiness in epilepsy patients. Neurology. 2001;57:879–84.

Chapter 9
Dissociation

Matthias Schmutz

Abstract Dissociative seizures represent a psychiatric symptom with a long tradition going back to the ancient Egyptian and Greek medicine. Due to their semiological similarity to epileptic seizures, establishing the proper diagnosis requires specialized neurological expertise. This chapter gives a short review of the relevant psychological theories about psychosomatic conversion and dissociation, which constitute the etiological and pathogenetic background of dissociative seizures. Furthermore, the major issues of the neurological differential diagnosis, the psychiatric and psychodynamic inclusion diagnosis, and the challenging clinical management of patients with dissociative seizures are comprehensively summarized and discussed. Finally, the current research data on treatment, outcome, and prognosis are critically reviewed. From a psychiatric point of view, dissociative seizures do not represent a disorder in the nosological sense, but merely an accompanying symptom of an underlying psychiatric disorder. Based on this perception, guidelines for clinical management and treatment can be improved. In addition, this shift in focus could foster future research by clarifying some methodological problems limiting the research findings so far.

Keywords Dissociative Seizures • Conversion Seizures • Psychogenic Non-Epileptic Seizures • Hysteric Seizures • Hysteria • Somatoform Disorder • Somatization • Dissociation • Trauma-Related Stress Disorder • Psychotherapy • Psychiatric Nosology • Differential Diagnosis

Introduction

Dissociative seizures represent a venerable psychiatric symptom with a long and sometimes controversial history pertaining to etiology, pathogenesis, diagnostic classification, and treatment. As paroxysms characterized by loss of consciousness

M. Schmutz, MA, PhD
Department of Psychiatry/Psychotherapy, Swiss Epilepsy Center, Bleulerstr. 60, Zurich 8008, Switzerland
e-mail: matthias.schmutz@swissepi.ch

M. Mula (ed.), *Neuropsychiatric Symptoms of Epilepsy*, Neuropsychiatric Symptoms of Neurological Disease, DOI 10.1007/978-3-319-22159-5_9

and motor signs they have formed—among other motor and sensory phenomena—the core symptoms of old hysteria since the ancient Egyptians and Greeks until the beginning of the twentieth century [1].

Displaying semiological features with oftentimes striking similarity to epileptic and other somatogenic seizures, dissociative seizures require profound medical and neurological expertise in order to achieve diagnostic certainty. Therefore, neurological examination to exclude epileptic seizures or other somatogenic paroxysms ranks first in the medical assessment, while psychiatric and psychotherapeutic interventions follow secondary. This succession of neurological and psychiatric involvement corresponds to the illness behavior of most patients with dissociative seizures, who actively seek neurological advice first and only reluctantly (if at all) accept referral to a mental health specialist. Most probably, this subordinate status is a major reason for the rather poor scientific contribution of contemporary psychiatry, compared to the abundant neurological literature in the field. To fill the psychiatric void, neurological contributions pertain—nolens volens—far beyond their differential diagnostic expertise and cover genuine psychiatric issues like etiology, treatment, outcome, and prognosis of dissociative seizures.

This chapter covers the topic of dissociative seizures in adolescent and adult patients. Dissociative seizures also occur in younger patients. Many of the following issues may apply to children with dissociative seizures as well. For specific information, however, the specialized pediatric literature is authoritative.

Definition

Dissociative seizures are defined as paroxysmal events with alterations of consciousness, emotions, motor body control, and/or sensory functions. They are psychogenic, i.e., internal and/or external stress and the psychological mechanisms of dissociation and conversion play a crucial role in their etiopathogenesis. In regard to semiology they tend to mimic epileptic seizures, however, electroencephalography during dissociative seizures does not show epileptiform activity. From a nosological point of view, dissociative seizures represent an accompanying symptom of an underlying psychiatric disorder.

Terminology

To begin with, some remarks related to naming and terminology may be helpful. Dissociative seizures are often circumscribed by a number of different terms in current scientific literature: non-epileptic attack disorder, pseudo-seizures, psychogenic non-epileptic seizures, non-epileptic seizures of non-organic origin, and functional seizures—just to mention a few [2–7]. In the last decades, most research papers on dissociative seizures have been written by neurologists and published in neurological or even epilepsy-centered journals. The main basing point is obviously the differentiation from epilepsy, and the selected terms to circumscribe dissociative seizures very well reflect this approach by emphasizing on what dissociative seizures are not. However, a "non-symptom" is hard to communicate to patients and even harder to treat. Therefore, let us focus next on how they are named in the authoritative psychiatric diagnostic manuals. Some very short medico-historic remarks will help to understand the current concepts and theories about dissociative seizures. The relevant differential diagnoses will be discussed in the sections on "Differential diagnosis" and "Diagnosing dissociative seizures".

Psychiatric Background

Conversion

DSM-V, the current version of the diagnostic and statistical manual of mental disorders of the American Psychiatric Association [8], subsumes "conversion disorder" (or "functional neurological symptom disorder") under the chapter "somatic symptom and related disorders" (a renaming of the "somatoform disorder" of DSM-IV). Conversion disorder (code 300.11) includes motor and/or sensory symptoms indicating an abnormal functioning of the somatic nervous system, though clear evidence of incompatibility with any neurological disease is required. Psychological or physical stress or trauma in close temporal relationship to symptom manifestation is an additional feature supporting the diagnoses. Among different sensory and motor symptoms, seizures or attacks may be specified as symptom type. Dissociative disorders like identity disorders, amnesia, depersonalization, derealization, and trance are dealt with in a separate chapter, thereby emphasizing their common focus on disruption and discontinuity of normal integration of consciousness (in contrast to conversion disorder with its focus on somatic symptoms).

The concept of conversion, which the DSM definition relates to, goes back to Freud. In 1894 he coined the term "conversion" as the main pathognomonic feature of hysteria, assuming a transformation of psychic arousal into a physical symptom [9]. In the very same year the German psychiatrist Sommer coined the term "psychogenic states." Though avoiding the term hysteria, he described a similar mechanism of generating physical symptoms by (mental) ideas [10]. While the concepts of conversion and hysteria kept closely connected in the first decades of psychoanalytic development, as from the 1960s conversion disorder was conceptualized completely uncoupled from both hysteria and hysterical personality traits [11]. Instead of "Hysteria," which was disposed from the official psychiatric discourse, Briquet's mid-nineteenth-century findings on hysteric symptomatology were revitalized by the St. Louise group of Guze in the early 1960s [12–14]. The so-called Briquet syndrome subsequently formed the basis for the introduction of the "somatization disorder" into the DSM-III in 1980. While keeping a prominent role in the somatoform disorders, conversion concurrently mutated into an unspecific intra-psychic mechanism to be found in the whole spectrum of mental disorders. By generating a psychologically meaningful physical symptom through the psychic mechanisms of repression, isolation, and dissociation, the process of conversion yields relief from internal or external stress.

As from the 1950s, a rich literature evolved, pursuing a psychosomatic approach and delivering clinical and therapeutic considerations that are useful still today [15–19]. Due to the common theoretical ground mentioned above, the terms "functional neurological symptoms," "psychogenic symptoms," and "conversion symptoms" are used synonymously by many clinicians today.

Dissociation

The term "dissociative seizures," which is preferred in this chapter, is used by the ICD-10, the International Classification of Diseases of the World Health Organization WHO [20]. ICD-10 does not distinguish conversion disorder from dissociative disorder. Both terms are used synonymously; hence, chapter F44 includes both the conversion symptoms and the dissociative symptoms of DSM. Dissociation is characterized by a partial or complete loss of the normal integration between consciousness, memory, awareness of identity and immediate sensations, perception, body representation, and control of body movements. The authors assume that dissociative mechanisms play the key role not only in the consciousness-related disorders like multiple identity disorder, amnesia or derealization and depersonalization, but also in the formation of physical conversion symptoms.

The concept of dissociation, which the ICD-10 relates to, goes back to the second half of the nineteenth century. Inspired by Charcot's studies on hysteria at the Salpêtrière in Paris, a lot of empirical research was done in order to decode the underlying mechanisms. While Charcot basically kept the idea of an organic, though still unknown origin of hysteria until his death [10], Janet—like Freud and some other contemporary researchers—assumed a psychogenic etiology. In contrast to Freud, who understood the hysteric symptom formation as a pathologic defense mechanism in the framework of intra-psychic conflict management, Janet originally coined the term "dissociation" as a weakness of the ego's capacity to synthesize mental processes of memory, sensory functions, and motor control. He emphasized the pivotal role of traumatic experience in the etiopathogenesis of dissociative symptoms, pointing at the same time to their close connection to non-pathological phenomena like hypnotic and trance states or somnambulism [1, 10, 21]. After decades of low reception, Janet's ideas on dissociation have experienced a fulminant revival as from the 1970s [22], promoting the still growing psychiatric field of post-traumatic stress disorders, dissociative disorders, and their interdependence. The majority of the recent research literature assumes that trauma and dissociation are intimately connected with each other [23]. Peri-traumatic dissociation as an adaptive mental survival strategy in a situation of overwhelming physical or psychological danger may lead to continuing dissociative symptoms as defined by the diagnosis of posttraumatic stress disorder. The concept of "structural dissociation" seems to be a useful theoretical framework for understanding and treating trauma-related dissociative long-time effects on personality development [24]. Furthermore from a clinical point of view, two subtypes of dissociation have been proposed recently [25, 26]. The core characteristic of "detachment" is an alteration in consciousness (as seen, e.g., in states of derealization or depersonalization), while "compartmentalization" is characterized by an inability to control and integrate mental processes otherwise regulated intentionally on a conscious level (as typically seen in conversion disorder). This dichotomous concept of dissociation may help to clarify the slight terminological confusion between DSM-V and ICD-10 by emphasizing both the common ground and the differences between conversion and dissociation.

A last remark in this paragraph pertains to the role of trauma in the etiopathogenesis of dissociative symptoms. Besides the mainstream of the current psychiatric theory, which clearly favors an almost obligatory relationship between trauma and dissociation [23], some serious research indicates that the correlation might not be as strong as suggested and, moreover, the causal link might also operate in the other direction than assumed [27–29]. Clinical evidence from the psychotherapeutic treatment of neurotic patients also shows that a significant part of dissociative symptomatology does not relate to prior severe anamnestic trauma [30]. It seems that the etiological role of internal stressors—as conceptualized for instance in the theory of intra-psychic neurotic conflict—is rather underestimated in the current scientific discussion on dissociative symptomatology. At this point, the issue shall not be further elaborated; an in-depth discussion is to be found in [31].

Epidemiology

The annual incidence of new cases is approximately three patients with dissociative seizures per 100,000 inhabitants [32]. The overall prevalence of patients with dissociative seizures is estimated to be 2–33 per 100,000 inhabitants [33]. For obvious reasons, patients with dissociative seizures are seen more frequently in epilepsy treatment settings than indicated by the average rates above. It is assumed that 5–20 % of all outpatients with the diagnosis of epilepsy with therapy-refractory seizures in fact suffer from dissociative seizures [34]. Likewise, 10–40 % of all patients with epilepsy admitted to intensive monitoring units for evaluation of neurosurgical treatment options turn out to have dissociative seizures only [34]. These figures clearly demonstrate that dissociative seizures represent a significant problem for health care providers.

Considering all patients with dissociative seizures regardless of their underlying psychiatric morbidity, some further epidemiological characteristics are particularly noteworthy.

The quota of woman patients amounts to 70–80 %. From the very beginning in old Egyptian and Hippocratic Greek medicine, hysteria was seen as a women's disease, characterized by the migrating womb inside the woman's body. This original etiological theory has certainly exerted a significant influence on the constant status of hysteria as a woman's disease throughout history, whatever other reasons for the female preponderance might have been and still are [1, 10].

Furthermore, initial manifestation seems to occur in a bimodal distribution. A first peak is observed in late adolescence from the age of 19–22, a second peak in early adulthood between 25 and 35 years of age [35]. The findings on socio-economic characteristics of patients with dissociative seizures are mostly normal, marital status is on average compared to the general population, and vocational training and professional qualification seem to be slightly lower-than-average.

There are an abundant number of studies comprehensively covering epidemiological and differential diagnostic topics pertaining to the group of patients with dissociative seizures. Several reviews—published both recently and over the last decade—provide excellent summaries [36–44].

Differential Diagnosis

Dissociative seizures oftentimes display a striking similarity to epileptic or other somatogenic seizures. Already Sydenham, the clinically gifted English seventeenth-century physician very accurately observed the "multiformity of the shapes" which hysteria puts on. "Few of the maladies of miserable mortality are not imitated by it … Hence, without skill and sagacity the physician will be deceived; so as to refer the symptoms to some essential disease of the part in question and not to the effects of hysteria" [1]. Making a proper diagnosis of dissociative seizures, therefore, requires the exclusion of epileptic or other somatogenic seizures that might come into differential diagnostic question.

In the field of somatogenic paroxysms, epileptic seizures (and particularly those of frontal lobe origin) constitute the most important and most difficult differential diagnosis to be considered. The specific features to be taken into account in these cases are discussed separately in the section on "Diagnosing dissociative seizures" below. Other relevant somatogenic differential diagnoses are listed in the left column of Table 9.1 [45].

In the field of psychogenic paroxysmal events, a number of differential diagnoses have to be considered likewise. They are listed in the right column of Table 9.1.

Diagnosing Dissociative Seizures

In the first step, establishing the diagnosis of dissociative seizures requires the exclusion of somatogenic and particularly epileptic seizures. Especially seizures of frontal lobe origin and some bilateral convulsive seizures may convey a strong psychogenic appearance and, therefore, mislead the intuitive judgment of even proven specialists [46].

Table 9.1 Non-epileptic differential diagnosis of dissociative seizures [45]

Somatogenic non-epileptic paroxysms	Psychogenic non-epileptic paroxysms
Syncope	Panic attack
Toxic or drug-induced events	Dissociative fugue
Transient ischemic attack	Dissociative stupor
Migraine attack	Psychogenic hyperventilation
Vertigo attack	Psychotic catatonia
Sleep-associated disorders, e.g., narcolepsy, parasomnias	Psychotic stupor
Movement disorders, e.g., choreoathethosis	Artificial paroxysmal events
Hyperekplexia	Simulation of paroxysmal events
Hypoglycemic events	

Reprinted with kind permission from Springer Science+Business Media and Springer Medizin Verlag Heidelberg, Germany from Schmutz et al. [45], © 2009

The combined video-EEG recording of a typical seizure remains the gold standard to confirm the diagnosis [36]. Ictal EEG findings with no activity typical for epilepsy in combination with semiological features suggestive for dissociative seizures do provide a high diagnostic certainty. However, home-based long-term EEG registration or Video-EEG registration in telemetry unit are expensive examinations usually reserved to tertiary centers. In many cases, the diagnosis has to be based on a normal standard EEG, the reported seizure history, and the reported semiological characteristics. However, no single semiological sign featuring a clear and unambiguous pathognomonic significance has been identified so far. The "*arc de cercle*," the posture of opisthotonus with a reclination of the head and an overextension of the trunk, used to be one of the prevalent seizure signs of the female hysterics in the era of Charcot and Freud. Occasionally, it can be observed in both men and women still today. It is a semiological feature, which is certainly unusual in epilepsy and rather indicative for dissociative seizures.

Some seizure signs (see Table 9.2) are diagnostically suggestive. Together with the anamnestic data and the EEG-findings they may facilitate a comprehensive clinical judgment.

There are some studies indicating that psychometric findings pertaining to personality features might differentiate between patients with dissociative seizures and patients with epileptic seizures [47, 48]. The limited accuracy, though, does not allow a reliable diagnostic classification, and the results remain indicative.

A micro-linguistic approach focusing on patient's spontaneous seizure narratives proves to reveal most interesting results, from both a differential diagnostic and a psychological point of view [49]. Patients with epileptic seizures use complex and repeating pattern of phrasing to describe their seizures; furthermore, they frequently mention attempts to stop their seizures by specific countermeasures. In contrast, dissociative patients basically omit their seizures in their spontaneous seizure narrative, thereby using simple and stereotype patterns of phrasing. Some promising empirical validation studies show that the method features quite powerful differential diagnostic properties [50]. A broader clinical application, however, will be limited by complexity and costs.

Table 9.2 Clinical characteristics of epileptic versus dissociative seizures [45]

Sign	Epileptic seizure	Dissociative seizure
Duration	<5 min	>5 min
Occurrence	No regularity	With bystanders, seldom alone
Motor signs	Tonic-clonic	Asynchronous
Automatisms	Stereotypical, oro-alimentary	Varying, bizarre
Injury	Stereotype pattern of injury	Severe self-injury possible
Tongue bite	Lateral, cheek bite	None or tip of tongue
Eyes	Initially open	Closed, squinting
Amnesia	Total	Partial, resolvable
Postictal	Slow reorientation	Sudden reorientation, astonished, rubbing the eyes
Enuresis, enkopresis	Possible	Enuresis possible, enkopresis seldom

Several attempts have been made to classify dissociative seizures according to their observable motor features [2, 51]. The value of these classifications for treatment or prognosis has yet to be shown. Referring to the concept of symbolic significance of somatic conversion symptoms, one of these classification systems tries to combine motor features and psychodynamic constellations [2]. From a clinical perspective, the practical feasibility can be taken for granted; however, the assumed connection between specific motor features and specific psychodynamics still remains to be demonstrated.

A last remark in this section pertains to the findings of neuroimaging studies. A number of MRI studies try to shed light on the pathophysiology of dissociative seizures [52–54]. The findings, though providing interesting insights in brain functioning, have no practical relevance for differential diagnosis or treatment so far. Furthermore, the authors often ignore the fundamental difference between causal and correlative connection in the interpretation of their findings. In fact, it remains unclear whether the identified neurobiological correlates have any etiological or pathogenic significance. Lastly, the group under investigation is most heterogeneous. As shown in the section on "Psychiatric and psychodynamic diagnosis" below, dissociative seizures represent a mere symptom, but not a disorder in the nosological sense. The group of patients with dissociative seizures includes a broad spectrum of psychiatric disorders. Therefore, any findings pertaining to this symptom group have to be appraised very cautiously.

Forcing Diagnostic Clarification

The time elapsed between the initial seizure manifestation and its diagnostic identification as dissociative is rather long. According to recent studies it amounts to 4–7 years [37–44]. Often, many medical examinations without conclusive findings, tentative treatments with anticonvulsive drugs, seizure-related inability to work, and, last but not least, a lot of social stress in families and friendships are the negative milestones of this interim time. Enabling early diagnostic clarification has become a relevant issue in the health care management of dissociative seizures in order to minimize their adverse socio-medical implications (or, psychologically speaking: their accessory symptoms). Many specialized epilepsy centers around the world apply provocation techniques for seizure induction (e.g., the injection of NaCl) so as to facilitate ictal registration. The ethical pros and cons have been (and still are) substantially debated [55–57] and both positions (in short: the potential damaging of the patient-physician relation by a deceiving medical procedure versus the prevention of future seizure-related and iatrogenic harm by forcing diagnostic clarification) merit full respect.

From a psychological point of view, however, the controversy is of minor significance. If a patient is ready to have a seizure during inward EEG monitoring and thereby allows diagnostic identification, it actually means that he or she is ready to face the intra-psychic conflict and the related feelings of anxiety, shame, guilt, or whatever may constitute the psychological reasons for the seizures. It is, so to speak, a first step in psychotherapy. The openness and willingness to tread this path does not depend on the seizure induction technique, but primarily on the patient's conscious and unconscious motivational state. Secondarily, the neurologist responsible for the lead-up to the inward monitoring should prepare the patient in a most frank and natural way for possible diagnostic outcomes, including dissociative seizures. Whether explicitly or implicitly, the patient will get the message that the neurologist would accept dissociative seizures and not despise them as probably suspected. And last but not least, the whole neurological and nursing inward stuff may substantially support the diagnostic procedure by maintaining a sympathetic attitude and thus enabling the patient to feel secure and to move forward psychologically. Some very basic theoretical education on dissociative seizures is required. Furthermore, appropriate communication training will foster stuff's attitude and facilitate a successful diagnostic procedure.

Psychiatric and Psychodynamic Diagnosis

As shown in the previous sections, making the proper diagnosis of dissociative seizures requires profound neurological expertise and, in many cases, the possibility of an inward monitoring setting in a specialized neurological or epilepsy center. In the initial phase of the diagnostic work-up, psychiatric and psychodynamic considerations have no more than an indicative value. The occurrence of even severe intrapsychic or social stress per se cannot provide diagnostic certainty, because too many patients with epileptic seizures or with syncope also report strain and stress in their life. Only in combination with a clear exclusion of epileptic and other somatogenic seizures, psychiatric and psychodynamic findings are conclusive. Nevertheless, there are good reasons to involve mental health specialist in an early stage of the diagnostic work-up. Communicating the diagnosis of dissociative seizures is much easier when both exclusion and inclusion diagnosis are provided together.

When asked to give an account on their current life situation, a substantial number of patients with dissociative seizures initially describe a largely unremarkable and well-balanced condition in regard to emotions, relationships, and job situation. A regular psychiatric exploration primarily checking for severe psychopathologic signs will most probably yield inconspicuous findings. From a psychological point of view, we should not be surprised about that and, moreover, we should not think that patients are not telling the truth. Every successful formation of a conversion symptom tries to absorb the unbearable internal or external stress and results in an emotional relief. This is the rationale behind all neurotic symptoms: a distress is covered up and displayed at the same time. Acknowledging this psychodynamic background, it makes sense to take down the past psychological and medical history in two stages. In a first step, a detailed history of initial seizure manifestation and seizure semiology is taken, though without actively focusing on potential psychological and social circumstances that might be associated with the seizure genesis. In a second step, the patient is asked to disclose an overview on his or her biography including family of origin, adolescence, schooling, further education, professional situation, and social development in adulthood. Usually, patients do not match these two discourses (of symptom history and biography). But if *we* do so (and match the time of initial symptom manifestation with the corresponding biographical situation), we are able to establish a working hypothesis pertaining to the psychological reasons of the symptom formation in many cases. However, we should be aware at this point that the way from a psychological working hypothesis to a shared understanding with the patient has to be prepared carefully. An untimely communication may lead to rejection.

Along with the classical psychosomatic tradition, DSM refers to the constellation just described above as conversion disorder. However, dissociative seizures may also occur as accessory symptom of severe psychopathology.

Most current publications on dissociative seizures include some remarks on the so-called psychiatric "comorbidity," specifying co-occurring psychiatric diagnosis under this heading. The term "comorbidity" is actually misleading in this context, because it implies that dissociative seizures constitute an own morbidity, possibly occurring with other psychiatric morbidities. However, dissociative seizures do not represent a psychiatric disease per se, but a mere symptom. In other words they represent a symptomatic sign of an underlying disorder. The distinction between symptom and disorder is not trivial. A useful differential diagnostic category is mistaken for a nosological entity [58]. From a neurological point of view, patients with dissociative seizures may comprehensibly appear as a homogenous patient group, distinguished from patients with epilepsy or from patients with syncope. However, patients with dissociative seizures are part of most different psychiatric disorder groups, thus, from a psychiatric perspective, representing a most heterogeneous group with one common symptom. The consequences of this confusion are rather serious. A lot of current research papers report heterogeneous and unsatisfactory findings in regard to therapy and outcome prediction. The common research practice to pool dissociative seizures patients and handle them as though they constituted a nosological group most certainly account for at least some of the problems reported. The issue will be elaborated further below in the sections on "Clinical management" and "Therapy".

Some recent reviews on dissociative seizures provide useful information about the comorbid, or more precisely, underlying psychiatric disorders associated with dissociative seizures [40, 42, 59]. However, data on frequency are very heterogeneous.

From a clinical point of view, a number of psychiatric disorders are particularly prone to include dissociative seizures or other conversion symptoms as one of their pathognomonic symptoms:

- Disorders with predominant "somatoform dissociation" [60] or dissociative "compartmentalization" (see the section on "Terminology") like the somatization disorders or the conversion disorders, respectively. While somatization disorders seem to operate on a rather undifferentiated psychological level close to bodily functions, conversion disorders rather include more sophisticated psychological conflicts, often pertaining to dependency and autonomy in late adolescence and early adulthood or parenthood.
- Disorders with predominant "psychoform dissociation" [61] or dissociative "detachment" (see the section on "Terminology") like the borderline personality disorders and the trauma-related stress disorders.
- Adjustment disorders in patients with severe learning or mental disabilities. Due to comorbid mental and/or physical handicaps a number of these patients live in sheltered or assisted accommodations. Most often, they develop dissociative seizures as a reaction to social and environmental change or stress. Neighboring patients with epileptic seizures frequently serve as symptomatic role model.
- Epilepsy patients developing dissociative seizures after having achieved seizure freedom either by successful epilepsy surgery or by antiepileptic drug treatment. The "burden of normality" [62] weighs more than the benefit of living without epileptic seizures and the conversion symptom intends to maintain secondary gain from illness. Referring to the neurobiological concept of "*alternative psychosis*" in epilepsy [63], we might term this psychological process of failed adjustment as "*alternative neurosis.*"
- Epilepsy patients developing dissociative seizures in addition to their preexisting epileptic seizures. In reverence to Charcot, the co-occurrence of epileptic and dissociative seizures is sometimes called "hystero-epilepsy" (although Charcot actually used the term with different and partly conflicting meanings over the years [10]). The conversion symptom represents a dysfunctional coping with the epilepsy. Along with mentally impaired patients, severe borderline patients with comorbid epilepsy are particularly prone to this constellation, thereby complicating and sometimes even impeding adequate seizure treatment. In many cases, a proper classification of an acute seizure exacerbation is not possible and non-adherence to the anticonvulsive drug treatment may further obscure the situation. In general, the co-occurrence of dissociative and epileptic seizures is rather seldom; however, in specialized tertiary centers it is seen quite often. 5–10 % of all patients with confirmed dissociative seizures suffer from epileptic seizures as

well [64, 65]. Considering the general prevalence of epileptic and of dissociative seizures [33], we can conclude the other way around that about 0.15 % of all patients with epileptic seizures also suffer from dissociative seizures.

Clinical Management

The clinical management of patients with dissociative seizures is generally considered as challenging [66]. A significant number of patients are desperately seeking for an organic cause of their seizures. They perceive the diagnosis of dissociative seizures as disappointing and even offending and prefer to obtain another second opinion instead of being referred to psychotherapeutic treatment. Some major pitfalls in the clinical management are discussed in the following.

Countertransference

Patients with dissociative seizures frequently behave in a most challenging way during inward investigation. They are demanding and they quickly complain of not being taken seriously. Even on inquiry they remain very vague in the description of their seizure symptoms, and the degree of their psychological strain is surprisingly low in view of all the previous emergency admissions, the spectacular seizure-related disturbances in the social and professional environment, and last but not least the serious strain of their partners and close friends. Inward staff is regularly annoyed and complains about limited cooperation.

Focusing on the underlying psychiatric disorders and psychodynamics helps the neurologists and the nursing professionals to master these challenges. Countertransference is a most useful concept originally developed in psychoanalysis. It basically assumes that the therapist's emotional reactions to the patient reflect the patient's inner conflicts and psychodynamic [67]. The reflection may operate in a complementary or parallel way. A depressed patient can cause health professionals to either react in a very protecting and sparing or in a rather aggressive and impatient way. Both attitudes obviously refer to a basic problem of aggression management in the psychodynamic of depression. Likewise, somatoform patients tend to induce anger and subtle reproaches of aggravating or even feigning their symptoms. This reaction refers to the somatoform process of fully absorbing interpersonal and emotional distress and strain by somatic symptoms, therefore effectively impeding the development of empathy and compassion. The tendency of borderline patients to induce splitting and overt conflict in treatment teams is well-known, well described, and does not need further elaboration here. Patients with conversion disorder often display a most irritating unconcern or even airiness pertaining to the most serious medical and social implications and consequences of their dissociative seizures. Typically and in a pronounced contrast to patients with epileptic seizures, they do not express an urgent wish to get rid of the seizures. Rather they are interested to know the diagnosis and how to cope better with the seizures. These phenomena have been described as the hysteric "*belle indifference*" and refer to the gain of neurotic symptom formation (see the section on "Psychiatric and psychodynamic diagnosis").

Communicating the Diagnostic Findings

In the framework of a comprehensive diagnostic work-up, the neurologist's task does not only include to secure the exclusion of the somatogenic differential diagnoses, but also to communicate the diagnostic findings, to give a treatment recommendation, and to initiate a referral if wished by the patient.

It is widely acknowledged that the way the diagnostic findings are communicated may influence the chance of a successful psychotherapeutic referral and might even have an impact on the symptomatic outcome. A number of manuals and protocols have been proposed in order to facilitate the diagnostic disclosure talk [34, 68, 69]. A central theme of the recommendations is to emphasize several exclusion issues: no epilepsy, no anticonvulsive drugs, no simulation. The intention to focus on seemingly good news and to avoid the conflict-prone "psycho"-issue is understandable; however, the impact of this approach seems questionable. Instead of beating about the bush and talking about what the seizures are *not* and what they do *not* imply, why not tell the patients directly what their seizures are: fits with a high disintegrative impact on the control of bodily motor functions and consciousness (therefore called dissociative), originating from psychological and sometimes social distress and strain (i.e., a kind of cry for help in body language), that can be further identified and resolved in a psychotherapy (by learning to read and translate the body's language).

Identifying a somatic symptom as being dissociative in nature and disclosing the diagnosis to the patient is equivalent to making a strong psychological interpretation. The theory and clinical practice of psychoanalytic interpretation clearly show that preparation, timing, and wording are crucial. There is a considerable potential for failure. Patients with dissociative seizures may react to the diagnosis with anger, rage, and sometimes even with a sudden breakup of the hospitalization. Clinical experience suggests that mental health professionals should actively be involved at this point of the diagnostic work-up. Psychiatric and psychodynamic findings—while only indicative in the early stages of medical investigations—become most relevant now. From a patient's point of view, the presentation of a working hypothesis about the psychological background of the dissociative seizures will significantly increase the diagnostic plausibility. In other words, disclosing the diagnostic findings should preferably include both the psychological and the neurological results, presented jointly by the psychologist and the neurologist [70, 71]. Due to limited personal and financial resources a leaner procedure may be required, though it is still possible to implement the presented basic idea.

Therapy

In 1730, the English physician Mandeville published the "*Treatise of the hypochondriac and hysteric diseases.*" Somewhere he describes "*hysteric seizures*" of a female patient and, subsequently, the following dialog between the physician and this female patient: "[Physician:...] wherefore if the Lady's youth and strength be prudently assisted, I am of the opinion, Madam, that she'll certainly be cured. In order to it, in the first place, I would for one month prescribe a course of exercise, and no medicines at all. [Patient:] A course of Exercise? and no medicines at all?" [72] The lady's upset reaction to the treatment recommendation seems very modern and could easily come from a present-day patient. Likewise, present-day research literature on dissociative seizures rather consistently agrees with Mandeville, that psychotherapy is the treatment of choice [37, 39, 41, 72–74]. The widely recognized methods of cognitive-behavioral, psychodynamic, and systemic therapies [75–81] have proven their clinical worth, in general as well as in patients with dissociative seizures. From an empirical point of view, several studies [82, 83] and meta-analyses [84, 85] have investigated the effectiveness of the major psychotherapeutic methods and other psychological interventions like, e.g., hypnosis. Most studies report improved symptomatic outcomes under the applied intervention under investigation. However, there are methodological shortcomings significantly limiting the results. Only some few studies control the selection bias by randomization. Therefore, it remains unclear what kind of patients would accept psychotherapy and what kind of patients would refuse to do so. Even the question whether psychotherapy is more beneficial than the natural course itself [83] is unanswered.

A further and more basic methodological problem pertains to the psychiatric heterogeneity of patients with dissociative seizures. As shown in the section on "Psychiatric and psychodynamic diagnosis", dissociative seizures represent a mere symptom, but not a disorder. They do not constitute a meaningful nosological group. This means that studies investigating psychotherapeutic treatments in patients with dissociative seizures are in fact dealing with very different underlying psychiatric disorders. It can be assumed that this heterogeneity basically accounts for the inconsistent and unsatisfactory treatment research findings.

From a clinical point of view, the selection of the appropriate psychotherapeutic method and interventions should primarily relate to the operant underlying psychiatric disorder (and to the psychodynamic constellation of course). A short example may help to clarify this point. Different psychiatric disorders include insomnia as an accessory symptom, e.g., psychosis, depression, or anorexia—just to mention a few. It would not make sense to pool these patients in an insomnia group, to develop one joint insomnia treatment program, and to evaluate the effectiveness of this program. Of course, any meaningful treatment and research would primarily relate to the different underlying disorders and not to the mere symptom of insomnia. Likewise, there is no reason to develop or to apply specific therapy programs for dissociative seizures [74, 82–84, 86]. Rather, the neurologist should notice that there are already different clinically approved and evidence-based methods of psychotherapy, providing most helpful theoretical and practical tools for the treatment of patients with all the psychiatric disorders that include dissociative seizures as an accessory symptom [75–81]. Neurologists do not have to start from scratch and reinvent psychotherapy.

The psychotherapists, on the other hand, should recognize that the treatment of dissociative seizures and other conversion symptoms used to be—and still is—their very own professional business [87]. After all, Anna O. and the other hysterics in the case histories of Freud and Breuer served as important catalysts for the development of psychotherapy [88]. As with epileptic seizures, dissociative seizures generally have a high impact on body and motor functioning. Most psychotherapists though—be it psychiatrists or psychologists—are exclusively using verbal interactions as working tool. Occurring seizures may be perceived as a damage or even destruction of this verbal space of interaction and communication both in the literal and in the figurative sense. The patient needs physical support, the verbal communication is interrupted, and the time schedule of the consultation might get disturbed. We may assume that patients with dissociative seizures subtly elicit fear and discomfort particularly in psychotherapists who are not experienced in treating these patients. This fits in with the fact, that epilepsy centers or neurologists trying to refer patients with dissociative seizures to outpatient psychotherapy departments encounter striking reservations.

Seizure-Specific Therapeutic Considerations

Certainly, there are some specific seizure-related issues that the psychotherapist needs to know and to consider. The occurrence of a dissociative seizure does not require an emergency physician unless major injury is suspected. Also, there is no indication to apply sedative drugs. Even in the case of a prolonged dissociative seizure (sometimes referred to as "dissociative seizure status"), the use of benzodiazepines or similar drugs is not recommended. All dissociative seizures will finally cease, be it by exhaustion or by sleep. The condition of an underlying or indeed comorbid psychiatric disorder may certainly require the use of psychotropic medication; however, it should be clear for both the patient and the psychotherapist that there is no direct anti-dissociative seizure medication.

Some simple behavioral rules have proven to be effective for shortening a seizure. Too many bystanders and too much care will most probably aggravate the seizures; too little attention will do the same. In the case of a seizure occurring during consultation, it is up to the psychotherapist to react in a neither over- nor "under"-protective way. At home and at work, it is up to the patient himself or herself to inform family member and coworkers appropriately about reasonable reactions in case of a seizure. Many patients report difficulties to implement this kind of indirect coping behavior pertaining to the own seizures. For the most part, the patient's readiness to move forward in the therapy will decide about the success.

As with other conversion symptoms, dissociative seizures are particularly suitable for the rapid development of secondary gain from illness. Family members feel obliged to accompany and supervise the patient 24 h a day, general practitioners are pressured to confirm the incapacity for work, and claims for insurance benefits or even a disability pension may arise. Secondary gain from illness in neurosis has always a strong anti-therapeutic impact because it ensures the perpetuation of the symptom. Therefore, the issue has to be addressed therapeutically with priority. Most certainly, there are a number of patients with dissociative seizures who do need a permanent supervision, and who are incapable for work indeed, and who may even qualify for insurance benefits. However, it is not the mere symptom of dissociative seizures but the underlying psychiatric disorder that may give reason for that.

Another seizure-specific issue is the fitness to drive a car. In many countries there are legal regulations that apply to all seizures coming along with alteration of consciousness or with a shortened capacity to control motor functions—irrespective of seizure etiology. In other countries, epileptic and dissociative seizures are addressed separately by the legal requirements, and finally there are some countries with unclear or even missing legal regulations pertaining to dissociative seizures. Due to the need for medical certification, patients regularly raise the issue of fitness to drive. Of course the psychotherapist must encourage the patient to observe any existing legal regulations—be it nationwide or statewide. In case of missing regulations, the psychotherapist should give a well-founded advice. The prognostic assessment should take into consideration the previous symptomatic and therapeutic course and, of course, seizure-related issues like frequency and circumstances of occurrence and possible changes in semiological features like altered consciousness or impaired motor control. Furthermore the potential for autoaggressive and self-injurious behavior should be evaluated. In most cases it is possible to achieve a reasonable and mutually agreed arrangement with the patient.

Lastly, some remarks pertain to role of the neurologist after the referral is done and the psychotherapy is established. Along with all conversion patients, patients with dissociative seizures repeatedly tend to mistrust the diagnostic findings and to actively seek diagnostic reevaluation. Most interestingly, psychotherapists (especially psychiatrists) do the very same and express overt mistrust of the diagnostic validity of ictal video-EEG-registration [89]. This gap between differential diagnostic specialists and treatment specialists is remarkable, the more so as empirical findings since the 1970s clearly demonstrate a constantly low rate of only 4 % of misdiagnosis in the field of conversion symptoms [90]. When both the patient and the psychotherapist mistrust the referral diagnosis, treatment will not work well for sure. From a psychotherapeutic perspective, mistrusting the diagnosis may preferentially occur in early, vulnerable, or stuck stages of the psychotherapeutic process. Psychotherapists challenging the diagnosis should not hesitate to check with the neurologist, who in turn should be ready to explicate the diagnostic findings again. Sometimes a patient who has doubts about the diagnosis needs direct reassurance by the neurologist. A short consultation may prevent both a discontinuation of psychotherapy and further unnecessary and costly reevaluations.

Outcome and Prognosis

Patients with dissociative seizures have a rather poor symptomatic outcome. In about one-third of all patients seizures chronically persist. Another third do symptomatically improve, though without achieving seizure freedom. The last third finally get seizure-free in the long run [58, 91, 92]. Due to methodological reasons, the pertinent outcome studies are difficult to compare; however, estimates of two meta-analyses consistently reveal a rather poor overall trend [58, 92]. In order to enhance understanding and treatment, quite a number of psychiatric, psychological, medical, and socio-demographic features have been investigated with regard to their prognostic properties. So far, the prognostic value of most of the investigated variables is controversially appraised by different studies. Two meta-analyses show that some few characteristics seem to be relevant for prognosis [58, 92]. First, a short period of time between initial seizure manifestation and diagnostic clarification is associated with a better outcome. Second, severe personality pathology is associated with a worse outcome. Third and last, the clear identification of a stressful event preceding the initial seizure manifestation is again associated with a better outcome.

There are some problematic methodological issues like the multitude of merely correlative findings and the multitude of retrospective, but not prospective data analysis. As already explicated in regard to therapy above in the section on "Clinical management", a further and more basic methodological problem pertains to the psychiatric heterogeneity of patients with dissociative seizures. How should it be possible to identify common prognostic factors in a group of most different psychiatric patients? The prognostic features mentioned in previous paragraph are rather general and, therefore, might apply to different psychiatric disorders indeed.

The close interrelation between diagnosis, treatment, and prognosis is well-known in most fields of medicine. In a recently published clinical guide to epileptic syndromes and their treatments, it is put as follows: "Medical diagnosis is the identification of a disease by investigation of its symptoms and history, which provides a solid basis for the treatment and prognosis of the individual patient" [93].

To the best of my knowledge there is no outcome or prediction research on dissociative seizures based on the underlying psychiatric disorders in the last decades. In the 1960s, Guze and Perley published two studies on the Briquet syndrome (i.e., the later somatization disorder) and could clearly demonstrate the diagnostic validity of the syndrome and a chronic poor symptomatic course in the long run [12, 13]. Here we have an example "of the identification of disease by investigation of its symptoms and history, which provides a solid basis for … prognosis…" [93].

In the field of neurology, dissociative seizures remain a most challenging differential diagnostic task. With regard to treatment issues as well as research on outcome and prognosis, the psychiatric and psychotherapeutic community should get into gear and increase its involvement. A look back into the history of psychotherapy reveals its formerly close connection to seizures and other conversion symptoms. This tradition and expertise must be resumed and further elaborated in close cooperation with epilepsy centers and neurologist already working in the field.

Acknowledgment I am grateful to Martin Kurthen for his hints and critical comments.

References

1. Veith I. Hysteria: the history of a disease. Chicago: The University of Chicago Press; 1965.
2. Betts T. Psychiatric aspects of nonepileptic seizures. In: Engel Jr J, Pedley TA, editors. Epilepsy: a comprehensive textbook. Philadelphia: Lippincott; 1997. p. 2101–16.
3. Benbadis SR. Psychogenic nonepileptic "seizures" or "attacks"? It's not just semantics: attacks. Neurology. 2010;75(1):84–6.
4. LaFrance Jr WC. Psychogenic nonepileptic "seizures" or "attacks"? It's not just semantics: seizures. Neurology. 2010;75(1):87–8.
5. O'Hanlon S, Liston R, Delanty N. Psychogenic nonepileptic seizures. Time to abandon the term pseudoseizures. Arch Neurol. 2012;69(10):1349–50.
6. Sethi NK. Psychogenic nonepileptic seizuzures: the name matters. JAMA Neurol. 2013;70(4):528–9.
7. O'Hanlon S, Liston R, Delanty N. In reply. JAMA Neurol. 2013;70(4):529.
8. American Psychiatric Association. Diagnostic and statistical manual of mental disorders: DSM-V. Arlington: American Psychiatric Association; 2013.
9. Freud, S. Die Abwehr-Neuropsychosen. In: Gesammelte Werke, Erster Band, Werke aus den Jahren 1892–1899. Frankfurt am Main: S. Fischer Verlag; 1894/1991. S. 59–74. German.
10. Shorter E. From paralysis to fatigue: a history of psychosomatic illness in the modern era. New York: Free Press; 1992.
11. Stefánsson JG, Messina JA, Meyerowitz S. Hysterical neurosis, conversion type: clinical and epidemiological considerations. Acta Psychiatr Scand. 1976;53:119–38.
12. Perley MJ, Guze SB. Hysteria – the stability and usefulness of clinical criteria. N Engl J Med. 1962;266(9):421–6.
13. Guze SB, Perley MJ. Observations on the natural history of hysteria. Am J Psychiatry. 1963;119:960–5.
14. Guze SB. Studies in hysteria. Can J Psychiatry. 1983;28:434–7.
15. Alexander F. Psychosomatic medicine: its principles and applications. New York: Norton; 1950.
16. Engel GL. "Psychogenic" pain and the pain prone patient. Am J Med. 1959;26:899–918.
17. Ziegler F, Imboden JB. Contemporary conversion reactions. II. A conceptual model. Arch Gen Psychiatry. 1960;16(6):279–87.
18. Ziegler F, Imboden JB, Rodgers DA. Contemporary conversion reactions. III. Diagnostic considerations. JAMA. 1963;186(4):307–11.
19. Engel GL. Conversion symptoms. In: MacBryde CM, Blacklow RS, editors. Signs and symptoms. Applied pathologic physiology and clinical interpretation. 5th ed. Philadelphia: Lippincott; 1970. p. 650–68.
20. World Health Organization. International statistical classification of mental disorders and related health problems. V Mental and behavioural disorder. 10th revision. Version 2015. http://apps.who.int/classifications/icd10/browse/2015/en. Accessed 01 Feb 2015.
21. Janet P. L'automatisme psychologique. Paris: F. Alcan; 1903. French.
22. Nemiah JC. Conversion: fact or chimera? Int J Psychiatry Med. 1974;5(4):443–8.
23. Van der Hart O, Nijenhuis ERS. Dissociative disorders. In: Blaney PH, Millon T, editors. Oxford textbook of psychopathology. 2nd ed. Oxford: Oxford University Press; 2009. p. 452–81.
24. Steel K, van der Hart O, Nijenhuis ER. Phase-oriented treatment of structural dissocation in complex traumatization: overcoming trauma-related phobias. J Trauma Dissociation. 2005;6(3):11–53.

25. Holmes EA, Brown RJ, Mansell W, Fearon RP, Hunter EC, Frasquilho R, et al. Are there two qualitatively distinct forms of dissociation? A review and some clinical implications. Clin Psychol Rev. 2005;25(1):1–23.
26. Brown RJ. Different types of "dissociation" have different types of psychological mechanisms. J Trauma Dissociation. 2006;7(4):7–28.
27. Mulder RT, Beautrais AL, Joyce PR, Fergusson DM. Relationship between dissociation, childhood sexual abuse, childhood physical abuse, and mental illness in a general population sample. Am J Psychiatry. 1998;155(6):806–11.
28. Merckelbach H, Dekkers T, Wessel I, Roefs A. Amnesia, flashbacks, nightmares, and dissociation in aging concentration camp survivors. Behav Res Ther. 2003;41(3):351–60.
29. Merckelbach H, Horselenberg R, Schmidt H. Modeling the connection between self-reported trauma and dissociation in a student sample. Personal Individ Differ. 2002;32:695–705.
30. Fiszman A, Vieira Alves-Leon S, Gopmes Nunes R, Andrea ID, Figueira I. Traumatic events and posttraumatic stress disorder in patients with psychogenic nonepileptic seizures: a critical review. Epilepsy Behav. 2004;5:818–25.
31. Merckelbach H, Muris P. The causal link between self-reported trauma and dissociation: a critical review. Behav Res Ther. 2001;39(3):245–54.
32. Szaflarski JP, Ficker DM, Cahill WT, Privitera MD. Four-year incidence of psychogenic nonepileptic seizures in adults in Hamilton County, OH. Neurology. 2000;55(10):1561–3.
33. Benbadis SR, Hauser A. An estimate of the prevalence of psychogenic non-epileptic seizures. Seizure. 2000;9:280–1.
34. Krummholz A, Hopp J. Psychogenic (nonepileptic) seizures. Semin Neurol. 2006;26(3):341–50.
35. Lancmann EL, Lambrakis CC, Steinhardt MI. Psychogenic pseudoseizures. A general overview. In: Ettinger AB, Kanner AM, editors. Psychiatric issues in epilepsy. Philadelphia: Lippincott; 2001. p. 341–54.
36. LaFrance Jr WC, Baker GA, Duncan R, Goldstein LH, Reuber M. Minimum requirements for the diagnosis of psychogenic nonepileptic seizures: a staged approach: a report from the International League Against Epilepsy Nonepileptic Seizures Task Force. Epilepsia. 2013;54(11):2005–18.
37. LaFrance Jr WC, Reuber M, Goldstein L. Management of psychogenic nonepileptic seizures. Epilepsia. 2013;54 Suppl 1:53–67.
38. Dickinson P, Looper KJ. Psychogenic nonepileptic seizures: a current overview. Epilepsia. 2012;54(10):1679–89.
39. Reuber M, Mayor R. Recent progress in the understanding and treatment of nonepileptic seizures. Curr Opin Psychiatry. 2012;25:244–50.
40. Widdess-Walsh P, Mostacci B, Tinuper P, Devinsky O. Psychogenic nonepileptic seizures. Handb Clin Neurol. 2012;107:277–95.
41. Goldstein LH, Mellers JDC. Recent developments in our understanding of the semiology and treatment of psychogenic nonepileptic seizures. Curr Neurol Neurosci Rep. 2012;12:436–44.
42. Brown RJ, Syed TU, Benbadis S, LaFrance Jr WC, Reuber M. Psychogenic nonepileptic seizures. Epilepsy Behav. 2011;22:85–93.
43. Reuber M. Psychogenic nonepileptic seizures: answers and questions. Epilepsy Behav. 2008;12(4):622–35.
44. Blum AS, LaFrance Jr WC. Overview of psychological nonepileptic seizures. In: Ettinger AB, Kanner AM, editors. Psychiatric issues in epilepsy. 2nd ed. Philadelphia: Lippincott; 2007. p. 421–31.
45. Schmutz M, Ganz RE, Krämer G. Dissoziative Anfälle. Nervenarzt. 2009;4:475–84. German.
46. LaFrance Jr WC, Benbadis SR. Differentiating frontal lobe epilepsy from psychogenic nonepileptic seizures. Neurol Clin. 2011;29:149–62.
47. Reuber M, Pukrop R, Bauer J, Derfuss R, Elger CE. Multidimensional assessment of personality in patients with psychogenic non-epileptic seizures. J Neurol Neurosurg Psychiatry. 2004;75:743–8.

48. Bewley J, Murphy PN, Mallows J, Baker GA. Does alexithymia differentiate between patients with nonepileptic seizures, patients with epilepsy, and nonpatient controls? Epilepsy Behav. 2005;7:430–7.
49. Schwabe M, Reuber M, Schöndienst M, Gülich E. Listening to people with seizures: how can lingustic anaysis help in the differential diagnosis of seizure disorders? Commun Med. 2008;5(1):59–72.
50. Reuber M, Monzoni C, Sharrack B, Plug L. Using interactional and linguistic analysis to distinguish between epileptic and psychogenic non-epileptic seizures: a prospective blinded multi-rater study. Epilepsy Behav. 2009;16:139–44.
51. Gröppel G, Kapitany T, Baumgartner C. Cluster analysis of clinical seizure semiology of psychogenic nonepileptic seizures. Epilepsia. 2000;41(5):610–4.
52. Vuilleumier P, Chicherio C, Assal F, Schwartz S, Slosman D, Landis T. Functional neuroanatomical correlates of hysterical sensorimotor loss. Brain. 2001;124(Pt 6):1077–90.
53. Montoya A, Price BH, Lepage M. Neural correlates of 'functional' symptoms in neurology. Funct Neurol. 2006;21(4):193–7.
54. Li R, Liu K, Ma X, Li Z, Duan X, An D, et al. Altered functional connectivity patterns of the insular subregions in psychogenic nonepileptic seizures. Brain Topogr. 2014. doi:10.1007/s10548-014-0413-3.
55. Benbadis SR. Provocative techniques should be used for the diagnosis of psychogenic nonepileptic seizures. Epilepsy Behav. 2009;15:106–9.
56. Leeman BA. Provocative techniques should not be used for the diagnosis of psychogenic non-epileptic seizures. Epilepsy Behav. 2009;15:110–4.
57. Kanner AM, Benbadis SR, Leeman B. Rebuttals and a final commentary. Epilepsy Behav. 2009;15:115–8.
58. Schmutz M. Dissociative seizures – a critical review and perspective. Epilepsy Behav. 2013;29:449–56.
59. Bowman ES, Kanner AM. Psychopathology and outcome in psychogenic nonepileptic seizures. In: Ettinger AB, Kanner AM, editors. Psychiatric issues in epilepsy. 2nd ed. Philadelphia: Lippincott; 2007. p. 432–60.
60. Nijenhuis ERS. Somatoform dissociation: phenomena, measurement, and theoretical issues. New York: Norton; 2004.
61. Näring GWB, Nijenhuis ERS. Relationships between self-reported potentially traumatizing events, psychoform and somatoform dissociation, and absorption, in two non-clinical populations. Aust N Z J Psychiatry. 2005;39(11/12):982–7.
62. Ferguson SM, Rayport M. The adjustment to living without epilepsy. J Nerv Ment Dis. 1965;140:26–37.
63. Trimble MR, Schmitz EB. Forced normalization and alternative psychosis of epilepsy. Petersfield: Wrightson Biomedical; 1998.
64. Benbadis SR, Agrawal V, Tatum WO. How many patients with psychogenic nonepileptic seizures also have epilepsy? Neurology. 2001;57:915–7.
65. Martin R, Burneo JG, Prasad A, Powell T, Faught E, Knowlton R, et al. Frequency of epilepsy in patients with psychogenic seizures monitored by video-EEG. Neurology. 2003;61(12):1791–2.
66. Lacey C, Cook M, Salzberg M. The neurologist, psychogenic nonepileptic seizures, and borderline personality disorder. Epilepsy Behav. 2007;11:492–8.
67. Gabbard GO. Contertransference issues in psychiatric treatment. Washington, DC: American Psychiatric Press; 1999.
68. Hall-Patch L, Brown R, House A, Howlett S, Kemp S, Lawton G, et al. Acceptability and effectiveness of a strategy for the communication of the diagnosis of psychogenic nonepileptic seizures. Epilepsia. 2010;51(1):70–8.
69. NEST (Non-Epileptic Seizures Treatment) Group. Non-epileptic attacks. Information for patients, family and friends. 2006. http://www.shef.ac.uk/neuroscience/nest/downloads. Accessed 02 Feb 2015.

70. Thompson N, Connelly L, Peltzer J, Nowack WJ, Hamera E, Hunter EE. Psychogenic nonepileptic seizures: a pilot study of a brief educational intervention. Perspect Psychiatr Care. 2013;49(2):78–83.
71. Acton EK, Tatum WO. Inpatient psychiatric consultation for newly-diagnosed patients with psychogenic non-epileptic seizures. Epilepsy Behav. 2013;27:36–9.
72. LaFrance Jr WC, Devinsky O. The treatment of nonepileptic seizures: historical perspectives and future directions. Epilepsia. 2004;45 Suppl 2:15–21.
73. LaFrance Jr WC, Kanner SM, Berry JJ. Treating patients with psychological nonepileptic seizures. In: Ettinger AB, Kanner AM, editors. Psychiatric issues in epilepsy. 2nd ed. Philadelphia: Lippincott; 2007. p. 461–88.
74. Baslet G. Psychogenic nonepileptic seizures: a treatment review. What have we learned since the beginning of the millennium? Neuropsychiatr Dis Treat. 2012;8:585–98.
75. Craske MG. Cognitive-behavioral therapy. Washington, DC: American Psychological Association; 2010.
76. Linehan MM. Understanding borderline personality disorder: the dialectic approach program manual. New York: Guilford Press; 1995.
77. Koerner K. Doing dialectical behavior therapy. A practical guide. New York: Guilford Press; 2012.
78. Clarkin JF, Fonagy P, Gabbard GO, editors. Psychodynamic psychotherapy for personality disorders: a clinical handbook. Washington, DC: Amercian Psychiatric Publishing; 2010.
79. Levy RA, Ablon JS, Kächele H. editors. Psychodynamic psychotherapy research. Evidence-based practice and practice-based evidence. New York: Springer; 2012.
80. Winek JL. Systemic family therapy: from theory to practice. Thousand Oaks: Sage; 2010.
81. Goldenberg H, Goldenberg I. Family therapy. An overview. 7th ed. Thomson: Belmont; 2007.
82. Goldstein LH, Deale AC, Mitchell-O'Malley SJ, Toone BK, Mellers JDC. An evaluation of cognitive behavioral therapy as a treatment for dissociative seizures. A pilot study. Cogn Behav Neurol. 2004;17:41–9.
83. Mayor R, Howlett S, Grünewald R, Reuber M. Long-term outcome of brief augmented psychodynamic interpersonal psychotherapy for psychogenic nonepileptic seizures: seizure control and health care utilization. Epilepsia. 2010;51(7):1169–76.
84. Broocks JL, Goodfellow L, Bodde NMG, Aldenkamp A, Baker GA. Nondrug treatment for psychogenic nonepileptic seizures. What's the evidence? Epilepsy Behav. 2007;11:367–77.
85. Martlew J, Pulman J, Marson AG. Psychological and behavioural treatment for adults with non-epileptic attack disorder. Cochrane Database Syst Rev. 2014;2, CD006370. doi:10.1002/14651858.CD006370.pub2.
86. Baxter S, Mayor R, Baird W, Brown R, Cock H, Howlett S, et al. Understanding patient perceptions following a psycho-educational intervention for psychogenic non-epileptic seizures. Epilepsy Behav. 2012;23(4):487–93.
87. Benbadis S. The problem of psychogenic symptoms: is the psychiatric community in denial? Epilepsy Behav. 2005;6:9–14.
88. Breuer J, Freud S. Studien über Hysterie. Leipzig und Wien: Franz Deuticke; 1895. German.
89. Harden CL, Burgut FT, Kanner AM. The diagnostic significance of video-EEG-monitoring findings on pseudoseizure patients differs between neurologist and psychiatrist. Epilepsia. 2003;44:453–6.
90. Stone J, Smyth R, Carson A, Lewis S, Prescott R, Warlow C, et al. Systematic review of misdiagnosis of conversion symptoms and "hysteria". BMJ. 2005;331(7523):989–91.
91. Reuber M, Pukrop R, Bauer J, Helmstaedter C, Tessendorf N, Elger CE. Outcome in psychogenic nonepileptic seizures: 1 to 10-year follow-up in 164 patients. Ann Neurol. 2003;53:305–11.
92. Durrant J, Rickards H, Cavanna AE. Prognosis and outcome predictors in psychogenic nonepileptic seizures. Epilepsy Res Treat. 2011;2011:274736.
93. Panayiotopoulos CP. A clinical guide to epileptic syndromes and their treatment. Revised second edition. New York: Springer; 2010.

Chapter 10
Consciousness

Andrea E. Cavanna

Abstract The concept of consciousness is central to human experience in both health and pathology. Over the last few years, consciousness studies have featured translational approaches with multidisciplinary contributions from philosophy, psychology, and neuroscience. Transient alterations of consciousness characterize the clinical phenomenology of different types of epileptic seizure. The assessment of both the level of consciousness (arousal, clinically tested as responsiveness) and the contents of consciousness (awareness, clinically tested as patient report of subjective experiences) is of pivotal importance for the clinical characterization of the ictal state. Investigation of changes in brain activity during epileptic seizures resulting in complete loss of consciousness (e.g., absence and generalized tonic-clonic seizures) or specific alterations of the normal conscious state (e.g., focal seizures of temporal lobe origin) is likely to shed light on the so far elusive neural correlates of consciousness. In turn, in-depth understanding of the functional aspects of the neural networks sustaining consciousness can lead to the development of better strategies to improve seizure severity and health-related quality of life in patients with epilepsy.

Keywords Arousal • Awareness • Consciousness • Contents • Default Mode Network • Epilepsy • Experiences • Level • Responsiveness • Seizures

---

A.E. Cavanna, MD, PhD, FRCP
Michael Trimble Neuropsychiatry Research Group, BSMHFT and University of Birmingham, Birmingham, UK

School of Life and Health Sciences, Aston University, Birmingham, UK

Sobell Department of Motor Neuroscience and Movement Disorders, UCL and Institute of Neurology, London, UK
e-mail: Andrea.Cavanna@bsmhft.nhs.uk

M. Mula (ed.), *Neuropsychiatric Symptoms of Epilepsy*, Neuropsychiatric Symptoms of Neurological Disease, DOI 10.1007/978-3-319-22159-5_10

No better neurological work can be done than the precise investigation of epileptic paroxysms. John Hughlings-Jackson, 1889 [1]

The good physician is concerned not only with turbulent brain waves but with disturbed emotions. William G. Lennox and Charles H. Markham, 1953 [2]

Defining Consciousness in Epilepsy

From Philosophy of Mind to Consciousness Studies

The turn of the new millennium marked the beginning of a new era characterized by mushrooming of neuroscientific publications on consciousness, a concept traditionally confined to philosophical and psychological enquiry [3]. In 2004, the authors of the chapter "The neural correlates of consciousness" in the second edition of the classical textbook *Human brain function* explicitly stated that "In the first edition of this book there was a final chapter on the future of imaging in which use of the word consciousness was strictly avoided until very last sentence. Now that we have moved into a new millennium it has no longer been so easy to resist the Zeitgeist. That single sentence has become a whole chapter" [4]. Unprecedented advances in both clinical and experimental neurosciences led to heightened interest in the search for the neurobiological underpinnings ("neural correlates") of mental states including the qualitative features of subjective experience [5, 6]. These include the whole spectrum of feelings and emotions and are collectively referred to by philosophers of mind using the concept of "qualia," a Latin word which is the plural of quale and literally means "of what sort" or "of what kind." Sensory qualia are familiar to all of us when we enjoy the taste of chocolate (*that kind of* pleasure) or experience shivers through the spine when listening to Puccini's opera (*that kind of* emotion). American philosopher Daniel Dennett encapsulated the essence of qualia in his famous 1988 article titled "Quining Qualia": "an unfamiliar term for something that could not be more familiar to each of us: the ways things seem to us" [7].

The very concept of qualia is still at the center of a heated philosophical debate on the mind-body problem, as their very existence and nature can pose a serious challenge to reductionist or physicalist views of consciousness. Moreover, qualia were traditionally considered accessible only through introspection ("first person perspective"), and therefore resistant to scientific investigation in terms of objective approaches ("third person perspective"). Despite conceptual difficulties and theoretical uncertainties, the last few years have seen neuroscientists entering the arena of consciousness studies to offer a key contribution towards the search for the neurobiological mechanisms underlying qualia [8–10].

Level and Contents of Consciousness in Neuropsychiatry

Qualia are not the only feature of our consciousness. In medical textbooks, consciousness is typically mentioned in the context of conditions characterized by its suppression, ranging from physiological states (sleep-wake cycle) to chronic brain pathologies (coma and vegetative state) and pharmacologically induced anesthesia (e.g., propofol-induced unconsciousness) [11]. Subjects in these conditions share the characteristic of being unresponsive, suggesting impairment in a core aspect of consciousness. While qualia refer to subjective experiences (contents of consciousness), unresponsiveness is an objective measure of arousal (level of consciousness). The identification of two different components of consciousness suggested a multidimensional approach to the scientific study of consciousness, through the development of a bidimensional model (level versus contents) for the assessment of conscious states [5, 11]. Of note, the two components of consciousness show a degree of correlation (when we experience the world [contents], we usually are in a responsive state [level]). This can be better understood by comparing consciousness to television: when the television is switched on (level), different programs can be viewed (contents); on the other hand when the television is off, it is not possible to watch any program (Fig. 10.1). There are however a few instances in which subjects can experience vivid contents of consciousness despite being unresponsive (absent level of consciousness), as in the rapid eye movement (REM) sleep stage. The bidimensional model of consciousness acknowledges the different properties (and underlying neurobiological mechanisms) of the level and contents of consciousness [5].

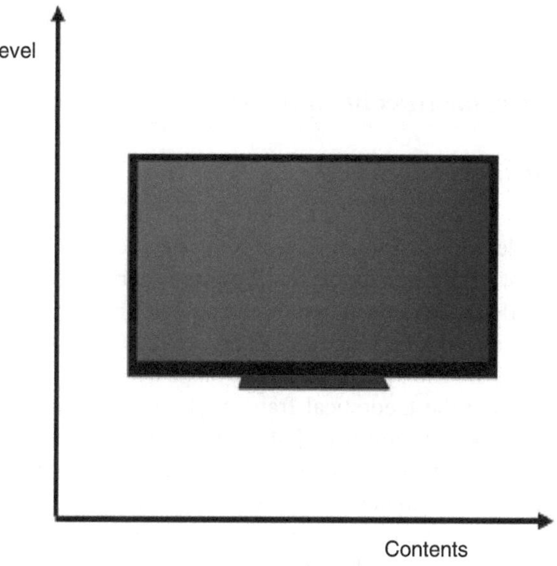

Fig. 10.1 Bidimensional model of consciousness and analogy with television: level of arousal (on-off) versus contents of awareness (television programs)

Over the last few years, the level-versus-contents bidimensional model has been successfully used to assess conscious states in chronic pathologies of consciousness and has been proposed and validated for use in transient pathologies of consciousness such as epilepsy [12–14]. Patients with epilepsy can present with different degrees of alterations in both the level and contents of consciousness, depending on the differential involvement of brain structures. This has crucial implications in terms of diagnosis, treatment, and prognosis for patients who suffer from epileptic seizures which affect consciousness. The clinical relevance of understanding the mechanisms responsible for the specific alterations of consciousness induced by different epileptic seizures cannot be underestimated, and it is not surprising that the international epilepsy community has recently developed a particular interest in consciousness studies. Over the last few years, two of the most important journals in the field of clinical neuropsychiatry devoted an entire special issue to the relationship between epilepsy and consciousness, with articles focusing on all relevant aspects of this relationship [15, 16]. In a sense, epilepsy is an open window on the neural correlates of consciousness, which in turn have the potential to inform clinical scientists about the most promising avenues to develop effective treatments to prevent epilepsy-induced alterations of consciousness and improve health-related quality of life of patients [17, 18]. The following section will review current strategies for the assessment of ictal conscious states in patients with epilepsy. This will be followed by an overview of the current understanding of the different alterations of consciousness in generalized seizures (complete black-out caused by absence and generalized tonic-clonic seizures) and focal seizures (especially experiential phenomena or epileptic qualia caused by temporal lobe seizures), along with their underlying brain mechanisms.

Assessing Consciousness in Epilepsy

Ictal Consciousness Inventory

Over the last decade a few instruments have been specifically developed to assist the clinical assessment of alterations of consciousness during epileptic seizures [19, 20]. These tools offer invaluable help to both clinicians and researchers who aim to systematically assess the ictal conscious state across different seizure types. The Ictal Consciousness Inventory (ICI) was developed in 2008 as the first of these instruments, following the theoretical framework of the bidimensional model for the evaluation of ictal consciousness [14]. This scale consists of 20 items which evaluate both arousal/responsiveness (level of consciousness: items 1–10) and qualia/subjective experiences (contents of consciousness: items 11–20) during epileptic seizures. The items focusing on the level of consciousness directly assess self-consciousness, general awareness of time, place and other people's presence, understanding of other people's words, verbal and nonverbal responsiveness, gaze control, forced attention, and voluntary action initiation. The items focusing on the contents of consciousness quantify the "vividness" of a range of subjective experiences: dreamy states, symptoms of derealization (with both temporal and spatial features), feeling of the presence of an absent person, illusions, hallucinations, déjà vu/vécu, unpleasant and pleasant ictal emotions. The results of the ICI development and validation study confirmed that the ICI is an accurate psychometric instrument for collecting retrospective accounts of the clinical phenomenology of seizure-induced alterations of consciousness, capturing the complexity of ictal experiential phenomena. Limitations are mainly related to the retrospective nature of self-report accounts of past seizures, which can be particularly relevant for seizures resulting in ictal and/or post-ictal amnesia.

Consciousness Seizure Scale

The Consciousness Seizure Scale (CSS) was developed in a 2009 study exploring the mechanisms underlying loss of consciousness during epileptic seizures arising from the temporal lobe [21]. This instrument assesses ictal consciousness across six different features (eight clinician-rated items): unresponsiveness (assessed in two ways), visual attention, consciousness of the seizure, adapted behavior, amnesia (assessed in two ways), global appreciation of consciousness by an experienced physician. The CSS was proposed as a valid tool for the assessment of the degree of consciousness impairment in temporal lobe seizures, based on the significant correlation between this index and objective measures of neural signal synchronization concomitant to ictal alterations of consciousness. The main limitation of this instrument is the methodology of its development, which was not based on standardized prospective testing, thus prompting the need for further research to fully evaluate its psychometric properties.

Responsiveness in Epilepsy Scale

The Responsiveness in Epilepsy Scale (RES) is the most recent addition to the instruments specifically developed for the assessment of consciousness in epilepsy [22]. This scale was modified from the JFK Coma Recovery Scale-Revised [23], with modifications which allow ictal responsiveness testing within the typical short timeframe of seizures in patients undergoing video-electroencephalography. The RES was developed in two multi-level versions: RES-I and RES-II. The RES-I consists of 12 items across three levels. The eight items in Level 1 include orientation questions, and other verbal questions and commands to test receptive and expressive language, visual processing, and motor praxis. The two items in Level 2 involve sensorimotor responses and visual tracking. Finally, the two items in Level 3 assess responses to visual threats and noxious tactile stimulation. The RES-I also includes additional tests for memory recall at seizures onset and post-ictal motor performance. Level 2 is scored only if patients score above a set threshold in Level 1, and Level 3 is scored dependent on patients' scores in Level 2. The results of the RES-I validation study showed that this scale yields an accurate measurement of consciousness impairment across different seizure types, with the possible limitations of the relatively small sample size and the requirement for skilled personnel for its administration. The RES-II scale is a more recent refinement of the RES-I, with a similar structure to the RES-I and the reduction of the number of items to ten plus the possibility to score an additional item assessing responsiveness to a painful stimulus, in case patients failed to respond to any of the other ten items [24]. Advantages of the RES-II include the improved user-friendliness and the shorter administration time compared to the RES-I, while maintaining the reliability of its predecessor.

Alterations of Consciousness in Epilepsy

Generalized Seizures

Generalized seizures (both convulsive seizures, such as generalized tonic-clonic seizures, and absence seizures) are the most common causes of epilepsy-induced loss of consciousness, as they are associated with disruption in both the level and the contents of consciousness [25–29]. The dramatic clinical phenomenology of generalized tonic-clonic seizures is characterized by rigid stiffening of the limbs (tonic phase), followed by violent bilateral spasms (clonic phase), which usually last for up to 2 min, during which consciousness is completely abolished. The ictal phase is typically followed by profound lethargy and confusion (i.e., decreased level of consciousness) persisting for a few hours. Most patients report complete amnesia for this type of seizures.

Ictal electroencephalographic recordings show widespread, low-voltage, fast or polyspike activity during the tonic phase, followed by polyspike-wave activity in the clonic phase, and generalized suppression in the post-ictal phase. Brain imaging during generalized tonic-clonic seizures is notoriously challenging because of obvious safety risks to the patients, as well as technical difficulties related to the presence of abundant muscle artifacts caused by the convulsions. Neuroimaging using single-photon emission computerized tomography (SPECT) has the advantage of allowing injection of radiotracers during the ictal phase: although imaging is performed over 45 min after administration, on medically stable patients, it is possible to map cerebral blood flow during the seizure as the radiotracers are taken up quickly by the brain after injection and do not redistribute [30]. SPECT imaging findings from both focal seizures with secondary generalization and tonic-clonic seizures induced by electroconvulsive therapy have shown substantial blood-flow changes, with bilateral increases in blood flow seen in the lateral fronto-parietal cortex, medial parietal cortex, thalamus, and upper brainstem, while ictal decreases have been observed in the medial frontal cortex and anterior cingulate cortex [25–29, 31]. These findings have generally been supported by positron emission tomography (PET) blood flow imaging studies [32].

During absence seizures patients experience complete loss of consciousness in terms of both level and contents. The behavioral picture features staring and unresponsiveness, plus occasionally eyelid fluttering or mild myoclonic spasms. The duration is short (a few seconds), with abrupt onset and termination, and patients tend to be amnestic for their transient "loss of contact" with the external environment [33]. This type of generalized seizures is most commonly seen in childhood absence epilepsy and its electroencephalographic correlate is characterized by generalized spike-wave discharges of 3–4 Hz lasting for up to 10 s, first described by Gibbs in 1935 [34].

High-resolution functional neuroimaging in absence seizures has been achieved in recent years with functional magnetic resonance imaging (fMRI), and most studies with simultaneous electroencephalography and fMRI during absence seizures have shown changes in brain activity in association with absence seizure-induced loss of consciousness. These studies have revealed increased activity in the thalamus and decreased activity in the medial frontal cortex, medial parietal cortex, anterior cingulate cortex, posterior cingulate cortex and lateral parietal cortex, as well as a mixture of increased and decreased activity in the lateral frontal cortex [25–29, 35, 36]. Interestingly, by using time-course analysis it has been shown that fMRI increases can begin in the medial frontal and parietal cortex up to 10 s before the electroencephalographic onset of absence seizures, and can be followed by complex changes in both cortical and subcortical activity, which cannot be measured by the standard hemodynamic-response function used for conventional fMRI analysis [37]. A summary of neurophysiological and neuroimaging findings during generalized seizures is presented in Table 10.1.

Focal Seizures

Temporal lobe epilepsy has long been associated with qualitative changes in the contents of the ictal conscious state, encompassing a wide range of experiential phenomena [38]. At phenomenological level, the assessment of these subjective symptoms is crucial for the diagnosis and classification of focal epileptic seizures, as the distinction between complex and simple seizures depends on whether the

Table 10.1 Summary of neurophysiological and neuroimaging findings during generalized seizures

Seizure type	Electrophysiological findings	Neuroimaging findings
Absence seizures	Widespread bilateral 3–4 Hz spike-wake discharges	Increased activity in the thalamus and midline cortical structures, followed by widespread decreases in the fronto-parietal association cortices
Generalized tonic-clonic seizures	Widespread high frequency polyspike discharges followed by rhythmic polyspike-wave discharges	Increased activity in the thalamus and fronto-parietal association cortices

level of consciousness is compromised ("complex partial seizures" in the traditional classification) or not ("complex partial seizures" in the traditional classification) [18, 39]. At neurobiological level, the investigation of the neurophysiological and neuroimaging correlates of ictal experiential phenomena induced by temporal lobe seizures has started to shed light on the brain mechanism underpinning pathophysiological states of altered contents of consciousness or "epileptic qualia" [12, 40, 41]. The most common alterations of the contents of consciousness during temporal lobe seizures encompass perceptual, dysmnesic, affective, and cognitive phenomena [42–45]. Reported perceptual phenomena include illusions and distortion of body image, as well as structured hallucinations. These later tend to present with the characteristic features of organic hallucinations (complex visual scenes, stereotyped, of short duration, and with preserved insight) [46]. See Case **10.1**.

Case 10.1: An Illustrative Case

A.B. was a 17-year-old male patient with a 1-year history of recurrent episodes characterized by visual hallucinations. He was originally referred to the Psychiatry Clinic for possible onset of schizophrenia and started on antipsychotic medications, without substantial benefits. His past medical history was unremarkable and there was no significant family history for psychiatric or neurological conditions. Routine tests including toxicological screening were unremarkable. On in-depth psychiatric assessment, it became clear that he had good insight into the nature of his hallucinatory experiences, which he described as vivid visual experiences of a hooded figure crossing his visual fields from left to right in slow motion for the duration of a couple of minutes (Fig. 10.2). He reported emotional distress associated with these experiences, although there was no communication between the hooded figure and him. These hallucinations were highly stereotyped and their frequency was weekly, sometimes leaving A.B. in a state of mild confusion.

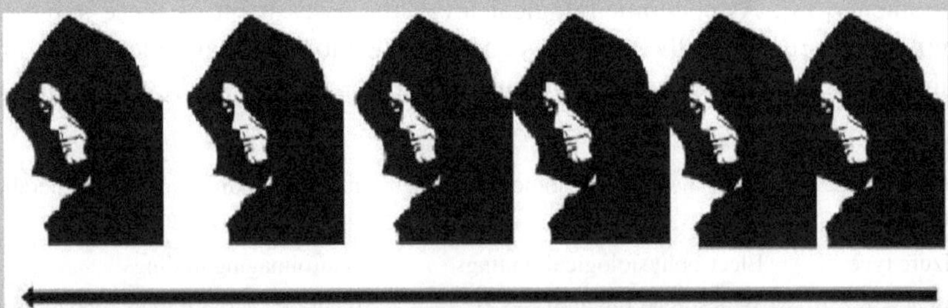

Fig. 10.2 Visual hallucination displayed by patient A.B. as a result of right temporal lobe epilepsy

An organic basis for these episodic symptoms was suspected and A.B. was referred to the Neuropsychiatry Clinic for a specialist assessment. A routine

EEG was unremarkable, but an ambulatory EEG was able to capture a typical clinical episode, showing focal epileptiform activity originating from the left temporal lobe. The diagnosis of temporal lobe epilepsy was explained to A.B. and a management plan consisting of medication review was agreed. The antipsychotic medication was therefore replaced with antiepileptic treatment (Carbamazepine monotherapy), to which the patient responded favorably with seizure remission.

Memory flashbacks and illusions of memory (déjà vu, déjà vécu, jamais vu, jamais vécu experiences, paramnesias, or false recollections) are the main types of dysmnesic ictal symptoms. Affective phenomena are more frequently sudden unexplained unpleasant emotions (e.g., fear, terror, anxiety, guilt, sadness, depression, anger, embarrassment), although pleasant or positive emotions have also been documented (exhilaration, mirth, blissful happiness, ecstasy, sexual excitement) [47, 48]. Ictal dissociative symptoms include transient derealization (alteration in one's sense of external reality) and depersonalization (alteration in one's sense of self), plus other forms of alteration in an individual's sense of personal reality and experience of self, such as autoscopy including out-of-body experiences and seeing one's double [49]. Finally, forced thinking and altered speed of thoughts are cognitive phenomena which are likely to be underreported and/or unrecognized [50]. In the clinical assessment of altered conscious states induced by focal seizures it is important to pay attention to a number of seizure-related factors: for example, forced attention and ictal dysphasia can affect the assessment of ictal responsiveness, whereas ictal and post-ictal amnesia can affect the retrospective recall of experiential phenomena [39, 50].

Scalp electroencephalographic recordings during temporal lobe seizures associated to altered contents of consciousness are characterized by epileptiform discharges over the temporal lobe, and the relationship between temporo-limbic activity and experiential phenomena has been known since Wilder Penfield's pioneering work in epilepsy surgery. Penfield's experiments marked a landmark in consciousness studies as they showed that similar subjective experiences can be elicited by electrical stimulation of temporal lobe structures [51].

An altered level of consciousness, assessed as decreased arousal and responsiveness, is the defining feature of complex partial seizures, which have been recently renamed as "focal seizures with impairment of consciousness" by a report from the International League Against Epilepsy [52]. The behavioral changes associated with complex partial seizures include arrest of voluntary behavior and onset of staring, often accompanied by automatisms, such as lip smacking, chewing, or repetitive semi-purposeful limb movements (e.g., fiddling with clothes), typically lasting for a couple of minutes. Decreased responsiveness in complex partial seizures can persist for several minutes into the post-ictal period, and patients are usually amnestic to events around the time of the seizure [53].

The development of specific instruments to assess the multifaceted spectrum of ictal experiences in complex partial seizures has recently improved our interpretation of the associated functional brain changes [54, 55]. Over the last few years, consistent findings across neurophysiological and neuroimaging studies have shown that alterations of consciousness during temporal lobe seizures correlate with large-amplitude slow EEG activity and neuroimaging signal decreases in fronto-parietal association networks [56]. These observations suggest an important role for extra-temporal structures in determining the nature and extent of ictal impairment of the level of consciousness in complex partial seizures of temporal origin ("network inhibition hypothesis") [57].

Temporal seizures are characterized by neuronal discharges that originate in the temporal lobe and propagate along networks interconnecting both cortical and subcortical regions. Alterations of consciousness caused by temporal love seizures can also be understood within the theoretical framework of the "global workspace" theory of consciousness [58, 59]. According to this model, information processing accesses consciousness through the synchronized activity of neuronal modules linked to widespread brain networks. Thalamo-cortical functional connectivity plays a crucial role in this dynamic system, as the deactivation of thalamic structures, along with fronto-parietal cortices, can impair conscious processing of information by preventing it from entering the global workspace [58, 59].

The Neural Correlates of Consciousness in Epilepsy

The reviewed data show that, although generalized (generalized tonic-clonic and absence seizures) and complex partial seizures differ in several ways, they all converge on the same set of anatomical structures to produce dysfunction in specialized cortical-subcortical network which has recently been termed the "consciousness system" [29, 60–62]. The cortical components of the consciousness system include the medial frontal, anterior cingulate, posterior cingulate, and medial parietal (precuneus and retrosplenial) cortices on the medial surface, and the lateral frontal, orbitofrontal, and lateral temporoparietal association cortices on the lateral surface, with a possible contribution from portions of the insula. The subcortical components are the basal forebrain, hypothalamus, thalamus, and upper-brainstem activating systems, plus possibly portions of the basal ganglia, cerebellum, and amygdala. Findings from neurophysiological and neuroimaging studies in epilepsy have consistently shown that involvement of the main components of the consciousness system result in alterations in the level of consciousness, whereas temporo-limbic structures appear to be selectively involved in the contents of consciousness [25–29]. Interestingly, there is a considerable overlap between the consciousness system and the "default mode network," a highly integrated network that is thought to sustain the level of consciousness and shows selective deactivations in both chronic and transient loss of consciousness [63–65]. A pivotal role in coordinating patterns of activation and deactivation within the default mode network seems to be played by midline structures such as the posteromedial parietal cortex [66–69].

These novel insights into the brain mechanisms that underlie alterations of consciousness during epileptic seizures have important implications for clinical practice in terms of diagnosis and management. The exact terminology for the description of ictal consciousness is regularly under review by the International League Against Epilepsy, in order to achieve a general consensus [70]. Arguably, the assessment of consciousness carries information which is potentially useful for the differential diagnosis of seizure types across epilepsy and non-epileptic attack disorder [71–75]. Moreover, the effects of transiently losing the ability to experience or respond have a huge impact on the health-related quality of life of patients with epileptic ranging from emotional distress to practical limitations such as driving [76, 77]. The importance of continuing to carry out research in order to fully elucidate the mechanisms whereby epileptic seizures can disrupt consciousness cannot be underestimated. A better understanding of the brain mechanisms underlying consciousness is relevant to both neuroscientists and epileptologists, as it could lead to improved treatment strategies to prevent impairment of consciousness and improve the well-being of patients with epilepsy [78–80].

References

1. Hughlings-Jackson J. On a particular variety of epilepsy ('intellectual aura'), one case with symptoms of organic brain disease. Brain. 1889;11:179–207.
2. Lennox WG, Markham CH. The socio-psychological treatment of epilepsy. J Am Med Assoc. 1953;152:1690–4.
3. Cavanna AE, Nani A. Consciousness: theories in neuroscience and philosophy of mind. Berlin: Springer; 2014.
4. Portas C, Maquet P, Rees G, Blakemore S, Frith C. The neural correlates of consciousness. In: Frackowiak RSJ, editor. Human brain function. 2nd ed. London: Academic Press; 2004. p. 269–302.
5. Cavanna AE, Shah S, Eddy CM, Williams A, Rickards H. Consciousness: a neurological perspective. Behav Neurol. 2011;24:107–16.
6. Cavanna AE, Seri S, Nani A. Consciousness and neuroscience. In: Cavanna AE, Nani A, Blumenfeld H, Laureys S, editors. Neuroimaging of consciousness. Berlin: Springer; 2013. p. 3–21.
7. Dennett DC. Quining qualia. In: Marcel AJ, Bisiach E, editors. Consciousness in contemporary science. Oxford: Oxford University Press; 1988. p. 44–77.
8. Searle JR. How to study consciousness scientifically. Philos Trans R Soc Lond B Biol Sci. 1998;353:1935–42.
9. Orpwood R. Neurobiological mechanisms underlying qualia. J Integr Neurosci. 2007;6:523–40.
10. Loorits K. Structural qualia: a solution to the hard problem of consciousness. Front Psychol. 2014;5:237.
11. Laureys S, Owen AM, Schiff ND. Brain function in coma, vegetative state, and related disorders. Lancet Neurol. 2004;3:537–46.
12. Monaco F, Mula M, Cavanna AE. Consciousness, epilepsy and emotional qualia. Epilepsy Behav. 2005;7:150–60.
13. Cavanna AE. Seizures and consciousness. In: Schachter SC, Holmes G, Kasteleijn-Nolst Trenite D, editors. Behavioral aspects of epilepsy: principles and practice. New York: Demos; 2008. p. 99–104.

14. Cavanna AE, Mula M, Servo S, Strigaro G, Tota G, Barbagli D, Collimedaglia L, Viana M, Cantello R, Monaco F. Measuring the level and contents of consciousness during epileptic seizures: the Ictal Consciousness Inventory. Epilepsy Behav. 2008;13:184–8.
15. Cavanna AE. Epilepsy and disorders of consciousness. Behav Neurol. 2011;24:1.
16. Cavanna AE. Epilepsy as a pathology of consciousness. Epilepsy Behav. 2014;30:1.
17. Monaco F, Mula M, Cavanna AE. The neurophilosophy of epileptic experiences. Acta Neuropsychiatr. 2011;23:184–7.
18. Cavanna AE, Ali F. Epilepsy: the quintessential pathology of consciousness. Behav Neurol. 2011;24:3–10.
19. Johanson M, Valli K, Revonsuo A. How to assess ictal consciousness? Behav Neurol. 2011;24:11–20.
20. Nani A, Cavanna AE. The quantitative measurement of consciousness during epileptic seizures. Epilepsy Behav. 2014;30:2–5.
21. Arthuis M, Valton L, Régis J, Chauvel P, Wendling F, Naccache L, et al. Impaired consciousness during temporal lobe seizures is related to increased long-distance cortical–subcortical synchronization. Brain. 2009;132:2091–101.
22. Yang L, Shklyar I, Lee HW, Ezeani CC, Anaya J, Balakirsky S, et al. Impaired consciousness in epilepsy investigated by a prospective responsiveness in epilepsy scale (RES). Epilepsia. 2012;53:437–47.
23. Giacino JT, Kalmar K, Whyte J. The JFK coma recovery scale revised: measurement characteristics and diagnostic utility. Arch Phys Med Rehabil. 2004;85:2020–9.
24. Bauerschmidt A, Koshkelashvili N, Ezeani CC, Yoo JY, Zhang Y, Manganas LN, et al. Prospective assessment of ictal behavior using the revised Responsiveness in Epilepsy Scale (RES-II). Epilepsy Behav. 2013;26:25–8.
25. Cavanna AE, Monaco F. Brain mechanisms of altered conscious states during epileptic seizures. Nat Rev Neurol. 2009;5:267–76.
26. Cavanna AE, Bagshaw AP, McCorry D. The neural correlates of altered consciousness during epileptic seizures. Discov Med. 2009;8:31–6.
27. Cavanna AE, Ali F. Brain mechanisms of impaired consciousness in epilepsy. In: Trimble MR, Schmitz B, editors. The neuropsychiatry of epilepsy. Cambridge: Cambridge University Press; 2011. p. 209–20.
28. Mann JP, Cavanna AE. What does epilepsy tell us about the neural correlates of consciousness? J Neuropsychiatry Clin Neurosci. 2011;23:375–83.
29. Blumenfeld H. Impaired consciousness in epilepsy. Lancet Neurol. 2012;11:814–26.
30. Kim SH, Zubal IG, Blumenfeld H. Epilepsy localization by ictal and interictal SPECT. In: Van Heertum RL, Tikofsky RS, Ichise M, editors. Functional cerebral SPECT and PET imaging. Philadelphia: Lippincott Williams & Wilkins; 2009. p. 131–48.
31. Paige L, Cavanna AE. Brain imaging and alterations of consciousness in epilepsy: generalized tonic-clonic seizures. In: Cavanna AE, Nani A, Blumenfeld H, Laureys S, editors. The neuroimaging of consciousness. Berlin: Springer; 2013. p. 81–97.
32. Takano H, Motohashi N, Uema T, Ogawa K, Ohnishi T, Nishikawa M, et al. Changes in regional cerebral blood flow during acute electroconvulsive therapy in patients with depression: positron emission tomographic study. Br J Psychiatry. 2007;190:63–8.
33. Bayne T. The presence of consciousness in absence seizures. Behav Neurol. 2011;24:47–53.
34. Gibbs FA, Davis H, Lennox WG. The EEG in epilepsy and in conditions of impaired consciousness. Arch Neurol Psychiatry. 1935;34:1134–48.
35. Seri S, Brazzo D, Thai NJ, Cerquiglini A. Brain mechanisms of altered consciousness in generalised seizures. Behav Neurol. 2011;24:43–6.
36. Bagshaw AP, Rollings D, Khalsa S, Cavanna AE. Multimodal neuroimaging investigations of alterations to consciousness: the relationship between absence epilepsy and sleep. Epilepsy Behav. 2014;30:33–7.
37. Bai X, Vestal M, Berman R, Negishi M, Spann M, Vega C, et al. Dynamic time course of typical childhood absence seizures: EEG, behavior, and functional magnetic resonance imaging. J Neurosci. 2010;30:5884–93.

38. Picard F, Craig AD. Ecstatic epileptic seizures: a potential window on the neural basis for human self-awareness. Epilepsy Behav. 2009;16:539–46.
39. Ali F, Rickards H, Cavanna AE. The assessment of consciousness during partial seizures. Epilepsy Behav. 2012;23:98–102.
40. Alvarez-Silva S, Alvarez-Rodriguez J, Cavanna AE. Epileptic aura and qualitative alterations of consciousness in focal seizures: a neuropsychiatric approach. Epilepsy Behav. 2012;23:512–3.
41. Hanoğlu L, Özkara C, Yalçiner B, Nani A, Cavanna AE. Epileptic qualia and self-awareness: a third dimension for consciousness. Epilepsy Behav. 2014;30:62–5.
42. Johanson M, Valli K, Revonsuo A, Wedlund JE. Content analysis of subjective experiences in partial epileptic seizures. Epilepsy Behav. 2008;12:170–82.
43. Johanson M, Valli K, Revonsuo A, Chaplin JE, Wedlund JE. Alterations in the contents of consciousness in partial epileptic seizures. Epilepsy Behav. 2008;13:366–71.
44. McCorry DJP, Cavanna AE. New thoughts on first seizure. Clin Med. 2010;4:395–8.
45. Mula M, Monaco F. Ictal and peri-ictal psychopathology. Behav Neurol. 2011;24:21–5.
46. Heydrich L, Marillier G, Evans N, Blanke O, Seeck M. Lateralising value of experiential hallucinations in temporal lobe epilepsy. J Neurol Neurosurg Psychiatry. 2015 (in press).
47. Picard F, Kurth F. Ictal alterations of consciousness during ecstatic seizures. Epilepsy Behav. 2014;30:58–61.
48. McCrae N, Whitley R. Exaltation in temporal lobe epilepsy: neuropsychiatric symptom or portal to the divine? J Med Humanit. 2014;35:241–55.
49. Medford N. Dissociative symptoms and epilepsy. Epilepsy Behav. 2014;30:10–3.
50. Johanson M, Revonsuo A, Chaplin J, Wedlund JE. Level and contents of consciousness in connection with partial epileptic seizures. Epilepsy Behav. 2003;4:279–85.
51. Penfield W, Rasmussen T. The cerebral cortex of man. New York: Macmillan; 1950.
52. Berg AT, Berkovic SF, Brodie MJ, Buchhalter J, Cross JH, van Emde Boas W, et al. Revised terminology and concepts for organization of seizures and epilepsies: report of the ILAE Commission on Classification and Terminology, 2005–2009. Epilepsia. 2010;51: 676–85.
53. Mula M. Epilepsy-induced behavioral changes during the ictal phase. Epilepsy Behav. 2014;30:14–6.
54. Cavanna AE, Rickards H, Ali F. What makes a simple partial seizure complex? Epilepsy Behav. 2011;22:651–8.
55. Bagshaw AP, Cavanna AE. Brain mechanisms of altered consciousness in focal seizures. Behav Neurol. 2011;24:35–41.
56. Englot DJ, Yang L, Hamid H, Danielson N, Bai X, Marfeo A, et al. Impaired consciousness in temporal lobe seizures: role of cortical slow activity. Brain. 2010;133:3764–77.
57. Englot DJ, Blumenfeld H. Consciousness and epilepsy: why are complex partial seizures complex? Prog Brain Res. 2009;177:147–70.
58. Bartolomei F, Naccache L. The global workspace (GW) theory of consciousness and epilepsy. Behav Neurol. 2011;24:67–74.
59. Bartolomei F, McGonigal A, Naccache L. Alteration of consciousness in focal epilepsy: the global workspace alteration theory. Epilepsy Behav. 2014;30:17–23.
60. Cavanna AE, Nani A, Blumenfeld H, Laureys S. Neuroimaging of consciousness. Berlin: Springer; 2013.
61. Foley E, Cerquiglini A, Cavanna A, Nakubulwa MA, Furlong PL, Witton C, Seri S. Magnetoencephalography in the study of epilepsy and consciousness. Epilepsy Behav. 2014;30:38–42.
62. Blumenfeld H. Epilepsy and the consciousness system: transient vegetative state? Neurol Clin. 2011;29:801–23.
63. Danielson NB, Guo JN, Blumenfeld H. The default mode network and altered consciousness in epilepsy. Behav Neurol. 2011;24:55–65.
64. Bagshaw AP, Cavanna AE. Resting state networks in paroxysmal disorders of consciousness. Epilepsy Behav. 2013;26:290–4.

65. Di Perri C, Stender J, Laureys S, Gosseries O. Functional neuroanatomy of disorders of consciousness. Epilepsy Behav. 2014;30:28–32.
66. Cavanna AE, Trimble MR. The precuneus: a review of its functional anatomy and behavioural correlates. Brain. 2006;129:564–83.
67. Cavanna AE. The precuneus and consciousness. CNS Spectr. 2007;12:545–52.
68. Cavanna AE, Bertero L, Cavanna S. The functional neuroimaging of the precuneus. Neurosci Imaging. 2008;2:161–75.
69. Cauda F, Geminiani G, D'Agata F, Sacco K, Duca S, Bagshaw AP, Cavanna AE. Functional connectivity of the posteromedial cortex. PLoS One. 2010;5:e13107.
70. Blumenfeld H, Jackson GD. Should consciousness be included in the classification of focal (partial) seizures? Epilepsia. 2013;54:1125–30.
71. Ali F, Rickards H, Bagary M, Greenhill L, McCorry D, Cavanna AE. Ictal consciousness in epilepsy and non-epileptic attack disorder. Epilepsy Behav. 2010;19:522–5.
72. Reuber M, Kurthen M. Consciousness in non-epileptic attack disorder. Behav Neurol. 2011;24:95–106.
73. Mitchell J, Ali F, Cavanna AE. Dissociative experiences and quality of life in patients with non-epileptic attack disorder. Epilepsy Behav. 2012;25:307–12.
74. Eddy CM, Cavanna AE. Video-electroencephalography investigation of ictal alterations of consciousness in epilepsy and non-epileptic attack disorder: practical considerations. Epilepsy Behav. 2014;30:24–7.
75. Roberts NA, Reuber M. Alterations of consciousness in psychogenic nonepileptic seizures: emotion, emotion regulation and dissociation. Epilepsy Behav. 2014;30:43–9.
76. Charidimou A, Selai C. The effect of alterations in consciousness on quality of life (QoL) in epilepsy: searching for evidence. Behav Neurol. 2011;24:83–93.
77. Chen WC, Chen EY, Gebre RZ, Johnson MR, Li N, Vitkovskiy P, Blumenfeld H. Epilepsy and driving: potential impact of transient impaired consciousness. Epilepsy Behav. 2014;30:50–7.
78. Koubeissi MZ, Bartolomei F, Beltagy A, Picard F. Electrical stimulation of a small brain area reversibly disrupts consciousness. Epilepsy Behav. 2014;37:32–5.
79. Blumenfeld H. A master switch for consciousness? Epilepsy Behav. 2014;37:234–5.
80. Gummadavelli A, Motelow JE, Smith N, Zhan Q, Schiff ND, Blumenfeld H. Thalamic stimulation to improve level of consciousness after seizures: evaluation of electrophysiology and behavior. Epilepsia. 2015;56(1):114–24.

Chapter 11
Emotion Recognition

Stefano Meletti

Abstract The recognition of emotional signals from all sensory modalities is a critical component of human social interactions. It is through the understanding of the affective states of others that we can guide our own behavioral responses. Notably, facial expression provides the greatest amount of emotional cues that are useful in recognizing emotions, such as joy, anger, and fear. The temporal lobe – and the amygdala in particular – plays a crucial role in processing the appropriate autonomic and behavioral responses to relevant emotional stimuli. Only in the past decade, however, the role played by the antero-medial temporal lobe region has been demonstrated in decoding the emotions, mental states, and beliefs of others. In the field of epilepsy, this knowledge has several clinical, as well as speculative, implications. Indeed, temporal lobe epilepsy (TLE) is the most common type of focal epilepsy. It is frequently characterized by lesions or gliosis/atrophy (hippocampal sclerosis) involving the medial temporal lobe region, and antero-medial temporal lobe resection is the standard treatment for drug-resistant medial TLE. Consequently, the investigation of emotional and social competence in TLE patients has been the focus of several studies. Such studies have extended the scope of neuropsychological evaluation in TLE beyond the traditional evaluation of memory, language, and executive functions.

Keywords Amygdala • Emotion Recognition • Emotional Prosody • Epilepsy • Facial Expression • fMRI • Temporal Lobe Epilepsy • Temporal Lobectomy • Social Cognition

S. Meletti, MD, PhD
Department of Biomedical, Metabolic, and Neural Science,
University of Modena e Reggio Emilia, Modena, Italy

Neurology Unit, NOCSAE Hospital – AUSL,
Via Giardini, 1355 – Nuovo Ospedale Civile, Modena, Italy
e-mail: stefano.meletti@unimore.it

M. Mula (ed.), *Neuropsychiatric Symptoms of Epilepsy*, Neuropsychiatric Symptoms of Neurological Disease, DOI 10.1007/978-3-319-22159-5_11

Introduction

Emotions are instinctive biological mechanisms that help us in the fundamental life tasks. Emotions are *provisions to act* in response to someone or something that is important to us. Probably, the entire, rich spectrum of human emotions has evolved from the behaviors of approach and avoidance, which represents the action tendencies of the simplest organisms.

Emotions have different independent purposes, albeit related. Emotions enrich our mental life; until the nineteenth century it was thought that this was the only function of the emotions, which were therefore considered as private experiences. Emotions facilitate social communication; Darwin first in 1872 (*The expression of emotions in man and animals*) understood that emotions have played an important role in evolution, have social functions and are adaptive [1]. Emotions affect our ability to act rationally; indeed emotions allow us to use the information obtained from autonomic bodily responses for planning decisions and complex actions [2]. Emotions, finally and probably the most important, help us to escape from dangerous situations and to approach potential sources of pleasure.

In this chapter, we will focus on one aspect of emotions, which is how emotions are perceived, recognized, and consciously categorized by people with epilepsy. In particular, researches of the last 20 years have provided a wealth of data on this topic, especially in patients affected by temporal lobe epilepsy (TLE).

TLE is a group of disorders that predominately involves dysregulation of amygdalo-hippocampal function caused by neuronal hyper-excitability [3, 4]. Medial TLE in particular, is perhaps the best-characterized electroclinical syndrome of all the epilepsies [5]. The inherent potential for the temporal lobe to be predisposed to focal seizures is based on the unique anatomic-functional networks that involve the amygdalo-hippocampal complex and entorhinal cortex. Beyond seizures, drug-resistant TLE is characterized by cognitive decline, especially involving memory functions, and by psychiatric co-morbidities [6–9]. Behavioral deficits in TLE have a great impact on the burden of the disease, and often contribute much more than seizures per se to deteriorate the patient's quality of life [10, 11].

The temporal lobe, and the *amygdala* in particular (Box 11.1), has been demonstrated to play a crucial role in the processing of the appropriate cognitive, autonomic, and behavioral responses to emotional relevant stimuli [12–17]. In particular, the role and importance of the antero-medial temporal lobe region in decoding emotions and in social cognition has been demonstrated by a number of lesion and functional imaging studies [18, 19].

Box 11.1: The Amygdala and the Evaluation of Emotional Stimuli
The amygdala plays a critical role in the neural system involved in the perception and coordination of emotions [13]. In particular, it is vital for the following aspects: (1) to learn the emotional significance of stimuli through

experience [20]; (2) to recognize the importance of this experience when it presents to us; (3) to coordinate the responses of the autonomic and endocrine systems in a appropriate manner; (4) to influence through emotion other cognitive functions, in particular perception, and decision making [2, 21].

The amygdala orchestrates the perception of emotional experience, both positive and negative. It does so by making us focused on emotionally significant stimuli. The amygdala also encodes both the valence of emotions (ranging from approach: positive; to avoidance: negative), as well as the degree of arousal induced by the stimulus [22, 23]. In reference to facial expressions, and in agreement with this view, the amygdala responds to a series of facial expressions, and not only to expressions of fear [24]. The amygdala plays a largely perceptual role in emotional response: it analyzes the incoming sensory information, classifies them, and then signals to other brain regions the appropriate response. In humans, the main consequence of damage to the amygdala is an inappropriate response to social ambiguous cues and the inability to effectively detect stimuli that are salient for the subject in relation to the context.

In the field of epilepsy, this knowledge has several clinical as well as speculative implications. Indeed, TLE is frequently characterized by lesions or gliosis/atrophy (hippocampal sclerosis) involving the medial temporal lobe region. Moreover, antero-medial temporal lobectomy (ATL) is the "standard" treatment for drug-resistant medial TLE [25]. Consequently, the investigation of emotional and social competence in TLE patients has been the focus of different studies [26–30].

After more than a decade of research it has been demonstrated that TLE patients show deficits in emotion recognition (ER) (either before or after ATL), especially for facial expressions, but also for different emotional stimuli such has prosody and music [31–34]. However, several questions are still open, in particular concerning the "specificity" of fear recognition impairment and the role of the right and left temporal lobes. These two questions are relevant and contribute to our understanding of how the brain processes emotions. Other important questions to be elucidated concern the impact of several disease variables on emotion recognition, as well as the effect of antiepileptic treatment, and temporal lobectomy procedures. These last issues are clearly relevant from a clinical perspective.

The aim of this chapter is therefore to describe the pattern of emotion recognition deficits in TLE through an appraisal of previous knowledge. In particular, we will consider whether differences in emotion recognition performance can be explained by disease-related factors, such as age of epilepsy onset, duration of disease, types and number of antiepileptic drugs, side of seizure focus, pre-/post-surgery status.

Recognition of Emotions in Chronic TLE

Before considering the features of emotions' recognition deficit in TLE we will briefly consider some methodological aspects concerning the patients' population that have been investigated, as well as the type of emotional stimuli used to assess emotion recognition.

Methodological Aspects

At present about 40 studies have been published since 2003 when we first investigated the recognition of *basic facial expression of emotions* (Box 11.2) in a group of chronic drug-resistant TLE patients [26].

Box 11.2: Basic Emotions and Darwin's Legacy
According to Darwin [1], along the continuum between approach and avoidance we can identify six universal components, which are reflected in facial expressions of emotion. These six components include two main primitive emotions: happiness (ranging from ecstasy to serenity) and fear (ranging from terror to anxiety). Between these two extremes, there are four other basic emotions: surprise, disgust, sadness, and anger. From these basic emotions can emerge, mingling, other emotions (such awe that comes from fear and trust) in which the role of learning and previous experience of the subject is crucial. Darwin assumed that facial expression is the primary social system of reporting human emotions and that consequently the expression of the face is crucial for social communication. Also, since all faces have a constant number of characteristics (two eyes, a nose, a mouth) sensory and motor aspects of emotional signals are universal and transcend culture. Furthermore, he stated that the ability to form facial expressions, as well as the ability to read facial expressions of another person, is innate.

Darwin's observation that the faces are the primary means of transmission of emotions has been extended a century later by the American psychologist Paul Ekman [35–37]. In a series of studies conducted at the end of the seventies. Ekman examined the recognition of facial expressions in a variety of cultures finding essentially the same six major facial expressions of emotions described by Darwin.

Neuroscientists have wondered: do the six universal emotions represent elementary biological systems, the "building blocks" of social cognition? Each discrete emotion is produced by a specific brain system or emotions have common components, overlapping, forming a continuum from positive to negative? Most scientists of emotions tend to agree that the six major emotions represent points along a continuum and that emotions have neural elements that are both distinctive than shared [38]. Moreover, most neuroscientists believed that emotions and their facial expressions are not entirely innate, but are partly determined by our previous experience with emotions and by our associations of certain emotions with certain contexts.

Since then, studies were drawn from a range of countries and ethnicities, including the United States, the United Kingdom, Italy, France, Canada, Japan, Spain, the Netherlands, India, Australia, and Switzerland. All of the studies compared patients' ER abilities with healthy volunteers matched for principal demographic variables (age, education, and sex). Some study included also a clinical control group (frontal or extra temporal lobe epilepsy, generalized epilepsy). The choice to compare medial TLE with other epilepsy patients is relevant to ascribe the specificity of the observed deficits to the medial temporal lobe region, and to exclude a generic effect of epilepsy per se. The rationale for using extra-TLE group is that people with extra-temporal lobe epilepsy live in a similar social and emotional environment with respect to people with TLE; they experiment epilepsy stigma and limitation in social and personal aspects due to epilepsy; they also are treated with antiepileptic drugs.

The majority of studies included at least one test of facial emotion recognition. The most commonly used stimuli were static black and white images from Ekman and Friesen series [35]. In some studies 60 pictures were used [39–42], with 10 stimuli for each basic emotion. In other studies 24–42 pictures, typically with four-five stimuli for each emotion, were used [12, 14, 15, 26–28, 33, 43–46]. Some authors excluded surprise, to avoid mistaking fear for surprise and vice versa [26–28, 33, 44]. In some studies, the recognition of emotion posed with different intensity was tested creating "morphed" facial stimuli from prototypical facial expressions [39, 42, 44, 47]. Other authors used tests composed by in-house made stimuli to test emotion recognition in children [48, 49]. Notably, few studies (only three to our knowledge) used dynamic stimuli realized by videos [43, 50, 51].

As far as emotional stimuli different from faces go, ten studies included tasks of emotion recognition in the auditory modality. The recognition of both short nonverbal vocal sounds (e.g., laughter and grows) as well as prosody from sentences with neutral meaning was evaluated [15, 33, 34, 47, 52, 53]. The emotions tested in most of studies were happiness, sadness, fear, anger, disgust, and surprise.

Finally, recently, three studies tested emotion recognition from music, using musical excerpts composed to induce fear, peacefulness, happiness, and sadness [31, 32, 54].

Emotion Recognition from Facial Expressions, Voices, Sounds, and Music

Considering facial expressions, data consistently demonstrates that patients with chronic TLE, as well as patients that underwent temporal lobectomy for curative drug-resistant TLE, were impaired in the recognition of facial expressions of others. Emotion recognition impairment was found across different stimuli: static pictures, "morphing" methods, and videos.

In Fig. 11.1 we reported for comparison the normalized performance from different patients' groups in nine studies: in all TLE patients were impaired with respect to the control population.

As far as the recognition of single emotional categories, fear recognition deficit was observed in each study.

In about 50 % of the studies fear recognition was selective, while in the remaining studies it was associated to deficits in the recognition of disgust, and sadness [28, 33, 42]. Impairment in anger recognition was reported only rarely, whereas deficit in the recognition of happiness was exceptionally observed. Notably, fear recognition deficits seem specific when comparing TLE/ATL patients with respect to extra-temporal lobe epilepsies. In this sense, fear recognition appears to be a good biological marker of chronic medial temporal lobe epilepsy.

Information about recognition of emotions via other sensory channels in TLE remains limited for firm conclusions to be drawn. However, at least for vocal

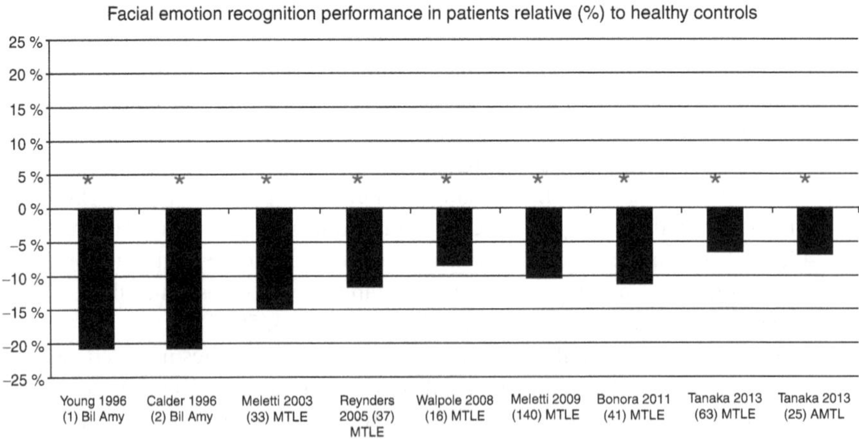

Fig. 11.1 Graphical representation of emotion recognition (composite performance across different emotions) in different studies relative to healthy controls scores. *Bars* represent the performance of TLE expressed as % of correct recognition relative to controls' norms. The *red asterisk* indicates $P<0.05$. Negative % indicates that TLE patients had a recognition score lower than controls. The x-axis reports the first authors of each study, the year of publication, and the sample of TLE patients

emotion recognition, the emerging picture is broadly convergent with the data obtained for facial expressions. The recognition of vocal fear was found consistently impaired, although recognition of vocal disgust and sadness were often defective [15, 29, 33, 34, 55]. Interestingly, the few studies that investigated emotion recognition from music suggest that TLE/ATL impairs also the emotional attributions to complex, and strongly emotional stimuli, as the music ones are [31, 32, 54]. In particular scary music recognition was consistently found to be impaired.

Importantly, patients with TLE appear to be impaired in categorizing negative emotional stimuli independently from the sensory channel. Indeed, TLE/ATL patients were impaired in both visual and auditory ER tasks. In particular, a fear recognition deficit, independently on the sensory channel, was reported in the studies where this issue has been specifically investigated [29, 32, 33].

Emotion Recognition and Brain Responses to Emotions in an Illustrative Case

The patient, LF, is a 38-years old right-handed male of average intelligence (full scale IQ, 100). He suffers from drug-resistant partial seizures since the age of 28 years. LF brain MRI demonstrated atrophy and gliosis of the left amygdala-hippocampal region, while noninvasive video-EEG monitoring showed an independent bilateral temporal lobe onset of seizures. LF was markedly impaired in memory functions, both verbal and visuo-spatial, as well as in attention and abstract reasoning. On the Benton test of unfamiliar face recognition, LF's performance was in the normal range [56]. Our test of emotion recognition used a forced-choice procedure in which the emotion conveyed by each of the faces was identified by selecting one label from a list (comprising a label for each emotion tested). The task used faces from the Ekman and Friesen series [35] and contained examples of five facial expressions (happiness, fear, sad, disgust, anger). Emotion labels were visible throughout testing.

Overall LF showed a very low accuracy in recognizing facial emotions (64 %) with respect to an age and education-matched healthy control group (96 % correct labeling). In particular, LF was significantly impaired in the recognition of sad, fear, and disgust from facial expression with accuracy scores that fall below three standard deviations from the controls' mean (Fig. 11.2) [57, 58].

The performance of LF appeared similar to the one of a clinical control group of patients with bilateral medial temporal lobe damage and epilepsy of comparable age and education [33]. These findings replicate previous results observed in patients with bilateral selective amygdala damage and in patients affected by drug-resistant bi-temporal lobe epilepsy [14, 59].

Interestingly, the patient's amygdala responses to facial expression were also tested during an intracranial EEG recording. Figure 11.2 shows the amygdala responses (intracranial event-related potentials, icERP) to facial expressions

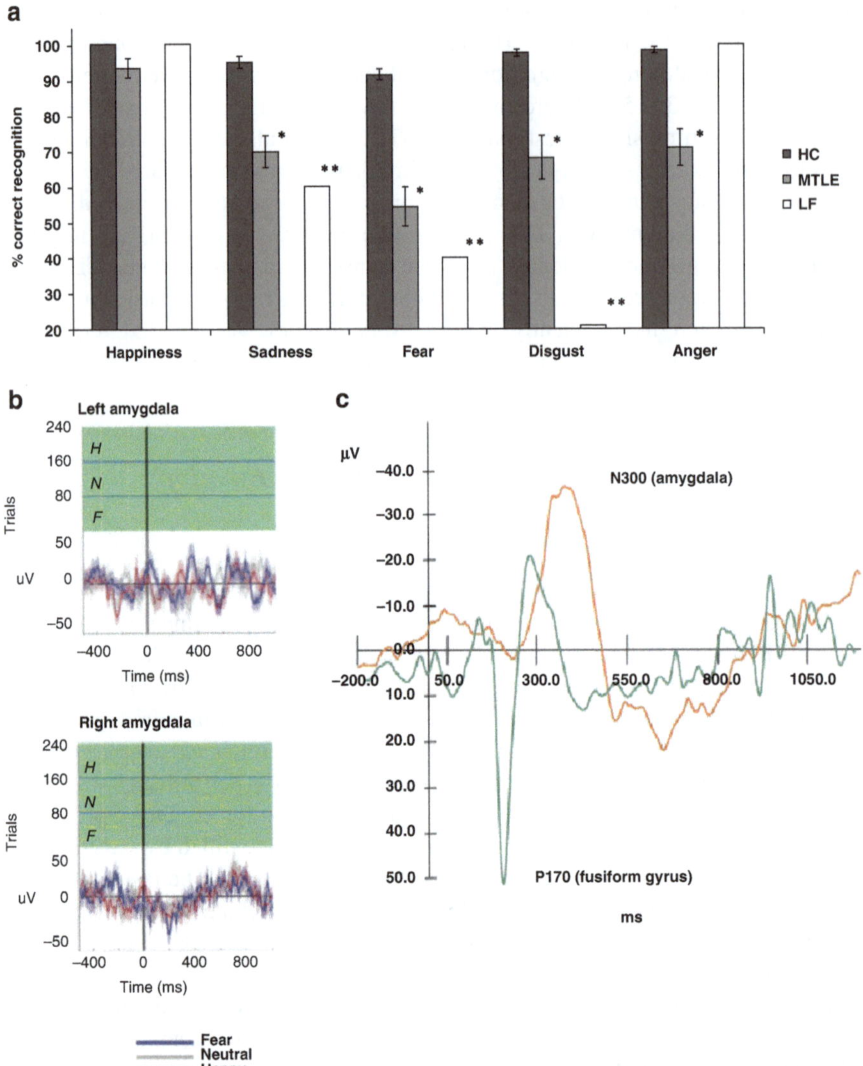

Fig. 11.2 (**a**) Accuracy of emotion recognition performance. Healthy controls (HC) ($n=12$) and the clinical control group with bilateral medial temporal lobe epilepsy and amygdala damage (MTLE) ($n=12$) were matched to LF for education and age. LF was severely impaired in the recognition of sadness (60 %), fear (40 %), and disgust (20 %) with respect to healthy subjects (**$p<0.001$). Facial emotion recognition of the MTLE group was significantly impaired compared to healthy controls for each emotion tested except happiness (*$p<0.001$). *Error bars* represent s.e.m. (**b**) IcERPs to facial expressions recorded from right and left amygdala in LF. No clear event related response was recorded in both amygdale; Stimuli consisted of briefly presented faces depicting different emotions (600 ms). *H* happy faces, *N* neutral faces, *F* fearful faces. (**c**) IcERPs in a patient with a normal amygdala. Note the high amplitude event-related potential in response to faces (with different emotions) between 200 and 500 ms post-stimulus. Note also that the temporo-occipital cortex showed a positive response to faces approximately a 170 mf from stimulus presentation representing the "fusiform face area" [57, 58]

signaling threat, happiness, and neutrality: no reproducible icERP was observed bilaterally. This negative finding is explained by the high number of pathological slow-wave and spikes recorded in the amygdala during the experimental procedure. The absence of an icERP in response to facial expressions represents the electrophysiological counterpart of the patient's severe impairment in decoding facial expressions, and especially fearful ones [60, 61].

Clinical Variables That Modulate Emotion Recognition Impairments

Side of Epilepsy/Lobectomy

The majority of studies have addressed the question of whether or not the ER deficit is lateralized to the right or left temporal lobe. The answer to this question has a dual significance. On one hand, it can contribute to our understanding of the role of the two temporal lobes in the perception of stimuli with emotional valence. On the other hand, it may indicate which patients are most at risk of developing deficits in emotion recognition. Present knowledge however, does not provide a framework for unambiguous interpretation. The majority of the studies demonstrated that right TLE/ATL patients had a worst performance compared with healthy controls and in few studies also with respect to left TLE/ATL. However, other works did not find a significant difference between right and left patients, and few studies found that only left-side patients were impaired in facial ER [45, 46, 50, 62]. Therefore it is not possible to give a definite answer. There are several possible explanations for these discordant results. Apart from methodological questions, regarding the type of stimuli and presentation, it must be considered that TLE is a complex disease. Moreover, in some cases the presumed lateralization of epilepsy may be incorrect – even if it is correct it can be misleading. For example, even in cases with unilateral hippocampal sclerosis, the epileptogenic network dysfunction might involve bi-temporal and extra-temporal regions [63–65]. It must be considered that adult TLE patients can present atrophy or dysfunctions that extend well beyond the medial temporal lobe, involving the cortical-sub-cortical regions that have been demonstrated to participate in processing different emotions. These brain regions include the anterior insula (which processes disgust), the orbital frontal cortex (anger and sadness), and somato-sensory cortices. Also in cases with early-onset seizures, plasticity phenomena may result in a remodeling of memory function, language, and emotions in the two temporal lobes [66, 67]. Finally, many studies are small series and probably underpowered to show statistically significant differences. For all these reasons, clearly the natural clinical variability may underlie many of the inter-study differences, meaning that where differences do exist, they are not necessarily contradictory.

Beyond side matters, an important and consistent finding is the observation that the patients showing the more severe and extended deficits were the ones with a bilateral dysfunction and a bilateral temporal lobe damage, often with the demonstration of a bi-temporal seizures onset zones [28, 33, 59].

Age of Epilepsy Onset and Duration of Epilepsy

There is an important question concerning the recognition of facial expressions. Does there exist a critical period of life for establishing the neural network underlying emotion processing? It has been hypothesized that early insults to the right medial temporal structures could play a crucial role in causing emotion recognition impairments [28]. Several studies tried to understand if there is a critical age of life that is important to develop a functional brain system(s) do recognize emotions. Despite different methodologies used there are convergent evidences demonstrating that the development of seizures in infancy (febrile or afebrile) correlates with a more severe deficit of emotion recognition. This issue was assessed in different ways. Authors compared the patients' groups, setting the age of 5 years as cut-off, finding that early-onset patients had impairment in ER, especially for fearful faces [26, 27, 33, 68]. Other authors considered the correlations between facial ER performance and the age of epilepsy onset: a positive correlation between the age at onset of epilepsy and ER performance was observed, supporting the hypothesis that earlier onset of temporal lobe seizures led to worse performances for recognition of facial expressions [12, 15, 26, 28, 40, 42, 48, 49, 51, 69]. Therefore, it is possible that inter-ictal/ictal seizure activity involving the right temporal lobe during the critical period of early childhood might affect the development of emotion recognition ability. This hypothesis was confirmed by a recent study in children with TLE. The study showed that emotion recognition deficits were already present during infancy in patients with early-onset seizures [48]. Altogether these data support the idea that the emotion recognition impairment observed in adults with early-onset TLE (surgical cases or otherwise) is a developmental disorder. In this line, a recent study investigated ER in a group of school-aged children that were exposed to febrile seizures in early infancy: a proportion of patients had ER deficits even if they had not (yet) developed overt epilepsy [70]. Taken together the evidence emerging from these studies suggests that recognition of various negative emotions may be affected from an early stage in TLE, and that impairments become more likely, more severe and more widespread across emotions as disease evolves. Indeed, also the duration of epilepsy was observed as a negative factor, able to influence ER performance: longer duration of epilepsy was related to worst performance in ER tasks, especially for fear recognition. Notably, it is important to emphasize that in TLE the term "exposure" does not mean a contact with a discrete event (that start and stop), but it means a damage/dysfunction that begins at a specific time-point and then continues chronically in subsequent years.

Effect of Antiepileptic Drugs

Only few studies reported information about the number and types of antiepileptic drugs (AED) used by patients during ER evaluation. Meletti et al. [28] grouped TLE patients according to the number of AED taken (one, two, three, and more-AED groups). No difference in ER scores was observed among the three groups. Then they analyzed ER in TLE patients using a given AED with respect to TLE patients that were not taking that particular AED observing that only the use of Phenobarbital had a negative effect on emotion recognition abilities. Hlobil et al. [71] described that fear recognition was significantly associated with the number of AED taken at time of testing.

Emotion Recognition and Measures of Intelligence

To date few studies have evaluated formally the relationship between global intelligence measures and emotion recognition in TLE. In these studies no significant correlation emerged at least concerning facial expressions. Two studies, on the other hand, documented a negative effect of low total and verbal IQ scores on auditory emotion recognition. Overall, the available literature is not sufficient to make a final judgment. At least with regard to the recognition of facial expressions, the overall level of intelligence and education do not seem to have an important role [28, 29, 33].

Emotion Recognition After Anterior Temporal Lobectomy

An important open question concerns the consequences (if any) of antero-medial temporal resections on ER abilities in patients with an enduring temporal lobe epileptic focus. Current literature shows that in patients with ATL there is a lack of emotion recognition skills, with qualitative and quantitative characteristics apparently similar to that observed in patients with pre-surgical TLE. Unfortunately, however, there are currently only few studies that have investigated the longitudinal changes before and after temporal lobectomy, that too in small groups or case reports [45, 46, 55, 72, 73]. For this reason, it is not possible to determine the real effect of temporal lobectomy in TLE patients. ER impairments, at least as facial emotion labeling is concerned, are "on average" similar in severity to those observed in patients with chronic TLE; however, the "average picture" observed after temporal lobectomy is likely the result of improvement in some patients and worsening in others. Indeed, some evidence exists that after lobectomy, and seizure-freedom, patients can improve in ER [45, 46, 73]. Finally, a weakness, observed in some of the studies, is the lack of clinical information pertaining to the surgical outcomes. In other words, if after temporal lobectomy the patients studied were recovered from epilepsy or not. This is a highly relevant issue in the analysis of neuropsychological outcomes. Longitudinal, prospective studies are needed to shed light on this issue.

Finally, another important issue concerns the ER ability of ATL patients seen at long follow-up intervals. Since several factors can contribute to the interpretations of neuropsychological findings in TLE and in ATL patients (i.e., etiology, side of focus/surgery, age of epilepsy onset, post-operative seizure freedom), we recently evaluated ER in an homogenous cohort of ATL patients (undergone to surgery at around 40 years of age) with: (a) more than 5 years of follow-up and (b) complete seizure-freedom status. We found that deficits in the evaluation of facial expressions were still present at long follow-up intervals in seizure-free patients [74]. This finding should prompt researchers to investigate in future studies whether this picture changes in relation to the age of ATL surgery, especially if the patients operated earlier can better compensate or implement plasticity mechanisms leading to recover the deficit.

Facial Expression Processing in TLE: Evidences from FMRI

Beyond neuropsychological and behavioral tasks, functional magnetic resonance imaging (fMRI) has been used to evaluate the brain processing of emotional stimuli in patients with TLE/ATL. Experiments have been performed to understand the consequences of pathological amygdala tissue (in the case of chronic medial TLE), or of the absence of the amygdala (in the case of ATL), on the processing of emotional material. Knowledge from fMRI experiments in healthy subjects consistently demonstrated that facial expressions, and particularly fearful faces, induce a robust response in the amygdala [75, 76]. The amygdala response to facial expression can be modulated by different variables (type of stimulus, type of response, type of task) but is highly reproducible. Moreover, the perception of emotional faces induces a higher fMRI response over the extra-striate visual cortical areas (such as the fusiform face area) with respect to the vision of neutral faces [77]. This means that the perception of emotional stimuli enhances cortical activity in associative areas. This is one of the ways through which emotions affect and enhance cognition. In the case of chronic medial TLE, different authors have reported two main results. First, the medial temporal lobe region ipsilateral to the epileptogenic zone does not show a reproducible response to facial expression, and especially to fearful ones; this result is the direct consequence of the pathological tissue affecting the amygdala/temporal pole region. This effect, or loss of fMRI responses to fearful faces, has also been used in chronic TLE to obtain information at single-subject level to lateralize the side of the epileptogenic focus [78–81]. Moreover, activation of the right amygdala preoperatively was predictive of emotional disturbances following right anterior temporal lobectomy [79].

Second, and probably most importantly, it has been demonstrated that amygdala pathology prevents the increased response in distant cortical areas as instead has been observed in healthy subject while viewing emotional facial expressions [44,

77]. These fMRI findings are an important demonstration of the role of the amygdala in the processing of emotional stimuli and of its relevance in the orchestration of perceptual responses to external stimuli that are salient for the individual. Very recently, the same evidence has been observed also for the processing of emotional voices. Indeed, emotional cues embedded in vocalizations receive enhanced decoding in sensory cortical areas of the auditory system. In subjects with TLE treated by ATL, this effect was lost [82].

Future Directions and Conclusions

From the perspective of the individual patient with TLE, present knowledge clearly shows that TLE is associated with impaired recognition of negative emotions, especially fear. One key implication is that emotion recognition could potentially serve as a biomarker of disease onset and progression in TLE. Emotion scores (both composites and individual emotions) are indeed a part of the neuropsychological deficits of patients with chronic TLE and further work should demonstrate how sensitive emotion recognition is at tracking decline over time, relative to other potential markers. There is however, little formal evidence concerning the impact of emotional deficits on the social functioning of people with TLE. The studies that investigated measures of wellbeing such as QOLIE-31 failed to demonstrate a correlation between measures of ER and measures of global and emotional wellbeing or depression. This is one important question that needs to be elucidated in future studies. Indeed, the possibility exists that the studies carried out so far have not documented a correlation because patients with TLE have little awareness of their own social difficulties. Therefore, future studies should use different measures, and not only subjective ones, to quantify the difficulty that patients have in everyday life.

Actual knowledge suggests certain directions for further work. There is a need for large, longitudinal studies of emotion comprehension in TLE (and especially before and after ATL) that are informed by emerging neurobiological data and which use consistent measures of disease stage and severity. In future studies it will be important to compare emotion processing in different sensory modalities and at different levels of response (autonomic as well as cognitive) and to extend the assessment to include more ecological kinds of emotion processing beyond the relatively artificial scenario of the forced-choice recognition protocols. There is also a need to understand how these deficits impact on patients' cognitive abilities. Like other diseases, TLE will almost certainly benefit from the progress currently being made in the basic neuroscience of human emotion. The structural and functional anatomical bases for altered emotion processing in TLE should be addressed in hypothesis-driven studies motivated by the neuropsychological data.

Acknowledgments I want to thank all the friends and colleagues that promoted the research in this field during the years, in particular Carlo Alberto Tassinari, Gaetano Cantalupo, Francesca Benuzzi, Giulia Monti, and Paolo Nichelli.

References

1. Darwin C, Ekman P, Prodger P. The expression of the emotions in man and animals. 3rd ed. London: Harper Collins; 1998.
2. Damasio A. The somatic marker hypothesis and the possible functions of the prefrontal cortex. Proc R Soc. 1996;B351:1420–31.
3. Schwartzkroin PA. Hippocampal slices in experimental and human epilepsy. Adv Neurol. 1986;44:991–1010.
4. Graebenitz S, Kedo O, Speckmann EJ, Gorji A, Panneck H, Hans V, et al. Interictal-like network activity and receptor expression in the epileptic human lateral amygdala. Brain. 2011;134:2929–47.
5. Wieser HG, ILAE Commission on Neurosurgery of Epilepsy. ILAE Commission Report, Mesial temporal lobe epilepsy with hippocampal sclerosis. Epilepsia. 2004;45:695–714.
6. Hermann BP, Seidenberg M, Schoenfeld J, Davies K. Neuropsychological characteristics of the syndrome of mesial temporal lobe epilepsy. Arch Neurol. 1997;54:369–76.
7. Jokeit H, Ebner A. Long term effects of refractory temporal lobe epilepsy on cognitive abilities: a cross sectional study. J Neurol Neurosurg Psychiatry. 1999;67:44–50.
8. Helmstaedter C, Kurthen M. Memory and epilepsy: characteristics course and influence of drugs and surgery. Curr Opin Neurol. 2001;14:211–6.
9. Helmstaedter C, Kurthen M, Lux S, Reuber M, Elger CE. Chronic epilepsy and cognition: a longitudinal study in temporal lobe epilepsy. Ann Neurol. 2003;54:425–32.
10. Hermann B, Seidenberg M, Jones J. The neurobehavioural comorbidities of epilepsy: can a natural history be developed? Lancet Neurol. 2008;7:151–60.
11. Helmstaedter C, Witt JA. Multifactorial etiology of interictal behavior in frontal and temporal lobe epilepsy. Epilepsia. 2012;53:1765–73.
12. Anderson AK, Spencer DD, Fulbright RK, Phelps EA. Contribution of the anteromedial temporal lobes to the evaluation of facial emotion. Neuropsychology. 2000;14:526–36.
13. Anderson AK, Phelps EA. Lesions of the human amygdala impair enhanced perception of emotionally salient events. Nature. 2001;411:305–9.
14. Adolphs R, Tranel D, Damasio H, Damasio A. Impaired recognition of emotion in facial expressions following bilateral damage to the human amygdala. Nature. 1994;372:669–72.
15. Adolphs R, Tranel D, Damasio H. Emotion recognition from faces and prosody following temporal lobectomy. Neuropsychology. 2001;15:396–404.
16. Adolphs R. Neural systems for recognizing emotions. Curr Opin Neurobiol. 2002;12:169–77.
17. Adolphs R. Fear faces and the human amygdala. Curr Opin Neurobiol. 2008;18:166–72.
18. Adolphs R. What does the amygdala contribute to social cognition? Ann N Y Acad Sci. 2010;1191:42–61.
19. Adolphs R. Cognitive neuroscience of human social behavior. Nat Rev Neurosci. 2013;4:165–78.
20. LeDoux JE. The emotional brain: the mysterious underpinnings of emotional life. New York: Touchstone; 1996.
21. Harrison NA, Gray MA, Gianaros PJ, Critchley HD. The embodiment of emotional feelings in the brain. J Neurosci. 2010;30:12878–84.
22. Phelps EA. Emotion and cognition: insights from studies of the human amygdala. Annu Rev Psychol. 2006;57:27–53.
23. Salzman CD, Fusi S. Emotion, cognition, and mental state representation in amygdala and prefrontal cortex. Annu Rev Neurosci. 2010;33:173–202.
24. Winston JS, O'Doherty J, Dolan RJ. Common and distinct neural responses during direct and incidental processing of multiple facial emotions. Neuroimage. 2003;20:84–97.
25. Wiebe S, Blume WT, Girvin JP, Eliasziw M. A randomized controlled trial of surgery for temporal-lobe epilepsy. N Engl J Med. 2001;345:311–8.

26. Meletti S, Benuzzi F, Rubboli G, Cantalupo G, Stanzani Maserati M, et al. Impaired facial emotion recognition in early-onset right mesial temporal lobe epilepsy. Neurology. 2003;60:426–31.
27. Meletti S, Benuzzi F, Nichelli P, Tassinari CA. Damage to the right hippocampal-amygdala formation during early infancy and recognition of fearful faces. Neuropsychological and fMRI evidence in subjects with temporal lobe epilepsy. Ann N Y Acad Sci. 2003;1000:385–8.
28. Meletti S, Benuzzi F, Cantalupo G, Rubboli G, Tassinari CA, Nichelli P. Facial emotion recognition impairment in chronic temporal lobe epilepsy. Epilepsia. 2009;50:1547–59.
29. Broicher SD, Kuchukhidze G, Grunwald T, Kramer G, Kurthena M, Jokeit H. "Tell me how do I feel" – emotion recognition and theory of mind in symptomatic mesial temporal lobe epilepsy. Neuropsychologia. 2012;50:118–28.
30. Giovagnoli AR, Franceschetti S, Reati F, Parente A, Maccagno C, et al. Theory of mind in frontal and temporal lobe epilepsy: cognitive and neural aspects. Epilepsia. 2011;52: 1995–2002.
31. Gosselin N, Peretz I, Noulhiane M, Hasboun D, Beckett C, et al. Impaired recognition of scary music following unilateral temporal lobe excision. Brain. 2005;128:628–40.
32. Gosselin N, Peretz I, Hasboun D, Baulac M, Samson S. Impaired recognition of musical emotions and facial expressions following anteromedial temporal lobe excision. Cortex. 2011;47:1116–25.
33. Bonora A, Benuzzi F, Monti G, Mirandola L, Pugnaghi M, et al. Recognition of emotions from faces and voices in medial temporal lobe epilepsy. Epilepsy Behav. 2011;20:648–54.
34. Dellacherie D, Hasboun D, Baulac M, Belin P, Samson S. Impaired recognition of fear in voices and reduced anxiety after unilateral temporal lobe resection. Neuropsychologia. 2011;49:618–29.
35. Ekman P, Friesen WV. Pictures of facial affect. Palo Alto: Consulting Psychologist Press; 1976.
36. Ekman P. The argument and evidence about universals in facial expressions of emotion. In: Wagner H, Manstead A, editors. Handbook of psychophysiology: emotion and social behavior. London: Wiley; 1989.
37. Ekman P. Facial expression and emotion. Am Psychol. 1993;48:384–92.
38. Calder AJ, Young AW. Understanding the recognition of facial identity and facial expression. Nat Rev Neurosci. 2005;6:641–51.
39. Calder A, Young AW, Rowland D, Perrett DI, Hodges RJ, Etcoff NL. Facial emotion recognition after bilateral amygdala damage: differentially severe impairment of fear. Cogn Neuropsychol. 1996;13:699–745.
40. Reynders HJ, Broks P, Dickson JM, Lee CE, Turpin G. Investigation of social and emotion information processing in temporal lobe epilepsy with ictal fear. Epilepsy Behav. 2005;7:419–29.
41. Walpole P, Isaac CL, Reynders HJ. A comparison of emotional and cognitive intelligences in people with and without temporal lobe epilepsy. Epilepsia. 2008;49:1470–4.
42. Sedda A, Rivolta D, Scarpa P, Frigerio E, Burt M, Zanardi G, et al. Ambiguous emotions recognition in temporal lobe epilepsy: the role of expression intensity. Cogn Affect Behav Neurosci. 2013;13:452–63.
43. Young AW, Hellawell DJ, Van deWal C, Johnson M. Facial expression processing after amygdalotomy. Neuropsychologia. 1996;34:31–9.
44. Benuzzi F, Meletti S, Zamboni G, Calandra-Buonaura G, Serafini M, Lui F, et al. Impaired fear processing in right mesial temporal sclerosis: a fMRI study. Brain Res Bull. 2004;63:269–81.
45. Yamada M, Muraib T, Satoa W, Namikib C, Miyamotoc T, Ohigashi Y. Emotion recognition from facial expressions in a temporal lobe epileptic patient with ictal fear. Neuropsychologia. 2005;43:434–41.
46. Shaw P, Lawrence E, Bramham J, Brierley B, Radbourne C, David AS. A prospective study of the effects of anterior temporal lobectomy on emotion recognition and theory of mind. Neuropsychologia. 2007;45:2783–90.

47. Brierley B, Medford N, Shaw P, David AS. Emotional memory and perception in temporal lobectomy patients with amygdala damage. J Neurol Neurosurg Psychiatry. 2004;75:593–9.
48. Golouboff N, Fiori N, Delalande O, Fohlen M, Dellatolas G, Jambaqué I. Impaired facial expression recognition in children with temporal lobe epilepsy: impact of early seizure onset on fear recognition. Neuropsychologia. 2008;46:1415–28.
49. Pinabiaux C, Bulteau C, Fohlen M, Dorfmuller G, Chiron C, Hertz-Pannier L, et al. Impaired emotional memory recognition after early temporal lobe epilepsy surgery: the fearful face exception? Cortex. 2013;49:1386–93.
50. Ammerlaan E, Hendriks PH, Colon AJ, Kessels RPC. Emotion perception and interpersonal behavior in epilepsy patients after unilateral amygdalohippocampectomy. Acta Neurobiol Exp. 2008;68:214–8.
51. Tanaka A, Akamatsu N, Yamano M, Nakagawa M, Kawamura M, Tsuji S. A more realistic approach using dynamic stimuli to test facial emotion recognition impairment in temporal lobe epilepsy. Epilepsy Behav. 2013;28:12–6.
52. Scott SK, Young AW, Calder AJ, Hellawell DJ, Aggleton JP, Johnson M. Impaired auditory recognition of fear and anger following bilateral amygdala lesions. Nature. 1997;385:254–7.
53. Fowler H, Baker GA, Tipples J, Hare DJ, Keller S, Chadwick DW, Young AW. Recognition of emotion with temporal lobe epilepsy and asymmetrical amygdala damage. Epilepsy Behav. 2006;9:164–72.
54. Khalfa S, Guye M, Peretz I, Chapon F, Girard N, Chauvel P, Liegeois-Chauvel C. Evidence of lateralized anteromedial temporal structures involvement in musical emotion processing. Neuropsychologia. 2008;46:2485–93.
55. Sanz-Martin A, Guevara MA, Corsi-Cabrera M, Ondarza-Rovira R, Ramos-Loyo J. Differential effect of left and right temporal lobectomy on emotional recognition and experience in patients with epilepsy. Rev Neurol. 2006;42:391–8.
56. Benton AH, Hamsher K, Varney N, Spreen O. Contribution to neuropsychological assessment. New York: Oxford University Press; 1983.
57. Kanwisher N, McDermott J, Chun MM. The fusiform face area: a module in human extrastriate cortex specialized for face perception. J Neurosci. 1997;17:4302–11.
58. Allison T, Puce A, Spencer DD, McCarthy G. Electrophysiological studies of human face perception. I: potentials generated in occipitotemporal cortex by face and non-face stimuli. Cereb Cortex. 1999;9:415–30.
59. Meletti S, Cantalupo G, Santoro F, Benuzzi F, Marliani AF, Tassinari CA, Rubboli G. Temporal lobe epilepsy and emotion recognition without amygdala: a case study of Urbach-Wiethe disease and review of the literature. Epileptic Disord. 2014;16:518–27.
60. Krolak-Salmon P, Henaff MA, Vighetto A, Bertrand O, Mauguiere F. Early amygdala reaction to fear spreading in occipital, temporal, and frontal cortex: a depth electrode ERP study in human. Neuron. 2004;42:665–76.
61. Meletti S, Cantalupo G, Benuzzi F, Mai R, Tassi L, Gasparini E, et al. Fear and happiness in the eyes: an intra-cerebral event-related potential study from the human amygdala. Neuropsychologia. 2012;50:44–54.
62. Carvajal F, Rubio S, Martin P, Serrano JM, Garcia-Sola R. Perception and recall of faces and facial expressions following temporal lobectomy. Epilepsy Behav. 2009;14:60–5.
63. Bernasconi N, Bernasconi A, Caramanos Z, Antel SB, Andermann F, Arnold DL. Mesial temporal damage in temporal lobe epilepsy: a volumetric MRI study of the hippocampus amygdala and parahippocampal region. Brain. 2003;126:462–9.
64. Chassoux F, Semah F, Bouilleret V, Landre E, Devaux B, Turak B, et al. Metabolic changes and electro-clinical patterns in mesio-temporal lobe epilepsy: a correlative study. Brain. 2004;127:164–74.
65. Lee SK, Kim DW, Kim KK, Chung CK, Song IC, Chang KH. Effect of seizure on hippocampus in mesial temporal lobe epilepsy and neocortical epilepsy: an MRS study. Neuroradiology. 2005;47:916–23.
66. Saykin AJ, Gur RC, Sussman NM, O'Connor MJ, Gur RE. Memory deficits before and after temporal lobectomy: effect of laterality and age of onset. Brain Cogn. 1989;9:191–200.

67. Davies KG, Hermann BP, Dohan Jr FC, Foley KT, Bush AJ, Wyler AR. Relationship of hippocampal sclerosis to duration and age of onset of epilepsy and childhood febrile seizures in temporal lobectomy patients. Epilepsy Res. 1996;24:119–26.
68. McClelland III S, Garcia RE, Peraza DM, Shih TT, Hirsch LJ, et al. Facial emotion recognition after curative nondominant temporal lobectomy in patients with mesial temporal sclerosis. Epilepsia. 2006;47:1337–42.
69. Palermo R, Schmalzl L, Mohamed A, Bleasel A, Miller L. The effect of unilateral amygdala removals on detecting fear from briefly presented backward-masked faces. J Clin Exp Neuropsychol. 2010;32:123–31.
70. Cantalupo G, Meletti S, Miduri A, Mazzotta S, Rios-Pohl L, Benuzzi F, et al. Facial emotion recognition in childhood: the effects of febrile seizures in the developing brain. Epilepsy Behav. 2013;29:211–6.
71. Hlobil U, Rathore C, Alexander A, Sarma S, Radhakrishnan K. Impaired facial emotion recognition in patients with mesial temporal lobe epilepsy associated with hippocampal sclerosis (MTLE-HS): Side and age at onset matters. Epilepsy Res. 2008;80:150–7.
72. Amlerova J, Cavanna AE, Bradac O, Javurkova A, Raudenska J, Marusic P. Emotion recognition and social cognition in temporal lobe epilepsy and the effect of epilepsy surgery. Epilepsy Behav. 2014;36:86–9.
73. Benuzzi F, Zamboni G, Meletti S, Serafini M, Lui F, Baraldi P, et al. Recovery from emotion recognition impairment after temporal lobectomy. Front Neurol. 2014;5:92. doi:10.3389/fneur.2014.00092.
74. Meletti S, Picardi A, De Risi M, Monti G, Esposito V, et al. The affective value of faces in patients achieving long-term seizure freedom after temporal lobectomy. Epilepsy Behav. 2014;36:97–101.
75. Morris JS, Frith CD, Perrett DI, Rowland D, Young AW, et al. A differential neural response in the human amygdala to fearful and happy facial expressions. Nature. 1996;383:812–5.
76. Breiter HC, Etcoff NL, Whalen PJ, Kennedy WA, Rauch SL, Buckner RL, et al. Response and habituation of the human amygdala during visual processing of facial expression. Neuron. 1996;17:875–87.
77. Vuilleumier P, Richardson MP, Armony JL, Driver J, Dolan RJ. Distant influences of amygdala lesion on visual cortical activation during emotional face processing. Nat Neurosci. 2004;7:1271–8.
78. Schacher M, Haemmerle B, Woermann FG, Okujava M, Huber D, Grunwald T, et al. Amygdala fMRI lateralizes temporal lobe epilepsy. Neurology. 2006;66:81–7.
79. Bonelli SB, Powell R, Yogarajah M, Thompson PJ, Symms MR, et al. Preoperative amygdala fMRI in temporal lobe epilepsy. Epilepsia. 2009;50:217–27.
80. Broicher S, Kuchukhidze G, Grunwald T, Krämer G, Kurthen M, Trinka E, Jokeit H. Association between structural abnormalities and fMRI response in the amygdala in patients with temporal lobe epilepsy. Seizure. 2010;19:426–31.
81. Labudda K, Mertens M, Steinkroeger C, Bien CG, Woermann FG. Lesion side matters – an fMRI study on the association between neural correlates of watching dynamic fearful faces and their evaluation in patients with temporal lobe epilepsy. Epilepsy Behav. 2014;31:321–8.
82. Frühholz S, Hofstetter C, Cristinzio C, Saj A, Seeck M, et al. Asymmetrical effects of unilateral right or left amygdala damage on auditory cortical processing of vocal emotions. Proc Natl Acad Sci U S A. 2015;112(5):1583–8.

Chapter 12
Neuropsychiatric Symptoms in Learning Disability

Anagha A. Sardesai and Howard Ring

Abstract This chapter commences with a brief introduction to the concept of learning disability, including its definition, causes, and manifestations. Issues around the co-occurrence of epilepsy and learning disability, including prevalence, etiological factors, and diagnosis are then introduced. The consequences of significant learning disability for the manifesation and diagnosis of abnormal mental states are considered. This chapter then progresses with accounts of the manifestation, diagnosis and management of affective, psychotic, and behavioral psychopathological states in people with epilepsy and a learning disability, including how to consider particular issues arising in those with severe intellectual disabilities and significant communication deficits. Accounts are also provided of specific comorbidities of epilepsy with autism and with Down syndrome.

Keywords Learning Disability • IQ • Diagnosis • Depression • Anxiety • Psychosis • Autism • Down Syndrome • Dementia

What Is LD?

Learning disability (or intellectual disability) used to be known as mental handicap or mental retardation. Sometimes the term general or global developmental delay is used. People meeting diagnostic criteria for a learning disability find it more difficult to learn, understand, and develop skills compared to others. The degree of disability can vary greatly. Some with greater degrees of disability will need life-long

A.A. Sardesai, MBBS, MRCPsych
Department of Learning Disability Psychiatry, Cambridgeshire and Peterborough NHS Foundation Trust, Ida Darwin Hospital, Block 11, Fulbourn CB21 5EE, UK
e-mail: sardesai1@aol.com

H. Ring, MD (✉)
Department of Psychiatry, University of Cambridge,
Douglas House, 18b Trumpington Road, Cambridge CB2 8AH, UK
e-mail: har28@cam.ac.uk

M. Mula (ed.), *Neuropsychiatric Symptoms of Epilepsy*, Neuropsychiatric Symptoms of Neurological Disease, DOI 10.1007/978-3-319-22159-5_12

help for most or almost all activities including basic self-care such as feeding, dressing, or going to the toilet. On the other hand, others may have a disability that is mild and compatible with living independently. Internationally three criteria are required to be met before a learning disability can be diagnosed. These are:

- Intellectual impairment (IQ)
- Social or adaptive dysfunction associated with low IQ (difficulty in everyday functioning or being able to flexibly adapt to everyday situations, for example, bus being late, change in model of washing machine, etc.)
- Onset during the developmental period

The prevalence of learning disability in the UK general population is reported as 3.7 per 1000 of the population [1] and in 2010, it was estimated [2] that 1,198,000 people in England had a learning disability. This included:

- 298,000 children (188,000 boys, 110,000 girls) age 0–17
- 900,000 adults aged 18+ (526,000 men and 374,000 women), of whom 191,000 (21 %) were known to learning disabilities services

How Is Learning Disability Different from Specific Learning Difficulty?

A global learning *disability* is distinct from a specific learning *difficulty*. The former describes a global impairment that limits an individual's ability to reach the average range of intellectual and functional achievements. The latter term is used to describe difficulties in circumscribed areas of intellectual achievement in an otherwise typically developing individual; for example, a specific learning difficulty in reading, writing or arithmetic, but with no problems learning skills in other areas of functioning.

Causes of Learning Disability

There are three critical periods when potential causes of learning disability may disturb development:

- Prior to birth: for instance – genetic disorders, metabolic disorders, and maternal factors
- During birth: for instance – hypoxia associated with birth complications
- After birth but during development – particularly during critical periods of early development in the first 2 years of life: for instance as a consequence of traumatic brain injury, infection, or effects of therapeutic intervention such as radiotherapy for malignant disease

The causes of learning disability include:

- Genetic factors:

  1. Chromosomes make up the genetic blueprint of every individual and each of us usually has 46 chromosomes. Sometimes there can be an abnormality in an individual's chromosomes, which can lead to learning disability. The commonest and most widely known example of this is Down's syndrome where there is extra chromosomal material of chromosome 21 (trisomy 21). It is estimated that this affects 1 in 650–1000.
  2. There could also be mutations in a single gene rather than a chromosome. Mutations of FMR1 gene cause Fragile X syndrome. Fragile X syndrome occurs in approximately 1 in 4000 males and 1 in 8000 females.
  3. Some conditions, for instance autism, appear to develop as a consequence of the result of multiple effects from many genes.

- Infections or exposure to harmful chemicals before birth:

  1. Some infections caught by the mother, for example, TORCH (Toxoplasma, Rubella, Cytomegalovirus, Herpes) and others, for instance syphilis and varicella zoster may be passed on to the unborn child, and may lead to learning disability.
  2. The mother may also have dietary deficiencies, or consume substances which can be detrimental to the developing brain of the fetus.
  3. Exposure to alcohol leading to Fetal Alcohol Syndrome or Fetal Alcohol Spectrum Disorder

- Brain injury or damage at birth: A learning disability may result if the baby's oxygen supply is interrupted for a significant length of time. Significantly premature birth also increases the risk of subsequent developmental disability
- Brain infections or brain damage after birth:

  1. Some childhood infections can affect the brain, causing learning disability; the most common of these are encephalitis and meningitis.
  2. Severe head injury, for example from a road accident, may result in learning disability.

- Metabolic disturbances in early life that if detected can be corrected – for instance hypothyroidism
- Idiopathic – For many people diagnosed with a learning disability the cause is unknown. It has also been established that adverse social and environmental factors, such as poor housing conditions, poor diet and health care, malnutrition, lack of stimulation, and all forms of child abuse may contribute to an exacerbation of learning disability, although the mechanisms of these effects are largely unknown

Why Do Epilepsy and LD Often Occur Together?

Epilepsy is common in those with a learning disability (LD). The prevalence of epilepsy in learning disability overall is said to be 20–30 % [3]. Its frequency increases progressively with more severe intellectual impairment. Overall lifetime prevalence of epilepsy in those with mild to moderate learning disability (IQ 35–70) has been estimated at 15 % while in those with severe to profound learning disability (IQ less than 50) a prevalence of 30 % has been reported [4], and overall, those with more significant learning disability are also likely to have more severe epilepsy [5–11]. Conversely, research in people presenting with epilepsy has demonstrated that up to a quarter also have a learning disability [12].

While, as indicated above, there are many causes of learning disability, some etiologies are associated with high rates of comorbid epilepsy. This is particularly the case for some genetically determined neurodevelopmental syndromes, where consideration of the underlying genetic defect is already starting to shed light on pathophysiological processes that underlie the development of intellectual disability, epilepsy, and the relationship between them. For instance, in Fragile X syndrome, resulting from expansion of a CGG-repeat beyond 200 triplets in the 5′-untranslated region of the FMR1 gene, prevalence of seizures is 11.8–13.1 %; in Rett syndrome, an X-linked disorder involving mutations in the MeCP2 gene the prevalence of seizures is higher [13], with reported prevalence of seizures varying between 60 and 94 %; and in Angelman syndrome, resulting from loss of expression of the maternal copy of the imprinted UBE3A gene, generally following microdeletion of the 15q11–q13 region, seizures are reported in 86 % of affected individuals. These genetic disturbances and the associated metabolic consequences result in different presentations of epilepsy. In most children with fragile X syndrome who develop epilepsy it starts between the ages of 4 and 10, while in those with Rett syndrome seizures typically develop between 3 and 5 years of age with decreasing seizure rates by adolescence, while in those with Angelman syndrome seizures often persist throughout childhood and tend to be more severe, with more seizure types. Considering treatment response, seizures in Fragile X syndrome tend to respond more readily to AEDs than is the case in Rett syndrome and Angelman syndrome. Learning Disability can also arise as a secondary consequence of severe epilepsy during a critical development period, for example, Lennox–Gastaut syndrome.

Diagnosing Epilepsy in People with LD

Diagnosis in patients with learning disability is complex as patients are frequently unable to provide any history themselves and the family carers or paid support workers who accompany them may not always be well informed. It is important to note that misdiagnosis of epilepsy among people with learning disabilities is relatively frequent – with an estimated rate of misdiagnosis of 32–38 %. Reasons for high misdiagnosis rates include misinterpretation of behavioral, physiological, syndrome-related and medication-related events by parents, paid support workers, and healthcare professionals [14]. There can often be diagnostic overlap and overshadowing, for instance the presence of stereotyped and self-stimulatory behaviors, expressions of pain or frustration and periods of drowsiness or withdrawal of engagement with the environment have all been misdiagnosed as seizures in people with a learning disability. Therefore, in England, National Institute for Clinical Excellence (NICE) clinical guidelines state that diagnosis of epilepsy should be established by a specialist medical practitioner with training and expertise in epilepsy. They further advise that diagnosis should be based upon a detailed history and (where possible) eyewitness reports of events usually supplemented with EEG. Where diagnosis cannot be clearly established, further investigations (e.g., blood tests, sleep EEG, neuroimaging, and 12-lead ECG) and/or referral to a tertiary center is recommended.

How Is Epilepsy Manifest in LD?

Compared to epilepsy in the general population, epilepsy in people with an LD is more likely to be refractory to antiepileptic drug (AED) treatment, with prognosis for seizure control in people with learning disability and epilepsy poorer than for those with epilepsy without learning disability [15]. These higher rates of inadequately controlled epilepsy bring increased rates of morbidity and also mortality [16]. In a Swedish study of over 1400 patients with learning disability, followed up for 7 years, the standardized mortality ratio (SMR) for those with learning disability without epilepsy was 1.6 but the SMR increased to 5.0 in those with concomitant epilepsy [17]. As is also the case for those with epilepsy in the absence of an associated learning disability, it is among those with ongoing seizures that the risk of neuropsychiatric symptoms is greatest.

How Is Psychopathology Diagnosed in People with LD?

There are particular and very important challenges to consider when diagnosing neuropsychiatric symptoms in people with a significant learning disability.

People with more severe learning disabilities often lack the language abilities to verbally describe their psychological experiences. In these circumstances history taking should focus on asking carers about observable changes in presentation that may be signs of the development of psychopathology. For instance, possible biological features of depression such as sleep disturbance and change in appetite should be discussed with carers. Behavioral changes such as decreased social interaction, loss of interest in activities previously engaged in, apparent agitation or distress, tearfulness, and a decrease in previous levels of functional abilities may all suggest significant lowering of mood. However, people with a learning disability often already lead relatively restricted lives and it can be harder to identify change in functioning at an early stage. Diagnosing delusions and hallucinations may be particularly difficult as manifestation of these symptoms generally requires well-developed speech. Thought disorder may also be difficult to identify in somebody whose behavior and communications may already be difficult to follow. It should also be kept in mind that the same symptom can present differently in patients depending on the level of their learning disability.

There is also the complex issue of equivalence of diagnoses to consider. For instance, how might somebody with severely impaired language and understanding experience auditory hallucinations or persecutory delusions. Thus for those with the most severe learning disabilities, it remains unclear whether behavioral disturbances that appear to indicate psychological distress are indicating mental states such as depression or psychosis that are equivalent to such states as experienced by those with higher IQs. The diagnosis of psychotic states may be particularly problematic in this context and this may relate to the observation that there are increased rates of depression and psychosis in those with moderate compared to those with severe or profound LD.

Particularly in the context of these challenges it is of *critical importance* to remain alert for signs and symptoms suggestive of psychiatric states in people with LD and epilepsy. At the same time it is equally important to consider whether the presentations of apparently psychiatric states are either manifestations of other illnesses and/or pain, or are psychiatric consequences of physical illness that has not been diagnosed. Similarly, adverse effects of AEDs and other medications are not uncommon and in people not able to report these verbally, clinicians should remain alert to such effects as the cause of behavioral or emotional symptoms. This issue can be addressed through careful and thorough history taking and searching for physical adverse effects of treatment that may go alongside psychiatric effects.

The role of informants: Collateral history takes on the utmost importance for patients who cannot tell the clinician what the problem is. While they might communicate "something is not quite right" it might be only someone close to them who is able to articulate "what" is not right. How robust the collateral history is depends on how long the carers have worked with the patient, how well versed they are in their observations of the patient and also what facets they see. Different carers often have different ways of working and different perspectives to offer which can lead to quite different collateral histories regarding nature, onset, duration and progression of the difficulties stated. The skill of the clinician lies in being able to fit in the different pieces of the jig-saw offered so as to form a coherent picture, arrive at a formulation and then come up with a management plan that can be effectively shared with the patient and carers so as to enable the patient to be supported effectively.

Mood Disorders in People with LD and Epilepsy

The association between epilepsy and affective disorders is well known [18, 19].

Prevalence

Patients with LD and epilepsy are at high risk for depression because of an incompletely understood combination of factors that may be both psychosocial and neurological. Research has shown that lifetime rates of depression and suicidal ideation in patients with epilepsy is at least twice as high as that of the general population. Mood disorders are also more common in patients with LD when compared to the general population.

Diagnosis and Presentation

It may be helpful to consider the different ways in which presentations of affective symptoms can relate to different stages in seizure manifestation. Some reports describe seizure prodromes, lasting for several hours or occasionally days and these states can be manifest as distinct changes in mood or behavior before an epileptic event, characterized for instance by increased lability of emotion or irritability. During the period after a seizure, the post-ictal period, during which a person is in the process of returning to their normal inter-ictal state, reports of symptoms of depression are relatively common. While this post-ictal depression may be short-lived – lasting for minutes to hours, it can be intense and at times associated with suicidal thoughts. Affective symptoms, as well as psychotic sates and behavioral disturbances, have also been reported in the context of period of reduced clinical and EEG seizure activity – described as "forced normalization." Such episodes may develop spontaneously but are also recognized to have occurred following introduction of an AED that has reduced seizure frequency. The factors that determine which psychiatric symptoms may arise during such an episode remain unclear. It is also interesting to note that depression appears to be much more common than manic or bipolar states in patients with a learning disability and epilepsy. This could be due to the fact that many of the most widely used AEDs also have mood stabilizing properties (for instance carbamazepine, lamotrigine, sodium valproate), while some others are associated with development of depressive symptoms (for instance, phenobarbitone and vigabatrin).

In the presence of communication difficulties, particularly in those with more severe learning disability, clinical presentation and diagnostic observations are, as described above in the section How is Psychopathology Diagnosed in People with LD, likely to involve observations of somatic symptoms such as psychomotor retardation/agitation, loss of appetite and weight, sleep disturbance, and withdrawal from environment or activities which were previously enjoyable.

Patients with a learning disability, particularly those with more severe disabilities, may also present with "Challenging behavior." This term describes behavior likely to challenge those providing support and care and may include repeated self-injurious or aggressive behaviors. The development of challenging behavior may indicate the presence of a developing mood or other psychiatric state, but can also occur as a response to pain or discomfort, fear, boredom, frustration or distress at environmental changes such unexpected alterations in established routines, the departure of a known carer or the introduction of a new one.

Management of Mood Disorders

It is important to know that the presence of a learning disability most definitely does not preclude successful treatment of a mood disorder. The NICE guidelines advocate person centered care in the treatment of all mood disorders. This holds particularly true for patients with learning disability with comorbid epilepsy who rely on carers for help. In the past there has been reluctance to treat depression that arises in patients with epilepsy due to concerns about affecting seizure threshold. With the availability of selective serotonin reuptake inhibitors (SSRIs), which have minimal effect on seizure threshold, it is no longer such a worry and consensus guidelines describing approaches to treatment have been published [20].

When treating depression the first consideration should always be to check the patients' anticonvulsant regimen for potential drug-induced depression (e.g., vigabatrin and phenobarbitone are particularly known to affect mood as a side effect). It may well be that the patient would benefit from changing the anticonvulsant to another agent with a more favorable effect on mood rather than adding in an antidepressant.

While the risk of seizures with SSRIs is low, no drug information leaflet lists it at "zero" and patients and carers should be made aware of this when prescribing. It is important to note that the risk of seizures increases with increasing doses.

SSRIs are considered the first line antidepressant option in patients with epilepsy. Fluoxetine is not the best choice due to its long half-life, a possibly greater incidence of seizures and an increased risk of drug interactions. Citalopram or sertraline may be considered the better options due to safety and reduced interaction potential with the anticonvulsants. Moclobemide is a good alternative, as it has a low incidence of seizures but due to limited data it should be reserved as a second choice.

Tricyclic antidepressants (TCAs) should be used cautiously in patients with epilepsy and reserved for patients who poorly respond to or are intolerant of other antidepressants. Where a TCA is needed, doxepin is possibly of lowest risk of adverse drug interactions and therefore the agent of choice. This is in keeping with the guidelines drawn up by the UK Medicines Information pharmacists.

There is always the possibility of interactions between antidepressants and anticonvulsants and clinicians should monitor carefully patients with epilepsy who are prescribed antidepressants. The old adage of "start low and go slow" holds particularly true when managing patients with learning disability. Introducing the antidepressant with a low dose, gradually increasing to therapeutic dose and not exceeding the maximum recommended dose may reduce the risk of a seizure as well as other side effects. If seizures occur or if the incidence of seizures increases, a clinical decision needs to be taken on whether the antidepressant should be discontinued and an alternative tried after the washout phase. Patients and carers also need to be made aware of the fact that it can often take 4–6 weeks for the benefits of treatment to be apparent.

In patients with mild learning disability, cognitive behavioral therapies (CBT) and other psychological treatments can be used as first line to manage depressive symptoms particularly if it appears that the symptoms arise in response to a known trigger such as bereavement or loss. Music therapy and Art therapy as well as environmental changes with removal of demand can be of help in treating affective and behavioral symptoms in patients with moderate/severe learning disability but tend to be more effective as an adjunct to pharmacological intervention rather than on their own.

In keeping with NICE guidance after achieving recovery and return to baseline, patients should continue on the medication at the appropriate dose for at least 2 years to minimize risk of relapse. Often in clinical practice it becomes apparent that a longer duration of treatment is needed particularly if the mood disorder was of a severe nature.

Discontinuation of the antidepressant should also be attempted extremely slowly allowing plenty of time (for instance 4–6 weeks) between each step to allow carers and patients to pick up any deterioration from decrease in dose of medication.

While a patient continues treatment with anti-depressants it is important to monitor for side effects in addition to monitoring for any change in seizure frequency. SSRIs are known to decrease bone density and predispose to osteoporosis. This is of particular importance in patients with learning disability and epilepsy who have an increased incidence of osteoporosis and Vitamin D deficiency. NICE recommends that Vitamin D levels are measured in patients receiving AEDs and they are of particular importance in patients treated with SSRIs in addition to AEDs. Significant SSRI induced hyponatremia is rare but can occur particularly in the elderly. This is particularly important if they are on anticonvulsants such as carbamazepine, eslicarbazepine, and oxcarbazepine, which are known to induce hyponatremia as a side effect, themselves. It may be difficult to elicit these symptoms, so consider ordering serum electrolytes if patients complain of fatigue, dizziness or cramping, or if carers report listlessness in patients.

Anxiety in People with LD and Epilepsy

Anxiety is a complex disorder, characterized by a combination of mood, thought, and autonomic system symptoms.

Prevalence

Next to depression, anxiety is the most prevalent condition in patients with epilepsy [21]. Anxiety seen as a direct manifestation of the seizure tends to be brief (a span of a few minutes to hours) as compared to primary anxiety disorders, which tend to be much more long lasting.

Anxiety occurring just before a seizure can be part of an aura and in patients with severe to profound LD may be a symptom recognized by the parents or carers who also sometimes report that a seizure appears to relieve the anxiety and fearfulness seen prior to its occurrence. Ictal anxiety is considered to be common with up to a third of patients with partial seizures reporting fear as part of their aura, particularly those with a right temporal foci. In patients with learning disability the figures are harder to determine as communication difficulties can often lead to difficulties with naming emotions. At times anxiety may be the only sign of a seizure noticed by carers who might not notice other features of seizure phenomena such as short-term loss of awareness or arrest of activity. Post-ictal anxiety is not particularly common but may be seen in someone who experiences post-ictal confusion and therefore gets anxious. Anxiety has also been reported following temporal lobe surgery in epilepsy in the first 6–12 weeks [22].

Diagnosis

It is important to establish whether the anxiety symptoms relate to seizure activity and therefore are best treated by pursuing adequate seizure control or whether they form a comorbid psychiatric illness that needs to be treated in its own right. Panic disorder, generalized anxiety, agoraphobia, social phobia, and obsessive compulsive disorder can occur in patients with LD and epilepsy and diagnostic criteria are the same as that of general population. However, obsessive behaviors and rituals are also seen in people with learning disabilities and autism and, as described below, there is an increased rate of epilepsy in people with autism and learning disability. It is important to note that psychosocial difficulties, social stigma, and unpredictable seizures may also contribute to anxiety symptoms. Diagnosis is based on clinical history and presentation after ruling out thyroid, other endocrine and medication side effects as causes.

Presentation

- Patients often present with a sense of fear, unease, or panic.
- Problems sleeping.
- Cold or sweaty hands and/or feet.

- Shortness of breath.
- Heart palpitations.
- Dry mouth.
- Inability to sit still and be calm.
- Tingling and numbness or altered sensation in their hands or feet.
- Carers occasionally report agitation or behavior difficulties. Often the behavior difficulties are described as "challenging behavior."

As with other disorders, as the degree of learning disability and communication difficulties increases the clinician has to rely more on the observable symptoms, as it can be difficult for the person with LD to effectively communicate their emotions and thoughts. Also, it is not always possible to gain cooperation for a physical examination.

Management

Attempting adequate seizure control and excluding other medical causes mentioned above are of utmost importance in managing the symptoms of anxiety.

Psychological treatments, for example, CBT play an important part in the management of anxiety symptoms and can be very effective particularly in patients with mild learning disability particularly when used alongside pharmacological intervention.

Pharmacological intervention is by using SSRIs as first line of medication with doses as per the appropriate guidelines, starting low and increasing slowly to titrate to good effect while carefully monitoring for side effects. Any SSRI may be used though it is helpful to avoid paroxetine, which can cause end dose anxiety. As mentioned above it is important to monitor carefully for side effects and possible increase in seizure activity.

Benzodiazepines and antipsychotics are not used for first line management of anxiety and benzodiazepines where used are limited to managing short-term crisis of no more than a week or so in duration.

Psychosis in People with LD and Epilepsy

Prevalence

Prevalence rates of schizophrenia in people with learning disabilities are thought to be about three times greater than the general population. Epilepsy has long been considered a risk factor for psychosis. A systematic review [23] recently concluded that 6 % of individuals with epilepsy have a comorbid psychotic illness and patients with epilepsy have almost an eightfold increased risk of psychosis with the prevalence rate being highest in temporal lobe epilepsy (7 %). Prevalence rates of psychosis in patients with LD range from 14–50 % depending on the assessment methods used and the degree of learning disability in the patients being screened. There are also reported cases of psychosis developing in patients being treated with antiepileptic drugs particularly with levatiracetam, vigabatrin, and topiramate. Inter-ictal psychosis is reported in up to 10 % of patients with temporal lobe epilepsy [24–26].

Diagnosis and Presentation

As noted above, it can be difficult to make a diagnosis of psychosis as people who have a learning disability often behave in a way that could make others think, incorrectly, that they are hearing voices, or experiencing some of the other symptoms of psychosis. The task is to work out whether someone's behavior is normal for them, or whether they are acting in a certain way because they are experiencing an episode of psychosis.

Talking to oneself or talking to imaginary friends, for example, may be developmentally appropriate for someone who has a learning disability. People who have a learning disability sometimes express their thoughts in a way that appears to be jumbled, which can be misattributed to disordered thinking as a symptom of psychosis. Also, people who have a learning disability are sometimes very concerned about what other people think – often because they have been treated unkindly, rejected or discriminated against in the past. This could be misinterpreted as paranoid thinking.

It is even more difficult to distinguish the symptoms of psychosis in people who have more severe learning disabilities and who are often unable to communicate properly. When making a diagnosis, it is crucial to look for changes in the way people normally behave, or changes in their personality. For example, socially inappropriate or disturbed behavior that is out of character could be an early sign of psychosis or, as noted above, of an affective disorder.

Patients with epilepsy and a learning disability who suffer from psychotic symptoms can present with negative symptoms – lack of energy, lack of motivation, loss of interest in themselves and other people, loss of interest in personal appearance, memory problems, and becoming socially withdrawn. These can seriously affect people's quality of life and also need to be distinguished from symptoms of a comorbid mood disorder such as depression. It is not always easy to clarify presence or absence of pervasive low mood that would aid in suggesting the presence of a mood disorder. As noted above, challenging behaviors in people with a learning disability can result from a variety of causes, among which can also be included the experiencing of psychotic symptoms.

Management

In general, similar approaches to the management of psychosis operate for people with a learning disability and epilepsy as for those with epilepsy without a learning disability. However, as noted above, it is particularly important to consider the differential diagnosis of the patient's presentation, considering issues such as environmental changes or stresses, physical illness and affective illness, and medication-related adverse effects including consideration of not only AEDs and psychotropic agents but also other medications. Patients with mild LD may be able to access mainstream mental health services for management of their psychosis, but those with a more severe learning disability are likely to do better with specialist services.

All patients suspected of having a psychotic illness should have access to a comprehensive multidisciplinary assessment. This should include assessment by a psychiatrist, a psychologist, or a professional with expertise in the psychological treatment of people with psychosis or schizophrenia.

Once the diagnosis, or working diagnosis – which in the context of severe learning disability may be the appropriate position to take as definitive diagnosis may not be possible – of psychotic disorder has been established it is important to intervene early. The mainstay of treatment is antipsychotic medication (preferably given orally) accompanied by psychological intervention and support to carers.

The choice of antipsychotic medication should where possible be made collaboratively with the individual and their carers taking into account likely drug interactions, benefits, and possible side effects of each drug including:

- Metabolic (including weight gain and diabetes)
- Extrapyramidal (including akathisia, dyskinesia, and dystonia)
- Cardiovascular (including prolonging the QT interval)
- Hormonal (including increasing plasma prolactin)
- Other (including unpleasant subjective experiences)

It is recommended by NICE that before starting antipsychotic medication the following baseline investigations are undertaken:

- Weight (plotted on a chart)
- Waist circumference
- Pulse and blood pressure
- Fasting blood glucose, glycosylated hemoglobin (HbA1c), blood lipid profile, and prolactin levels
- Assessment of any movement disorders
- Assessment of nutritional status, diet, and level of physical activity
- ECG

Particularly where a working diagnosis has been made, when it has not been possible to reach a definite diagnosis of psychosis, treatment with antipsychotic medication should be considered as an explicit individual therapeutic trial – with clear outcome goals identified at the start of treatment and against which the patient's progress should be regularly assessed. Management should include the following:

- Where possible discuss and record the side effects that the person is most willing to tolerate.
- Record the indications and expected benefits and risks of oral antipsychotic medication, and the expected time for a change in symptoms and appearance of side effects.
- Describe the pre-treatment investigations and likely treatment-related adverse effects and discuss with the aim of identifying with the patient and their carers anything that the patient may find it particularly hard to tolerate. This may lead to the need to reconsider the choice of antipsychotic. For instance some patients may not tolerate blood tests, blood pressure measurement, or other physical intrusions. In others, increased appetite and weight gain may present particular challenges.
- At the start of treatment give a dose at the lower end of the licensed range and slowly titrate upwards within the accepted dose range.
- Record the rationale for continuing, changing or stopping medication, and the effects of such changes.
- Carry out a trial of the medication at optimum dosage for 4–6 weeks.

Treatment guidelines generally recommend the following monitoring and recording regularly and systematically throughout treatment, but especially during titration:

- Response to treatment, including changes in symptoms and behavior
- Side effects of treatment, taking into account overlap between certain side effects and clinical features of schizophrenia (e.g., the overlap between akathisia and agitation or anxiety) and impact on functioning
- The emergence of movement disorders
- Weight, weekly for the first 6 weeks, then at 12 weeks, at 1 year, and then annually (plotted on a chart)
- Waist circumference annually (plotted on a chart)
- Pulse and blood pressure at 12 weeks, at 1 year, and then annually
- Fasting blood glucose, HbA1c, serum prolactin, and blood lipid levels at 12 weeks, at 1 year, and then annually
- Adherence to medication
- Overall physical health

It *must* be kept in mind that individuals with more severe learning disability will lack capacity to give informed consent to medication and in such cases it is important to deliver treatment in the best interests of the patient, following discussion with others including family, paid carers, patient advocates, other involved members of the clinical team, etc. It is important to maintain dialogue and to support the patient and their carers throughout the treatment. At times it may be appropriate to consider whether an in-patient assessment would be of use in supporting diagnosis and if indicated initiation of medication.

Despite medication patients can be left with residual psychotic symptoms, and psychological treatments such as modified CBT, art therapy, and music therapy can help them manage the impact of their symptoms better. Appropriate support is crucial. It is also imprtant to consider patients' adherence to oral medication regimens. If it appears that medication is helpful but the individual fails to adhere to it, consider treatment with depot. However, it is important to bear in mind that if adherence to antipsychotics is in question, then adherence to antiepileptics may well be in question too.

Autism and Epilepsy in People with LD

Prevalence

There appears to be an increased rate of epilepsy in people with autism, with estimates in children with autism ranging from 5 to 40 %. However, the relationship between autism and epilepsy is not clearly understood. Epilepsy is associated with older age, lower cognitive ability, poorer adaptive and language functioning, history of developmental regression and more severe autistic spectrum disorder symptoms such that for every one standard deviation increase in IQ, the odds of having epilepsy decrease by 47 % [27]. Most studies indicate that prevalence of epilepsy in autism is around 30 %.

Diagnosis

Core symptoms of autism include impairment in reciprocity of social interaction, stereotyped repetitive behaviors and clear circumscribed or unusual interests, and for a diagnosis of autism to be made these symptoms need to have been present since early childhood. However, it is increasingly being recognized that in people with more severe learning disability, of various etiologies, a range of autistic traits may be recognized but that the presence of these do not necessarily confer a definitive diagnosis of autism.

Management

The management of autism itself is currently limited to various approaches to alleviating particular symptoms. The approach to managing epilepsy in those with autism does not differ from the management of epilepsy in the absence of autism.

As with any other patients it is important to monitor for side effects of antiepileptic drugs and this may be more difficult in patients with more severe LD due to difficulties in communication. Patients with autism may be particularly fearful of touch or any medical investigations. Often, this can be resolved by systemic desensitization approaches and gently introducing them to the equipment.

Down Syndrome, Dementia, and Epilepsy

Prevalence

Down syndrome is the most common chromasomal cause of intellectual disability with a prevalence of 1 in every 650–1000 live births. Three peak periods for development of epilepsy in people with Down syndrome have been described; early childhood when infantile spasms have been reported, early adulthood when epilepsy more often takes the form of partial seizures, and, most frequently, from around 40 years of age, when Alzheimer-type neuropathological changes and clinical symptoms of dementia develop at significantly higher rates and at earlier ages in those with Down syndrome than in the rest of the population [28]. Indeed, 40 % of people over 50 years with Down syndrome and 75 % of those aged over 60 are suffering from Alzheimer's disease. The prevalence of epilepsy increases significantly in association with these Alzheimer-type changes in middle age. In one recent study 74 % of people with Down syndrome and a clinical diagnosis of dementia had epilepsy, with the epilepsy developing on average about 6 months after the dementia was diagnosed [29].

Diagnosis

Standard assessments such as the mini-mental state exam are not appropriate. It is important to explicitly look for a change in the individual's own baseline. The reliance is on collateral history obtained from an informant but this can be challenging at times because a reliable informant history may not be available. Diagnosis is much harder in patients with moderate and severe LD due to limited communication skills and difficulties for carers to notice and clinicians to interpret change. These individuals already receive a significant level of support with their day-to-day care and it can be difficult to notice any loss of skills particularly early on.

It is particularly important to rule out hypothyroidism and also sedation/seizure related confusion mimicking as cognitive decline in patients who have both Learning disability and epilepsy. It is also important to rule out other medical conditions such as pain, constipation, infections, and depression, which may present as behavioral and emotional problems.

Presentation of Dementia

Patients often do not complain of memory problems themselves, rather they may be brought to the attention of services due to a decline in their functioning or activities of daily living or due to emotional and behavioral changes. Onset of epilepsy may sometimes be the first sign of dementia.

Management

The mainstay in pharmacological management of dementia is by use of acetylcholinesterase inhibitors. However, it is important to note that these drugs may reduce seizure threshold, so it is important to monitor carefully for side effects alongside monitoring for any possible benefit.

As dementia is a progressive disease, it is important to work with carers supporting the patients to aid their understanding of the nature of the disease as well as environmental modifications that may be needed to aid the individual.

References

1. Morgan CL, Ahmed Z, Kerr MP. Health care provision for people with a learning disability. Record-linkage study of epidemiology and factors contributing to hospital care uptake. Br J Psychiatry. 2000;176:37–41.
2. Emerson E, Hatton C, Robertson J, Roberts H, Baines S, Glover G. People with learning disabilities in England: services and supports. Lancaster: Improving Health and Lives: Learning Disabilities Observatory; 2010.
3. National Institute for Health and Clinical Excellence (NICE). The epilepsies: the diagnosis and management of the epilepsies in adults and children. London: NICE; 2012.
4. Lhatoo SD, Sander JW. The epidemiology of epilepsy and learning disability. Epilepsia. 2001;42 Suppl 1:6–9; discussion 19–20.
5. McGrother CW, Bhaumik S, Thorp CF, Hauck A, Branford D, Watson JM. Epilepsy in adults with intellectual disabilities: prevalence, associations and service implications. Seizure. 2006;15:376–86.
6. Adachi N, Matsuura M, Okubo Y, et al. Predictive variables of interictal psychosis in epilepsy. Neurology. 2000;55:1310–55.
7. Deb S, Hunter D. Psychopathology of people with mental handicap and epilepsy: II. Psychiatric illness. Br J Psychiatry. 1991;159:826–30.
8. Espie C, Watkins J, Curtices L, et al. Psychopathology in people with epilepsy and intellectual disability: an investigation of potential explantory variable. J Neurol Neurosurg Psychiatry. 2003;74:1485–92.
9. Matsuura M, Adachi N, Muramatsu R, Kato M, Onuma T, Okubo Y, et al. Intellectual disability and psychotic disorders of adult epilepsy. Epilepsia. 2005;46 Suppl 1:11–4.
10. Rodin E, editor. The prognosis of people with epilepsy. Springfield: Charles C Thomas; 1968. p. 156–74.

11. Ring H, Zia A, Lindeman S, Himlok K. Interactions between seizure frequency, psychopathology, and severity of intellectual disability in a population with epilepsy and a learning disability. Epilepsy Behav. 2007;11(1):92–7.
12. de Boer HM, Mula M, Sander JW. The global burden and stigma of epilepsy. Epilepsy Behav. 2008;12(4):540–6.
13. Jian L, Nagarajan L, de Klerk N, Ravine D, Bower C, Anderson A, et al. Predictors of seizure onset in Rett Syndrome. J Pediatr. 2006;149(4):542–7.
14. Chapman M, Iddon P, Atkinson K, Brodie C, Mitchell D, Parvin G, Willis S. The misdiagnosis of epilepsy in people with intellectual disabilities: a systematic review. Seizure. 2011;20(2):101–6.
15. Sillanpaa M. Learning disability: occurrence and long-term consequences in childhood-onset epilepsy. Epilepsy Behav. 2004;5(6):937–44.
16. Nashef L, Fish DR, Garner S, Sander JW, Shorvon SD. Sudden death in epilepsy—a study of incidence in a young cohort with epilepsy and learning difficulty. Epilepsia. 1995;36(12):1187–94.
17. Forsgren L, Edvinsson SO, Nyström L, Blomquist HK. Influence of epilepsy on mortality in mental retardation: an epidemiologic study. Epilepsia. 1996;37(10):956–63.
18. Bredkjaer S, Mortensen P, Parnas J. Epilepsy and non-organic nonaffective psychosis: national epidemiologic study. Br J Psychiatry. 1998;172:235–8.
19. Vuilleumier P, Jallon P. Epilepsy and psychiatric disorders: epidemiological data. Rev Neurol. 1998;154:305–17.
20. Kerr M, Guidelines Working Group, Scheepers M, Arvio M, Beavis J, Brandt C, Brown S, Huber B, Iivanainen M, Louisse AC, Martin P, Marson AG, Prasher V, Singh BK, Veendrick M, Wallace RA. Consensus guidelines into the management of epilepsy in adults with an intellectual disability. J Intellect Disabil Res. 2009;53(8):687–94.
21. Jacoby A, Baker GA, Steen N, Potts P, Chadwick DW. The clinical course of epilepsy and its psychosocial correlates: findings from a U.K. community study. Epilepsia. 1996;37:148–61.
22. Ring HA, Moriarty J, Trimble MR. A prospective study of the early postsurgical psychiatric associations of epilepsy surgery. J Neurol Neurosurg Psychiatr. 1998;64(5):601–4.
23. Clancy MJ, Clarke MC, Connor DJ, Cannon M, Cotter DR. The prevalence of psychosis in epilepsy; a systematic review and meta-analysis. BMC Psychiatry. 2014;14:75. doi:10.1186/1471-244X-14-75.
24. Onuma T, Adachi N, Ishida S, Katou M, Uesugi S. Prevalence and annual incidence of psychosis in patients with epilepsy. Psychiatry Clin Neurosci. 1995;49(3):267–8.
25. Sachdev P. Schizophrenia-like psychosis and epilepsy: the status of the association [review]. Am J Psychiatry. 1998;155:325–36.
26. Kanemoto K, Tsuji T, Kawasaki J. Reexamination of interictal psychoses based on DSM IV psychosis classification and international epilepsy classification. Epilepsia. 2001;42:98–103.
27. Viscidi EW, Triche EW, Pescosolido MF, McLean RL, Joseph RM, Spence SJ, Morrow EM. Clinical characteristics of children with autism spectrum disorder and co-occurring epilepsy. PLoS One. 2013;8(7):e67797.
28. Menendez M. Down syndrome, Alzheimer's disease and seizures. Brain Dev. 2005;27:246–52.
29. McCarron M, McCallion P, Reilly E, Mulryan N. A prospective 14-year longitudinal follow-up of dementia in persons with Down syndrome. J Intellect Disabil Res. 2014;58(1):61–70.

Chapter 13
Attention, Executive Function, and Attention Deficit Hyperactivity Disorder

David W. Dunn and William G. Kronenberger

Abstract People with epilepsy have an increased risk of problems with attention and executive function. Approximately one third meet criteria for attention deficit hyperactivity disorder (ADHD). Also, children with ADHD have an increased risk for seizures. Risk factors for difficulties with attention and executive functioning are common genetic vulnerability or underlying central nervous system damage, early age of seizure onset, more severe and more frequent seizures, and adverse effect of antiepileptic drugs. Phenobarbital, benzodiazepine, and topiramate have been associated with attention problems. Problems with attention and executive function are associated with cognitive and academic disability. Methylphenidate is first choice medication to treat attention difficulties and rarely has a negative impact on seizure control. Atomoxetine is a second choice medication. Alpha-2 agonists, amphetamines, and low dose tricyclic antidepressants can be tried if neither methylphenidate nor atomoxetine are successful. Educational interventions may also be required.

Keywords Attention • Executive function • ADHD • Academic function • Epilepsy

Introduction

Epilepsy is a pervasive disorder characterized by seizures, cognitive difficulties, and behavioral problems. In this chapter we will review disturbances in attention and executive function and the comorbidity of attention deficit hyperactivity disorder (ADHD) and epilepsy. We will ask several questions. How are ADHD, attention,

D.W. Dunn, MD (✉)
Departments of Psychiatry and Neurology, Indiana University School of Medicine, Riley Child and Adolescent Psychiatry Clinic, 705 Riley Hospital Drive, ROC 4300, Indianapolis, IN 46202, USA
e-mail: ddunn@iupui.edu

W.G. Kronenberger, PhD
Section of Psychology, Department of Psychiatry, Indiana University School of Medicine, Riley Child and Adolescent Psychiatry Clinic, 705 Riley Hospital Drive, ROC 4300, Indianapolis, IN 46202, USA
e-mail: wkronenb@iupui.edu

M. Mula (ed.), *Neuropsychiatric Symptoms of Epilepsy*, Neuropsychiatric Symptoms of Neurological Disease, DOI 10.1007/978-3-319-22159-5_13

and executive function defined and measured? Is the risk of ADHD and difficulties with attention and executive function greater in people with epilepsy? What are the potential explanations for the comorbidity of ADHD, problems with attention and executive function in patients with epilepsy? What are the optimal treatments for ADHD or impairments in attention and executive function in patients with epilepsy? Are there changes over time in attention and executive function? Finally, what are the areas needing additional research?

Attention Deficit Hyperactivity Disorder (ADHD)

The current Diagnostic and Statistical Manual of Mental Disorders, 5th edition (DSM 5) lists ADHD as a neurodevelopmental disorder defined by the presence of six of nine symptoms of inattention and six of nine symptoms of hyperactivity and impulsivity, beginning prior to 12 years of age, and causing impairment of function in at least two settings [1]. For people over 17 years of age, only five symptoms of inattention or hyperactivity and impulsivity are needed to meet criteria for diagnosis. If both inattention and hyperactivity/impulsivity are present, the diagnosis is ADHD, combined presentation and if only one of the sets of symptoms meets the threshold of 6 symptoms, the ADHD is called predominantly inattentive presentation or predominantly hyperactive/impulsive presentation. ADHD occurs in 5–10 % of children and 3–5 % of adults and is twice as common in males compared to females, particularly when hyperactive-impulsive symptoms are present. In a child and adolescent psychiatry clinic, ADHD, combined presentation is most common. In children, ADHD is often comorbid with the disruptive behavior disorders, oppositional defiant disorder, and conduct disorder, and specific learning disorder also occurs more frequently when ADHD is present. Comorbidities in adults include substance-related disorders, mood disorders, and anxiety disorders.

Attention and Executive Functioning

Attention and executive functioning are multifaceted neuropsychological ability areas. While ADHD is a categorical measure with a diagnosis made once criteria are met, attention and executive functioning are dimensional measures with no exact demarcation between normal and abnormal. Attention includes the processes involved in perceiving and selecting stimuli, maintaining and shifting focus, and inhibiting responses to extraneous stimuli. Executive functioning is a broader term that encompasses multiple dimensions without a single well-accepted definition [2, 3]. One representative definition describes executive functions as the cognitive abilities "necessary to organize, control, and sustain the processing of information in a planned, goal-directed manner" [4]. The core components of executive functioning include shifting mental sets, updating and monitoring information in working memory, and inhibiting impulsive responses [5]. Other components of executive functioning that have been identified in some studies include self-regulation, planning, organization, concept formation, controlled attention, controlled cognitive fluency, emotional control, initiation, and self-monitoring [2, 6].

Attention depends on multiple, widely distributed networks within the central nervous system. The parietal lobe, basal ganglia, and cerebellum are components of the attentional systems with control of attention centered in the prefrontal cortex. The types of attention most often assessed in people with epilepsy include selective attention, divided attention, and sustained attention. Sustained attention is most frequently reported to be impaired in people with epilepsy [7]. Sustained attention is mediated by the frontoparietal networks, predominantly the right hemisphere. The anterior cingulate cortex is essential in selective and divided attention. The prefrontal cortex with its network connections to basal ganglia, limbic system, and cerebellum is the anatomic locus for executive functions. The networks for executive functioning develop gradually throughout childhood into early adult years.

Assessment for ADHD, Attention, and Executive Function

A diagnosis of ADHD is based on history, consideration of differential diagnosis, and rating scales. Practice parameters and best practices recommendations for evaluation of ADHD recommend several primary components: (1) clinical diagnostic interviews with the patient and parent, (2) review of background information (family history, social history, medical history, developmental history), (3) evaluation of possible comorbid or alternative psychiatric disorders, and (4) investigation of behavior and functioning at school or work [8, 9]. Behavior rating scales are not required for the diagnosis of ADHD but can be extremely valuable components because they provide structured, quantified data that can be obtained rapidly and easily from multiple sources.

Most behavior rating scales designed specifically for ADHD assessment use the 9 inattentive items and the 9 hyperactive impulsive items found in the DSM 5, worded for ratings on a 3- or 4-point scale by caregivers or other observers. Examples of rating scales include the ADHD Rating Scale IV [10] and the NICHQ Vanderbilt Assessment scales [11]. Broad scale measures that assess for ADHD and multiple other psychiatric disorders or symptoms are the Child and Adolescent Symptom Rating Scales [12], the Child Behavior Checklist (CBCL) [13], the Strengths and Difficulties Questionnaire (SDQ) [14], and the Behavior Assessment System for Children, Second Edition (BASC-2) [15]. Other rating scales focus on neurocognitive functions that are impaired in ADHD, such as executive functions; for example, the Behavior Rating Inventory of Executive Function (BRIEF) has been used to assess patients with epilepsy [6].

Numerous performance-based neuropsychological tests that assess attention and executive functioning have been used clinically and in research with patients with epilepsy [16], and neuropsychological assessment is a valuable clinical tool in evaluation and management of epilepsy [17]. Continuous performance tests measure vigilance, concentration, and inhibition by requiring patients to respond to target items and withhold response to nontarget items presented sequentially over time. Tests such as the Stroop Color-Word Test assess the ability to withhold prepotent responses in order to provide more effortful responses, reflecting controlled attention and inhibitory control. Large neuropsychological test batteries such as the Delis-Kaplan Executive Functioning System [18] consist of a number of neuropsychological tests to evaluate strengths and weaknesses across a wide variety of functions, including attention and executive functioning. Working memory tests present the patient with a stimulus (typically a series of verbal or visual stimuli) that must be remembered and recalled at the same time that another cognitive activity is taking place; for example, N-back working memory tests require the subject to indicate when a stimulus is the same as a prior stimulus presented N-times prior in a sequence. There are a large number of other neuropsychological tests and batteries that can be used to identify attention and executive function deficits in patients with epilepsy, some of which have been specifically designed for the assessment of neuropsychological functioning in epilepsy [17, 19].

Results of performance-based neuropsychological tests, which are administered in office settings, show only modest agreement with behavioral reports provided by parents, teachers, and patients [2, 3]. Formal neuropsychological testing generally does not add to the diagnostic accuracy of ADHD and is not a required part of practice parameters or best practice recommendations for ADHD diagnostic assessment. Rather, clinical interview, evaluation of history, and observation are generally considered to provide a more valid diagnostic assessment of ADHD [2, 8, 9]. Neuropsychological testing yields specific information about abilities under controlled conditions, whereas behavior checklists, interviews, and observations provide a more global assessment of behavior in day-to-day life [2].

Prevalence of ADHD in Epilepsy Samples

A wide range of prevalence rates has been reported for ADHD in people with epilepsy, depending on differences in methodology of ADHD assessment or differences in sample composition. One epidemiological study provides data on incidence of ADHD and epilepsy. Chou et al. [20] used a health insurance database of children and adolescents less than 19 years of age identifying samples with epilepsy, with a diagnosis of ADHD, and controls. Over a 7-year follow-up, the incidence of ADHD was 7.76 % in the sample with epilepsy and 3.22 % in the controls, a hazard ratio of 2.54 (95 % Cl 2.02–3.18). Several population-based studies have reported prevalence of ADHD in people with epilepsy. Reilly et al. [21] assessed behavior in a population-based sample of children 5–15 years of age with epilepsy and noted ADHD in 33 %. Cohen et al. [22] found ADHD in 27.7 % of people with epilepsy versus 12.6 % in the general population. Russ et al. [23] described a diagnosis of ADHD in 23 % of children with epilepsy or seizures compared to 6 % of controls.

Turkey et al. [24] noted ADHD in 44 %. Davies et al. [25] reported symptoms of ADHD in 12 % of patients with complicated epilepsy, 2 % of controls, and none of the patients with uncomplicated epilepsy. In a population-based survey, McDermott et al. [26] described 28.1 % of children with epilepsy as hyperactive compared to 5 % of controls, and Carlton-Ford et al. [27] noted impulsivity in 39 % of children with epilepsy compared to 11 % of controls, though neither study made a specific diagnosis of ADHD.

There are fewer reports of ADHD in adults with epilepsy. In three of four population-based surveys of psychiatric comorbidity in adults with epilepsy, the risk of ADHD has been found to be higher than in controls. In the Canadian Community Health survey, adults with epilepsy had an increased risk of anxiety and suicidal ideation, but symptoms of ADHD were apparently not assessed [28]. Ottman et al. [29] compared 3488 adults with epilepsy from the United States to a control group of 169,471. ADHD was reported by 13.2 % of adults with epilepsy and 5.5 % of controls for a prevalence ratio of 2.39 (2.03–2.81). Raj et al. [30] reported a population-based survey of psychiatric comorbidity in adults with epilepsy from England. They found symptoms of ADHD on a screening instrument in 15.4 % of adults with epilepsy for an adjusted odds ratio of 1.6 (0.9–3.0). Ettinger et al. [31] assessed adults with epilepsy using a 6-item screen for ADHD. They found that 18.4 % of the adults with ADHD had a positive screen for ADHD. They also noted that adults with a positive screen for ADHD had more symptoms of anxiety and depression, lower quality of life, and more social impairment than adults with epilepsy and no symptoms of ADHD.

The prevalence of ADHD in people with epilepsy is also higher in clinical samples, most often from tertiary epilepsy centers. In these studies, the ADHD diagnosis is most often based on psychiatric interview, rating scales, or structured interviews. The majority of studies report a prevalence of ADHD of 20–40 % in sample with epilepsy and 6–12 % rate in controls [32–42]. Two studies reported prevalence below the usual range. Freilinger et al. [43] noted symptoms of ADHD in the at-risk or clinical range in 12 % of children and adolescents with various epilepsy syndromes, and Benn et al. [44] found ADHD in 12.4 % of the epilepsy sample and 7.8 % of controls, a nonsignificant difference. Their sample consists of patients followed for 8–9 years after seizure onset and 65 % of the sample had been in remission for at least 5 years. In contrast, Sherman et al. [45] noted ADHD in 71 % of their sample. The seizure patients had severe epilepsy or were undergoing seizure surgery evaluation.

In the studies documenting ADHD type, three found more ADHD, predominantly inattentive type. Dunn et al. [34] noted ADHD, predominantly inattentive type in 24 %; ADHD, combined type in 11.4 %; and ADHD, predominantly hyperactive-impulsive type in 2.4 % of children with epilepsy. Hermann et al. [37] in a new-onset seizure sample found that 52 % had the inattentive type, 17 % hyperactive impulsive, 13 % combined type, and 17 % not specified. In a sample of children with severe epilepsy, 34.5 % had ADHD, predominantly inattentive type versus 34 % combined and 2.5 % hyperactive impulsive [45]. The one report that found more combined type (58 %) compared to inattentive type (42 %) was based on a sample referred for an ADHD medication trial and may have been biased toward more disruptive children [46].

Children with ADHD frequently have other comorbid psychiatric disorders. Few groups have commented on additional behavioral disorders in children with epilepsy and ADHD. Caplan et al. [47] assessed children with complex partial seizures and found ADHD with comorbid oppositional defiant disorder or conduct disorder in 17 % compared to 6 % of controls and ADHD with comorbid anxiety or depressive disorders in 23 % compared to 3 % of controls. Gonzalez-Heydrich et al. [46] noted ADHD with comorbid anxiety disorder in 36 % and oppositional defiant disorder in 31 %.

Summary

The data from studies of prevalence of ADHD in people with epilepsy consistently show that ADHD is 2–3 times more common in people with epilepsy than in controls. Demographic data generally show that the male–female ratio is equal in studies with ADHD and epilepsy, whereas males are more often affected in samples with isolated ADHD seen in psychiatric clinics. Though only a few of the studies report ADHD subtypes, there seems to be more ADHD predominantly inattentive presentation in the epilepsy groups and more ADHD, combined presentation in psychiatric samples. There are two things missing in the data. Impairment in at least two areas is a criterion for diagnosis in the DSM 5 but is not usually addressed in current studies of ADHD in epilepsy. Second, symptoms of ADHD persist into adulthood, but as of the time of this review, there is very little information on natural history of symptoms of ADHD in people with epilepsy and very few reports on ADHD in adults with epilepsy.

Prevalence of Problems with Attention and Executive Functioning

Problems with attention are consistently reported as higher in clinical samples of children or adolescents with epilepsy than in controls or normative data. Questionnaires such as the Child Behavior Checklist and the Strengths and Difficulties Questionnaire are often used as measures of attention problems, hyperactivity, and impulsivity. On the attention problems subscale of the CBCL or on the hyperactivity-inattention subscale of the SDQ, 30–42 % of children and adolescents with epilepsy have been found to score in the "at risk" or "clinical" range compared to 5–10 % of controls [35, 38, 40, 42]. Two studies reported values outside this range. Freilinger et al. [43] noted elevated attention problems scores on the CBCL in 11.2 % of a sample of patients with epilepsy 8–18 years of age. Dunn et al. [34] reported CBCL attention problem scores in the "at risk" or "clinical" range in 58 % of children and 42 % of adolescents with epilepsy. The higher prevalence reported by Dunn et al. [34] may be partially explained by the age of patients. Several other studies have found more attention or hyperactivity problems in younger patients with epilepsy [35, 41].

Though most studies have used parents as informants, there are reports that use teachers as informants. Teachers reported inattention in 42 % of children with epilepsy in the report by Holdsworth and Whitmore [48] and inattention or hyperactivity in 58 % of the children described by Sturniolo and Galletti [49]. Dunn et al. [50] prospectively followed children with new-onset seizures using teachers as raters of behavior. The ratings were obtained at baseline, 12, and 24 months. Teachers noted attention problems in 21 % of children with recurring seizures at baseline dropping slightly to 19 % at 24 months; attention problems were reported in 13 % of the children with a single episode of seizures.

Other studies have used computerized performance tasks to assess attention and impulsivity in children and adolescents with epilepsy. Again, most show more problems in children and adolescents with epilepsy than in controls or normative scores. In general, these studies have found more problems with attention than with impulsivity [51]. In one of the few studies to use as controls both an ADHD group and healthy peers, Semrud-Clikeman and Wical [52] found that children and adolescents with ADHD and complex partial seizures had more impaired attention than patients with complex partial seizures without ADHD or than patients with ADHD and no seizures. Both the patients with seizures and those with ADHD had more impairment than healthy controls.

Results of neuropsychological studies suggest differences in types of attention that are impaired in patients with epilepsy. Sánchez-Carpintero and Neville [7] reviewed studies of attention in patients with epilepsy and found that sustained attention was most consistently reported as impaired. Selective and divided attentions were affected less often. Triplett and Asato [53] evaluated patients 8–17 years of age with new-onset seizures and normal development prior to instituting antiepileptic drugs and found the lowest scores in tasks of complex attention. Similarly, Stiers et al. [54] found that complex attention but not simple attention was more impaired in patients with epilepsy and hippocampal malrotation than in patients with epilepsy without malrotation or in typically developing controls.

Studies of other components of executive functioning also frequently show deficits in children with epilepsy relative to healthy controls, particularly when ADHD is present. Bechtel et al. [55], for example, compared children with ADHD and epilepsy to those with ADHD alone and found comparable levels of working memory abilities. Because of the broad neuropsychological risks related to epilepsy, neuropsychological testing, including evaluation of attention and executive functioning, is an important component of epilepsy evaluation [17].

The specific prevalence of broad executive function impairment in children with epilepsy is difficult to characterize because there is no clear definition of executive function, multiple measures have been used, and for many tests there are no clear demarcations between normal and impaired. Parrish et al. [56] found that 48 % of 8–18 year old epilepsy patients had scores on the BRIEF in the "at risk" or "clinical" range versus 8 % of controls. Poor executive functioning was not predicted by age, gender, or seizure duration or type. Høie et al. [57] used five separate measures of executive functioning and defined abnormality as scores at or below the tenth percentile. They found executive function problems in 33 % of the 6–12 year old epilepsy patients and 11 % of controls. In a previous study, they showed that problems with executive functions were associated with early seizure onset, more frequent seizures, and use of multiple antiepileptic drugs and were found in patients with all seizures types except for benign epilepsy with centrotemporal spikes (BECTS). Campiglia et al. [58] found impaired executive function in children with frontal or temporal lobe epilepsies with few differences between the two seizure groups. In contrast, Longo et al. [59] found more executive function problems in youth with frontal lobe epilepsy than in those with temporal lobe seizures. Conant et al. [60] evaluated executive function in children with absence epilepsy compared to children with diabetes mellitus and controls. The children were similar in intelligence, memory, and processing speed, but the children with seizures were more impaired on multiple measures of executive function. Chowdhury et al. [61] assessed adults with idiopathic generalized epilepsy and found more impairment in executive function in patients than in first-degree relatives or healthy controls.

Most studies of attention or executive function in children with epilepsy are cross sectional and do not describe change over time. Williams et al. [33] followed 42 children 5–16 years of age with new-onset seizures and ADHD assessing symptoms at baseline and a mean of 7 months later. Inattention and hyperactivity-impulsivity were present in 31 % at baseline. At follow-up, 27 % were still inattentive and 24 % hyperactive-impulsive. Dunn et al. [50], using teacher ratings of attention in children with new-onset seizures, showed a minor drop in attention problems from 21 % at baseline to 19 % at 24 months. One study found an increase in attention problems as measured by a computerized performance task with 21 % having inattention at baseline prior to treatment with antiepileptic drugs and 42 % at 1-year follow-up [62]. Austin et al. [63] found attention problems in 22 % of children with new-onset seizures at baseline with a drop to 11 % at 36 months. Only 4.7 % had symptoms of ADHD at all follow-up visits.

Summary

Studies of attention and executive function in children and adolescents with epilepsy show a clear pattern of increased risk of problems in those with epilepsy with approximately 30–40 % having attention problems and executive function difficulties. There is a suggestion that sustained attention and complex attention may be impacted more than selective or divided attention or simple attention, but the data is limited. Problems with the literature include small sample sizes, few adult studies, and a multiplicity of measures for attention of attention or executive function restricting the ability to compare results across studies. There seems to be improvement over time but there are too few studies for a definite conclusion.

Risk Factors for ADHD in Children with Epilepsy

There are several potential explanations for the comorbidity of epilepsy and ADHD, disorders of attention, or deficits in executive functioning. There may be concurrent comorbidity in which both epilepsy and impaired attention and executive function are due to a common underlying problem. Alternatively, the association may be due to successive comorbidity in which either epilepsy or ADHD causes or creates a vulnerability to developing the other condition. There are several potential explanations for problems with attention and executive functioning (see Table 13.1).

Concurrent Comorbidity

Suggestive evidence for concurrent comorbidity comes from studies that show symptoms of ADHD present prior to or at the onset of seizures and from studies demonstrating a bidirectional association between epilepsy and ADHD. Population-based surveys have shown that children with ADHD have over twice the risk of developing seizures than controls. Chou et al. [20] followed 3664 children and adolescents with ADHD and 14,522 age matched controls for 3–3.5 years. The incidence of epilepsy was 3.24 % in the ADHD sample in 0.78 % in controls for a hazard ratio of 3.94 (95 % CI 2.58–6.03). Hesdorrfer et al. [64] noted that the association between ADHD and subsequent epilepsy existed for ADHD predominantly inattentive type but not for ADHD combined or hyperactive-impulsive types. Davis et al. [65] used data from the Rochester Epidemiology Project to compare children with ADHD to controls. The children found with ADHD were 2.7 times more likely to develop epilepsy than controls. The children with ADHD developed seizures earlier and had more severe seizures than controls with epilepsy, and the children with ADHD and epilepsy were less likely to receive treatment for ADHD than those with ADHD alone.

Several studies have obtained EEGs in patients with ADHD and found focal spikes in approximately 5–10 % of recordings [66–70]. Two studies of new-onset seizures found evidence of ADHD prior to first seizure. Austin et al. [71] noted symptoms of ADHD in 10.7 % of children with new-onset seizures compared to 3.0

Table 13.1 Risk factors for problems with attention and executive function and ADHD

Risk factors for problems with attention and executive function and ADHD
1. Common genetic vulnerability
2. Central nervous system damage
3. Early age of seizure onset
4. Severe or frequent seizures
5. Frequent epileptiform discharges
6. Adverse effect of antiepileptic drugs

% of sibling controls. Hermann et al. [37] found that 82 % of the children with new-onset seizures and ADHD had evidence of ADHD prior to first seizure.

One possible explanation for the association of epilepsy and ADHD is a common genetic vulnerability. The genetic bases of ADHD and epilepsy are being rapidly defined by use of genome-wide association studies. The rapid progress in genetics suggests possible links between epilepsy and ADHD. Lo-Castro and Curatolo [72] reviewed prior studies and found genes involved in synapse formation, neurotransmission, and DNA methylation and remodeling that conveyed vulnerability for epilepsy and ADHD. In a small sample of 16 mothers of children with epilepsy and ADHD, 8 of the 16 mothers had a current or past history of ADHD [73]. In contrast, Hesdorffer et al. [74] assessed family history of behavioral problems in first degree relatives of patients with seizures. They found a familial clustering of symptoms of multiple behavioral problems in patients with unprovoked seizures, but did not find an increase in attention problems or ADHD in relatives.

Underlying central nervous system damage may be a factor in both epilepsy and ADHD. One epidemiological study found that ADHD was significantly more common in children with complicated epilepsy compared to those with no additional neurological impairment [25]. The two clinical series reported on symptoms in children with severe epilepsy. Ferrie et al. [75] found hyperactivity in 77 % of children with intractable epilepsies and Sherman et al. [45] noted ADHD in 71 % of children being assessed for seizure surgery or having severe epilepsy.

Children with epilepsy and ADHD have been assessed with structural and functional imaging. One group initially found increased gray matter in the frontal lobes of children with epilepsy and ADHD, but later reported an association between symptoms of attention problems and decreased cortical thickness in the frontal and left parietal lobes and an association between higher ADHD scores and decreased cortical thickness in the frontal and occipital lobes [37, 76]. Functional magnetic resonance imaging (fMRI) has been used to assess attention and executive function. Bechtel et al. compared boys with epilepsy and ADHD and boys with ADHD alone. They found similar areas of reduced activation in response to a working memory task in the two groups [55]. Killory et al. [77] evaluated attention in children with absence epilepsy and found reduced activity in the medial frontal cortex and impaired connectivity between the medical frontal cortex and the right anterior insula/frontal operculum. Using fMRI, McGill et al. [78] studied the default mode network and found decreased functional connectivity between the cingulate cortex and frontal lobe similar to what would be found in patients with impaired attention.

Successive Comorbidity

Potential reasons for successive comorbidity could include impaired attention and executive function secondary to seizures, to adverse effects of antiepileptic drugs, or to psychological or social reactions to having seizures. Seizure-related variables could include age of onset, duration or severity of seizures, seizure type or locus, or epileptiform discharge on EEG. Antiepileptic drugs may have a negative impact on attention and executive functioning, or, alternatively, might be beneficial. The occurrence of ADHD is not secondary to psychosocial stressors, but severity of ADHD symptoms has been related to adverse circumstances of life. Epilepsy may be an additional stress that contributes to severity of ADHD or executive dysfunction.

Age of onset of seizures has been associated with cognitive problems but not emotional difficulties. Though it might be expected that early onset of seizures might negatively impact development of attention networks, age of onset has not been consistently associated with problems of attention or executive function in people with epilepsy. Tsai et al. [79] and Tanabe et al. [42] found an association between early age of onset and problems with attention. Black et al. [80] and Campiglia et al. [58] noted an association of early age of onset with executive function impairment. However, other studies have found no association with age of onset [37, 81]. This may be partially due to sample characteristics. Hermann et al. [37] assessed children with new-onset seizures starting after 8 years of age, and Cerminara et al [81] restricted their sample to children with BECTS, which typically starts after 3–4 years of age.

Duration of epilepsy, frequency of seizures, and severity of epilepsy may contribute to difficulties with attention and executive function. The prevalence of ADHD was highest in children with severe epilepsies and lowest in a sample that followed children after remission of seizures [44, 45]. In children with childhood onset absence epilepsy, Caplan et al. [40] found an association of ADHD with duration and frequency of absence seizures. Vega et al. [82] found that children with uncontrolled absence seizures were more impatient than those with controlled seizures, and Masur et al. [83] noted more attention difficulties in those children that continued to have absence seizures in spite of AED treatment. In the initial evaluation of childhood absence epilepsy, future attention problems were associated with duration of seizures but not seizure frequency on initial EEG.

The association of seizure type and focus of epileptiform discharge with attention and executive function has been assessed. Hernandez et al. [84] showed that children with frontal lobe epilepsy had more attention problems than those with temporal or generalized seizures, and Gottlieb et al. [85] found more impairment of executive function in children with frontal lobe seizures than in those with temporal lobe foci. In contrast, Dunn et al. [34], Hermann et al. [37], Jones et al. [39], and Almace et al. [86] found no association between seizure type or localization and attention/executive functioning, and Jackson et al. [87] found more executive function difficulties in children with idiopathic generalized than in those with idiopathic focal epilepsy. Hoie et al. [88] noted no problems with executive function in children with benign focal seizures, although it would seem likely that frontal lobe dysfunction would lead to inattention or executive function impairment.

Epileptiform discharges may be important in attention and executive function. In a study combining video-EEG with neuropsychological function, frequent nonconvulsive seizures were associated with attention and cognitive impairment [89].

Studies of children and adolescents with BECTS have found an association between frequency of EEG discharges and problems with attention. In addition, as the epileptiform discharges abate, attention returns to normal [90]. In a sample of children with frontal lobe seizures, Zhang et al. [91] found that 89 % of children with frontal spikes on the most recent EEG had ADHD compared to 25 % of children with a normal EEG. Ibrahim et al. [92] combined fMRI and magnetoencephalography to show that changes in intrinsic connectivity networks including default mode and dorsal attention networks secondary to epileptiform discharges were associated with cognitive impairment.

Both inattention and hyperactivity have been adverse side effects of phenobarbital and the benzodiazepines [93, 94]. Impaired attention and executive functioning and decreased speed of responsiveness have been related to use of topiramate [95]. Glauser et al. [96] showed that sodium valproic acid had more negative effect on attention than ethosuximide or lamotrigine in children with absence epilepsy. In contrast, one small study of children with ADHD and spikes on EEG found that when treatment with valproic acid reduced spikes, there was improvement in attention [97]. In an fMRI study, Wandschneider et al. [98] found normalization of deactivation of the default mode network in patients receiving levetiracetam.

Psychosocial stressors related to epilepsy are probably not a factor in causing problems with attention or executive function. Rodenberg et al. [99] performed a meta-analysis of 46 studies of psychopathology in children with epilepsy and other chronic illness. They found that attention problems were relatively specific to epilepsy whereas anxiety and depression were in part associated with the presence of chronic illness. It is possible that anxiety and depression, both common comorbidities in children, adolescents, and adults with epilepsy, could negatively impact the ability to attend and concentrate.

Treatment of Problems of Attention in Children with Epilepsy

Children with ADHD alone respond well to the stimulant medication. Biederman and Faraone [100] report effect sizes of 0.9–0.95 for stimulants and 0.6 for nonstimulants used to treat children, adolescents, and adults with ADHD. Consensus statements suggest starting with either methylphenidate or amphetamine, switching to the stimulant not previously used if patients fail to respond or have side effects and utilizing atomoxetine if stimulants are not effective or cause adverse effects [101]. Next choices are antidepressants such as bupropion or tricyclic antidepressants and adrenergic agents such as clonidine and guanfacine. A similar approach with some modifications can probably be used in patients with epilepsy. However, the data for this recommendation are much weaker for people with epilepsy and ADHD than for patients with ADHD alone. See Table 13.2 for treatment of attention problems with people with epilepsy.

For the most part, the old worries that stimulants might worsen seizures have abated. There is very little data to suggest that stimulants may lower the seizure

Table 13.2 Treatment of attention problems with people with epilepsy

Treatment of attention problems with people with epilepsy
1. Optimize seizure control
2. Review antiepileptic drugs for adverse effect on attention
3. Review history for possible learning disability, assess and treat if needed
4. Start methylphenidate if evidence of ADHD
5. If no effect or adverse effect from MPH, switch to atomoxetine
6. If no effect or adverse effect from atomoxetine, consider alpha-2 agonist
7. If no effect or adverse effect, consider amphetamine or low dose tricyclic antidepressant

threshold, and the data to support this concern are limited. Several studies assessed the effect of methylphenidate on symptoms of ADHD in children with reasonably well-controlled seizures. Feldman et al. [102] and Gross-Tsur et al. [103] gave children with ADHD and well-controlled epilepsy methylphenidate 0.3–0.6 mg/kg/day and found improvement in attention with no adverse effect on seizure control. Gucuyener et al. [70] treated 57 children with ADHD and epilepsy with methylphenidate 0.3–1 mg/kg/day and found no change in mean seizure frequency during the 12-month trial. Two recent studies evaluated response to methylphenidate in patients with more severe, persistent seizures. Fosi et al. [104], in a study of 18 patients, 6–18 years of age with intractable seizures, intellectual disability, and ADHD, found that 61 % responded favorably to methylphenidate 0.3–1 mg/kg/day, with no worsening of seizures. Santos et al. [105] assessed response to methylphenidate up to 1 mg/kg/day in 22 patients with severe seizures. They found that 73 % had significant improvement in symptoms of ADHD and also noted a reduction in seizure severity.

There is much less data on amphetamine to treat ADHD in children with epilepsy. In one retrospective study of 36 patients less than 18 years of age with epilepsy, the response to amphetamine in 17 patients was compared to methylphenidate in 19 patients [106]. There was a significant difference in improvement of ADHD symptoms with 63 % of patients on methylphenidate improved versus 24 % on amphetamine. Seizure-related factors and cognitive status did not predict response to stimulant. An increase in seizure frequency was seen in one patient on amphetamine and one on methylphenidate.

Gonzalez-Heydrich et al. [107] performed a placebo-controlled trial of methylphenidate OROS in 33 patients 6–18 years of age with epilepsy. Patients received 18, 36, or 54 mg of methylphenidate or placebo for 1 week and were monitored for seizures and for response of symptoms of ADHD using the CGI-ADHD-improvement scale. At each dose, patients receiving methylphenidate OROS showed a greater decrease in ADHD symptoms than those receiving placebo. The percent of patients improving was higher on 54 mg than on 18 or 36 mg, but there was a trend for increase in seizure number at the higher dose of methylphenidate.

Approximately 60–70 % of children with epilepsy and ADHD respond to methylphenidate. This may be less than seen in children with ADHD alone, though none of the above studies directly compared children with epilepsy and ADHD to children with ADHD alone. Conflicting data is present in the two studies that had groups with epilepsy and ADHD and ADHD alone. Semrud-Clikeman and Wical [52] compared the response of children with complex partial seizures and ADHD and children with ADHD alone to methylphenidate as measured by a computerized performance task. Both groups improved but the children with ADHD alone had normal scores after methylphenidate whereas the children with epilepsy and ADHD improved but remained 1.5 standard deviations below normal. Bechtel et al. [55] compared the response to methylphenidate of 17 boys with epilepsy and ADHD and 15 boys with ADHD alone. Both groups improved to near-normal scores.

Decisions on second choice medication to use for ADHD and epilepsy if stimulants are not effective or cause adverse effects are difficult. Atomoxetine, a norepinephrine reuptake inhibitor, is the next choice in ADHD treatment algorithms. It does not seem to lower seizure threshold. Wernicke et al. [108] reviewed company databases and postmarketing reports and noted rates of 0.1–0.2 % for seizures during trials of atomoxetine for ADHD and reports of seizures in 8/100,000 drug exposures after atomoxetine was approved for use. There was no statistically significant difference in occurrence of seizures in patients receiving atomoxetine, methylphenidate, or placebo. Torres et al. [109] reported a retrospective review of 27 patients with epilepsy that received atomoxetine. Atomoxetine was discontinued in 63 %, 7/17 for inadequate improvement in ADHD symptoms and 9/17 with adverse effects. There was no worsening in seizure control. In an abstract, Hernández and Barragán [110] reported on atomoxetine in 17 children with epilepsy and ADHD, noting improvement in symptoms of ADHD without an increase in seizure frequency.

Antidepressants and the alpha adrenergics, guanfacine and clonidine, are alternative agents, but should be used cautiously if at all. There is a high relative risk for seizures at high doses of bupropion and an intermediate risk at moderate or low doses. The risk of seizures is intermediate at moderate to high doses of tricyclic antidepressants [111]. Guanfacine and clonidine may cause sedation and there are no published reports of use in patients with ADHD and epilepsy. They remain possible choices if other medications provide inadequate benefits [112].

For ADHD without epilepsy, behavioral therapies have been demonstrated to be effective in clinical trials, although their effect size for short-term improvement in core ADHD symptoms is somewhat lower than the effect size for stimulant medication treatment [113]. The most widely used behavior therapy for ADHD is parent behavior training (PBT), in which parents are taught to apply behavioral principles such as ignoring, reinforcement, and contingency management to the specific behavior challenges associated with ADHD (impulsivity, inattention). Behavioral therapies for ADHD are also often implemented in the school setting, with teachers providing frequent, specific behavior feedback associated with target behaviors. Less often, behavior therapy may be delivered in intensive summer camps that include activities ranging from classroom work to sports, embedded within a strong system of behavioral goals, monitoring, and interventions [113].

Despite widespread research and clinical use of behavior therapies for ADHD alone, there has been relatively little research on the efficacy of behavior therapies for comorbid ADHD and epilepsy. Some authors have investigated cognitive rehabilitation interventions attempting to improve attention and executive functioning, with behavioral components such as rewards or repetition practice sometimes incorporated into treatment as well. Engelberts et al. [114] reported improvements in attention in adults with epilepsy after cognitive rehabilitation. In a small fMRI study of 17 children with epilepsy, Triplett et al. [115] showed improvement in inhibitory control with reward trials suggesting the potential beneficial effect of cognitive rehabilitation. Executive function deficits may respond only partially to medication and may require educational interventions.

Treatment of ADHD and related symptoms is essential for functional improvement and positive long-term outcomes. Williams et al. [116] found that after controlling for intelligence, attention was more important in predicting academic achievement than memory, self-esteem, or socioeconomic status. Similarly, Hermann et al. [117] noted that children with ADHD and new-onset epilepsy had more cognitive deficits at baseline and at 2-year follow-up than healthy controls or children with new-onset seizures and no evidence of ADHD. The children with symptoms of ADHD and epilepsy were significantly more likely to require special education service than children with epilepsy and no ADHD [37]. Fastenau et al. [118] found an association between ADHD and learning disability in children with epilepsy. Høie et al. [88] showed that impaired executive function was associated with worse school performance than seen in controls. Missing in the data is a demonstration that appropriate treatment of ADHD in children with epilepsy leads to significant improvement in academic functioning.

Just as academic achievement is negatively impacted by epilepsy and ADHD, quality of life is lower in people with epilepsy and ADHD than in those with epilepsy alone. Here there is one study showing that methylphenidate treatment of attention problems in children with epilepsy leads to significantly increased scores measuring quality of life [119].

Summary

There is reasonable data to support the use of methylphenidate for treatment of symptoms of ADHD in children and adolescents with epilepsy. If methylphenidate is not effective or if adverse effects occur, atomoxetine is a second option. Amphetamines and alpha adrenergics may be considered though there is limited data to support their use in children with epilepsy and symptoms of ADHD. Behavioral therapies and educational programming is essential for the child with epilepsy, symptoms of ADHD, and comorbid executive function difficulty and learning disability.

Conclusions

Several things now seem clear. First, there is good epidemiological and clinical data to conclude that people with epilepsy are at increased risk of having symptoms of ADHD and problems with attention. There is adequate data to suggest that problems with executive functioning exist in people with epilepsy, though the data are less compelling than that on problems with attention. The data on risk factors for ADHD, attention problems, and impairment in executive function in people with epilepsy are not as clear. There does not seem to be a gender difference in the occurrence of ADHD, inattention, or executive dysfunction in people with epilepsy. Severity and frequency of seizures seem to be a risk for attentional problems. Other than barbiturates, benzodiazepines, and topiramate, antiepileptic drugs do not seem to be a significant contributor to inattention or ADHD. Seizure type and location of epileptiform discharges have not been consistently found to be associated with ADHD, inattention, or executive dysfunction. Methylphenidate is a reasonable choice for treatment of ADHD and attention problems in people with epilepsy. Atomoxetine may be helpful or at least does not seem to lower seizures threshold significantly. Behavioral treatments are also likely to produce beneficial effects.

The body of research on epilepsy and combined ADHD, attention difficulty, and executive dysfunction also has significant limitations. Many of the studies report results using a very small sample size. This might be expected in fMRI studies, but larger samples are needed to comment on attention difficulties, executive function problems, and the risk factors for symptoms of ADHD. Multiple measures of attention and executive function are used, making comparison of studies difficult. Too few studies assess the youngest children or adults, and not enough studies measure change over time.

There are multiple areas that still need research. Longitudinal studies are needed of people with new-onset epilepsy that assess attention, executive function, and symptoms at onset of seizures and throughout the course of epilepsy. Infants and preschool age children with epilepsy should be included in studies and should be followed to determine risk factors for development of symptoms of ADHD. Adults with epilepsy need to be assessed for symptoms of ADHD, problems with attention, and executive dysfunction. Recent neuroimaging studies could be helpful in explaining the occurrence of problems with attention, and more information is needed in this area. Genetic studies may be able to improve the understanding of the comorbidity of epilepsy and symptoms of ADHD. In addition, pharmacogenomics studies may help with understanding the role of AEDs in impaired attention and executive function. Finally, options for treatment of attention and executive function difficulties other than methylphenidate should be explored. We need to know what type of attention problems or executive function difficulties will respond to medication and which need cognitive or behavioral therapies. There need to be trials demonstrating improvements in academic achievement, employment, social relationships, and quality of life with appropriate treatment of symptoms of ADHD in people with epilepsy.

References

1. American Psychiatric Association. Diagnostic and Statistical Manual of Mental Disorders. 5th ed. Arlington: American Psychiatric Association; 2013.
2. Barkley RA. Executive functions. New York: Guilford Press; 2012.
3. Brown TE. A new understanding of ADHD in children and adults. New York: Routledge; 2013.
4. Kronenberger WG, Beer J, Castellanos I, Pisoni DB, Miyamoto RT. Neurocognitive risk in children with cochlear implants. JAMA Otolarnygol Head Neck Surg. 2014;140:608–15.
5. Miyake A, Friedman NP, Emerson MJ, Witzki AH, Howerter A, Wager TD. The unity and diversity of executive functions and their contributions to complex 'frontal lobe' tasks: a latent variable analysis. Cogn Psychol. 2000;41:49–100.
6. Gioia GA, Isquith PK, Guy SC, Kenworthy L. BRIEF: behavior rating inventory of executive function professional manual. Lutz: Psychological Assessment Resources; 2000.
7. Sánchez-Carpintero R, Neville BGR. Attentional ability in children with epilepsy. Epilepsia. 2003;44:1340–9.
8. American Academy of Pediatrics. Subcommittee on Attention-Deficit/Hyperactivity Disorder. ADHD: clinical practice guideline for the diagnosis, evaluation, and treatment of attention-deficit/hyperactivity disorder in children and adolescents. Pediatrics. 2011;128:1007–22.
9. Plizka S. Practice parameter for the assessment and treatment of children and adolescents with attention-deficit/hyperactivity disorder. J Am Acad Child Adolesc Psychiatry. 2007;46:894–921.
10. DuPaul GJ, Power TJ, Anastopoulos AD, Reid R. ADHD rating scale – IV: checklists, norms, and clinical interpretation. New York: Guilford; 1998.
11. Wolraich ML, Lambert W, Doffing MA, Bickman L, Simmons T, Worley K. Psychometric properties of the Vanderbilt ADHD Diagnostic Parent Rating Scale in a referred population. J Pediatr Psychol. 2003;28:559–68.
12. Gadow KD, Sprafkin J. Child symptom inventory 4 norms manual. Stonybrook: Checkmate Plus, Ltd.; 1997.
13. Achenbach TM, Rescorla LA. Manual for the ASEBA school-age forms and profile. Burlington: University of Vermont, Research Center for Children, Youth, and Families; 2001.
14. Goodman R. Psychometric properties of the strengths and difficulties questionnaire. J Am Acad Child Adolesc Psychiatry. 2001;40:1337–45.
15. Reynolds CR, Kamphaus RW. Behavior assessment system for children. 2nd ed. Circle Pines: AGS; 2004.
16. MacAllister WS, Vasserman M, Rosenthal J, Sherman E. Attention and executive functions in children with epilepsy: what, why, and what to do. Appl Neuropsychol Child. 2014;3:215–25.
17. Jones-Gotman M, Smith ML, Risse GL, Westerveld M, Swanson SJ, Giovagnoli AR, et al. The contribution of neuropsychology to diagnostic assessment in epilepsy. Epilepsy Behav. 2010;18:3–12.
18. Delis D, Kaplan E, Kramer J. The Delis-Kaplan executive function system. San Antonio: The Psychology Corporation; 2001.
19. Witt JA, Alpherts W, Helmstaedter C. Computerized neuropsychological testing in epilepsy: overview of available tools. Seizure. 2013;22:416–23.
20. Chou IC, Chang YT, Chin ZN, Muo CH, Sung FC, Kuo HT, et al. Correlation between epilepsy and attention deficit hyperactivity disorder: a population-based cohort study. PLoS One. 2013;8:e57926.
21. Reilly C, Atkinson P, Das KB, Chin RF, Aylett SE, Burch V, et al. Neurobehavioral comorbidities in children with active epilepsy: a population-based study. Pediatrics. 2014;133:e1586–93.

22. Cohen R, Senecky Y, Shuper A, Inbar D, Chodick G, Shalev V, et al. Prevalence of epilepsy and attention-deficit hyperactivity (ADHD) disorder: a population-based study. J Child Neurol. 2013;28:120–3.
23. Russ SA, Larson K, Halfon N. A national profile of childhood epilepsy and seizure disorder. Pediatrics. 2012;129:256–64.
24. Turky A, Beavis JM, Thapar AK, Kerr MP. Psychopathology in children and adolescents with epilepsy: an investigation of predictive variables. Epilepsy Behav. 2008;12:136–44.
25. Davies S, Heyman I, Goodman R. A population survey of mental health problems in children with epilepsy. Dev Med Child Neurol. 2003;45:292–5.
26. McDermott S, Mani A, Krishnaswami S. A population-based analysis of specific behavior problems associated with childhood seizures. J Epilepsy. 1995;8:110–8.
27. Carlton-Ford S, Miller R, Brown M, Nealeigh N, Jennings P. Epilepsy and children's social and psychological adjustment. J Health Soc Behav. 1995;36:285–301.
28. Tellez-Zenteno JF, Patten SB, Jetté N, Williams J, Wiebe S. Psychiatric comorbidity in epilepsy: a population-based analysis. Epilepsia. 2007;48:2336–44.
29. Ottman R, Lipton RB, Ettinger AB, Cramer JA, Reed ML, Morrison A, et al. Comorbidities of epilepsy: results from the Epilepsy Comorbidities and Health (EPIC) survey. Epilepsia. 2011;52:308–15.
30. Raj D, Kerr MP, McManus S, Jordanova V, Lewis G, Brugha TS. Epilepsy and psychiatric comorbidity: a nationally representative population-based study. Epilepsia. 2012;53:1095–103.
31. Ettinger AB, Ottman R, Lipton RB, Cramer JA, Fanning KM, Reed ML. Attention-deficit/hyperactivity disorder symptoms in adults with self-reported epilepsy: results from a national epidemiologic survey of epilepsy. Epilepsia. 2015;56(2):218–24.
32. Hoare P, Mann H. Self-esteem and behavioural adjustment in children with epilepsy and children with diabetes mellitus. J Psychosom Res. 1994;38:859–69.
33. Williams J, Lange B, Phillips T, Sharp GB, Delos Reyes E, Bates S, et al. The course of inattentive and hyperactive-impulsive symptoms in children with new onset seizures. Epilepsy Behav. 2002;3:517–21.
34. Dunn DW, Austin JK, Harzlak J, Ambrosius WT. ADHD and epilepsy in childhood. Dev Med Child Neurol. 2003;45:50–4.
35. Thome-Souza S, Kuczynski E, Assumpção F, Rzezak P, Fuentes D, et al. Which factors may play a pivotal role on determining the type of psychiatric disorder in children and adolescents with epilepsy? Epilepsy Behav. 2004;5:988–94.
36. Keene DL, Manion I, Whiting S, Belanger E, Brennan R, Jacob P, et al. A survey of behavior problems in children with epilepsy. Epilepsy Behav. 2005;6:581–6.
37. Hermann B, Jones J, Dabbs K, Allen CA, Sheth R, Fine J, et al. The frequency, complications and aetiology of ADHD in new onset paediatric epilepsy. Brain. 2007;130:3135–48.
38. Hanssen-Bauer K, Heyerdahl S, Eriksson A. Mental health problems in children and adolescents referred to a national epilepsy center. Epilepsy Behav. 2007;10:255–62.
39. Jones JE, Watson R, Sheth R, Caplan R, Koehn M, Seidenberg M, et al. Psychiatric comorbidity in children with new onset epilepsy. Dev Med Child Neurol. 2007;49:493–7.
40. Caplan R, Siddarth P, Stahl L, Lanphier E, Vona P, Gurbani S, et al. Childhood absence epilepsy: behavioral, cognitive, and linguistic comorbidities. Epilepsia. 2008;49:1838–46.
41. Wagner JL, Wilson DA, Smith G, Malek A, Selassie AW. Neurodevelopmental and mental health comorbidities in children and adolescents with epilepsy and migraine: a response to identified research gaps. Dev Med Child Neurol. 2015;57:45–52.
42. Tanabe T, Kashiwagi M, Shimakawa S, Fukui M, Kadobayashi K, Azumakawa K, et al. Behavioral assessment of Japanese children with epilepsy using SDQ (strengths and difficulties questionnaire). Brain Dev. 2013;35:81–6.
43. Freilinger M, Reisel B, Reiter E, Zelenko M, Hauser E, Seidl R. Behavioral and emotional problems in children with epilepsy. J Child Neurol. 2006;21:939–45.

44. Benn EKT, Hesdorffer DC, Levy SR, Testa FM, DiMarco FJ, Berg AT. Parental report of behavioral and cognitive diagnoses in childhood-onset epilepsy: a case-sibling-controlled analysis. Epilepsy Behav. 2010;18:276–9.
45. Sherman EMS, Slick DJ, Connolly MB, Eyrl EKL. ADHD, neurological correlates and health-related quality of life in severe pediatric epilepsy. Epilepsia. 2007;48:1083–91.
46. Gonzalez-Heydrich J, Dodds A, Whitney J, MacMillan C, Waber D, Faraone SV, et al. Psychiatric disorders and behavioral characteristics of pediatric patients with both epilepsy and attention-deficit hyperactivity disorder. Epilepsy Behav. 2007;10:384–8.
47. Caplan R, Siddarth P, Gurbani S, Ott D, Sankar R, Shields WD. Psychopathology and pediatric complex partial seizures: seizure-related, cognitive, and linguistic variables. Epilepsia. 2004;45:1273–81.
48. Holdsworth L, Whitmore K. A study of children with epilepsy attending ordinary schools. 1: their seizure patterns, progress and behaviour in school. Dev Med Child Neurol. 1974;16:746–58.
49. Sturniolo MG, Galletti F. Idiopathic epilepsy and school achievement. Arch Dis Child. 1994;70:424–8.
50. Dunn DW, Austin JK, Caffrey HM, Perkins SM. A prospective study of teachers' ratings of behavior problems in children with new-onset seizures. Epilepsy Behav. 2003;4:26–35.
51. Mitchell WG, Zhou Y, Chavez JM, Guzman BL. Reaction time, attention, and impulsivity in epilepsy. Pediatr Neurol. 1992;8:19–24.
52. Semrud-Clikeman M, Wical B. Components of attention in children with complex partial seizures with and without ADHD. Epilepsia. 1999;40:211–5.
53. Triplett RL, Asato MR. Brief cognitive and behavioral screening in children with new-onset epilepsy: a pilot feasibility trial. Pediatr Neurol. 2015;52:49–55.
54. Stiers P, Fonteyne A, Wouters H, D'Agositno E, Sunaert S, Lagae L. Hippocampal malrotation in pediatric patients with epilepsy associated with complex prefrontal dysfunction. Epilepsia. 2010;51(4):546–55.
55. Bechtel N, Kobel M, Penner I-K, Specht K, Klarhöfer M, Scheffler K, et al. Attention-deficit/hyperactivity disorder in childhood epilepsy: a neuropsychological and functional imaging study. Epilepsia. 2012;53:325–33.
56. Parrish J, Geary E, Jones J, Seth R, Hermann B, Seidenberg M. Executive functioning in childhood epilepsy: parent-report and cognitive assessment. Dev Med Child Neurol. 2007;49:412–6.
57. Høie B, Sommerfelt K, Waaler PE, Alsaker FD, Skeidsvoll H, Mykletun A. The combined burden of cognitive, executive function, and psychosocial problems in children with epilepsy: a population-based study. Dev Med Child Neurol. 2008;50:530–6.
58. Campiglia M, Seegmuller C, Le Gall D, Fournet N, Roulin J-L, Roy A. Assessment of everyday executive functioning in children with frontal and temporal epilepsies. Epilepsy Behav. 2014;39:12–20.
59. Longo CA, Kerr EN, Smith ML. Executive functioning in children with intractable frontal lobe or temporal lobe epilepsy. Epilepsy Behav. 2013;26:102–8.
60. Conant LL, Wilfong A, Inglese C, Schwarte A. Dysfunction of executive and related processes in childhood absence epilepsy. Epilepsy Behav. 2010;18:414–23.
61. Chowdhury FA, Elwes RDC, Koutroumanidis M, Morris RG, Nashef L, Richardson MP. Impaired cognitive function in idiopathic generalized epilepsy and unaffected family members: an epilepsy endophenotype. Epilepsia. 2004;55:835–40.
62. Borgatti R, Picinelli P, Montirosso R, Donati G, Rampani A, Molteni L, et al. Study of attentional processes in children with idiopathic epilepsy by Conners' continuous performance test. J Child Neurol. 2004;19:509–15.
63. Austin JK, Perkins SM, Johnson CS, Fastenau PS, Byars AW, deGrauw TJ, et al. Behavior problems in children at time of first recognized seizure and changes over the following 3 years. Epilepsy Behav. 2011;21:373–81.

64. Hesdorffer DC, Ludvigsson P, Olafsson E, Gudmundsson G, Kjartansson O, Hauser WA. ADHD as a risk factor for incident unprovoked seizures and epilepsy in children. Arch Gen Psychiatry. 2004;61:731–6.
65. Davis SM, Katusic SK, Barbaresi WJ, Killian J, Weaver AL, Ottman R, et al. Epilepsy in children with attention-deficit/hyperactivity disorder. Pediatr Neurol. 2010;42:325–30.
66. Hemmer SA, Pasternak JF, Zecker SG, Trommer BL. Stimulant therapy and seizure risk in children with ADHD. Pediatr Neurol. 2001;24:99–102.
67. Richer LP, Shevell MI, Rosenblatt BR. Epileptiform abnormalities in children with attention-deficit-hyperactivity disorder. Pediatr Neurol. 2002;26:125–9.
68. Aydin K, Okuyaz Ç, Serdaroğlu A, Gücüyener K. Utility of electroencephalography in the evaluation of common neurologic conditions in children. J Child Neurol. 2003;18:394–6.
69. Holtmann M, Becker K, Kentner-Figura B, Schmidt MH. Increased frequency of rolandic spikes in ADHD children. Epilepsia. 2003;44:1241–4.
70. Gucuyener K, Erdemogly AK, Senol S, Serdaroglu A, Soysal S, Kockar I. Use of methylphenidate for attention-deficit hyperactivity disorder in patients with epilepsy or electroencephalographic abnormalities. J Child Neurol. 2003;18:109–12.
71. Austin JK, Harezlak J, Dunn DW, Huster GA, Rose DF, Ambrosius WT. Behavior problems in children prior to first recognized seizures. Pediatrics. 2001;107:115–22.
72. Lo-Castro A, Curatolo P. Epilepsy associated with autism and attention deficit hyperactivity disorder: is there a genetic link? Brain Dev. 2014;36:185–93.
73. Gonzalez-Heydrich J, Hamoda HM, Luna L, Rao S, McClendon J, Rotella P, et al. Elevated rates of ADHD in mothers of children with comorbid ADHD and epilepsy. Neuropsychaitry. 2012;2:385–91.
74. Hesdorffer DC, Caplan R, Berg AT. Familial clustering of epilepsy and behavioral disorders: evidence for a shared genetic basis. Epilepsia. 2012;53:301–7.
75. Ferrie CD, Madigan C, Tilling K, Maisey MN, Marsden PK, Robinson RO. Adaptive and maladaptive behaviour in children with epileptic encephalopathies: correlation with cerebral glucose metabolism. Dev Med Child Neurol. 1997;39:588–95.
76. Dabbs K, Jones JE, Jackson DC, Seidenberg M, Hermann BP. Patterns of cortical thickness and the Child Behavior Checklist in childhood epilepsy. Epilepsy Behav. 2013;29:198–204.
77. Killory BD, Bai X, Negishi M, Vega C, Spann MN, Vestal M, et al. Impaired attention and network connectivity in childhood absence epilepsy. Neuroimage. 2011;56:2209–17.
78. McGill ML, Devinsky O, Kelly C, Milham M, Castellanos FX, Quinn BT, et al. Default mode network abnormalities in idiopathic epilepsy. Epilepsy Behav. 2012;23:353–9.
79. Tsai FJ, Liu ST, Lee CM, Lee WT, Fan PC, Lin WS, et al. ADHD-related symptoms, emotional/behavioral problems, and physical conditions in Taiwanese children with epilepsy. J Formos Med Assoc. 2013;112:396–405.
80. Black LC, Schefft BK, Howe SR, Szaflarski JP, Yeh H, Privitera MD. The effect of seizures on working memory and executive functioning performance. Epilepsy Behav. 2010;17:412–9.
81. Cerminara C, D'Agati E, Lange KW, Kaunziger I, Tucha O, Parisi P, et al. Benign childhood epilepsy and with centrotemporal spikes and the multicomponent model of attention: a matched control study. Epilepsy Behav. 2010;19:69–77.
82. Vega C, Vestal M, DeSalvo M, Berman R, Chung M, Blumenfeld H, et al. Differentiation of attention-related problems in childhood absence epilepsy. Epilepsy Behav. 2010;19:82–5.
83. Masur D, Shinnar S, Cnaan A, Shinnar RC, Clark P, Wang J, et al. Pretreatment cognitive deficits and treatment effects on attention in childhood absence epilepsy. Neurology. 2013;81:1572–80.
84. Hernandez M-T, Sauerwein HC, Jambaqué I, de Guise E, Lussier F, Lortie A, et al. Attention, memory, and behavioral adjustment in children with frontal lobe epilepsy. Epilepsy Behav. 2003;4:522–36.
85. Gottlieb L, Zelko FA, Kim DS, Nordli D. Cognitive proficiency in pediatric epilepsy. Epilepsy Behav. 2012;23:146–51.

86. Almane D, Jones JE, Jackson DC, Seidenberg M, Hermann BP. The social competence and behavioral problem substrate of new- and recent-onset childhood epilepsy. Epilepsy Behav. 2014;31:91–6.
87. Jackson DC, Dabbs K, Walker NM, Jones JE, Hsu DA, Stafstrom CE, et al. The neuropsychological and academic substrate of new/recent-onset epilepsies. J Pediatr. 2013;162: 1047–53.
88. Høie B, Mykletun A, Waaler PE, Skeidsvoll H, Sommerfelt K. Executive functions and seizure-related factors in children with epilepsy in western Norway. Dev Med Child Neurol. 2006;48:519–25.
89. Aldenkamp A, Arends J. The relative influence of epileptic EEG discharges, short nonconvulsive seizures, and type of epilepsy on cognitive function. Epilepsia. 2004;45(1):54–63.
90. Kavros PM, Clarke T, Strug LJ, Halperin JM, Dorta NJ, Pal DK. Attention impairment in rolandic epilepsy: systemic review. Epilepsia. 2008;49:1570–80.
91. Zhang DQ, Li FH, Zhu XB, Sun RP. Clinical observations on attention-deficit hyperactivity disorder (ADHD) in children with frontal lobe epilepsy. J Child Neurol. 2014;29:54–7.
92. Ibrahim GM, Cassel D, Morgan BR, Smith ML, Otsubo H, Ochi A, et al. Resilience of developing brain networks to interictal epileptiform discharges is associated with cognitive outcome. Brain. 2014;137:2690–702.
93. Kwan P, Brodie MJ. Neuropsychological effects of epilepsy and antiepileptic drugs. Lancet. 2001;357:216–22.
94. Loring DW, Meador KJ. Cognitive side effects of antiepileptic drugs in children. Neurology. 2004;62:872–7.
95. Cirulli ET, Urban TJ, Marino SE, Linney KN, Birnbaum AK, Depondt C, et al. Genetic and environmental correlates of topiramate-induced cognitive impairment. Epilepsia. 2012;53:e5–8.
96. Glauser TA, Cnaan A, Shinnar S, Hirtz DG, Dlugos D, Masur D, et al. Ethosuximide, valproic acid, and lamotrigine in childhood absence epilepsy. N Engl J Med. 2010;362:790–9.
97. Kanemura H, Sano F, Tando T, Hosaka H, Sugita K, Aihara M. EEG improvements with antiepileptic drug treatment can show a high correlation with behavioral recovery in children with ADHD. Epilepsy Behav. 2013;27:443–8.
98. Wandschneider B, Stretton J, Sidhu M, Centeno M, Kozák LR, Symms M, et al. Levetiracetam reduces abnormal network activations in temporal lobe epilepsy. Neurology. 2014;83:1508–12.
99. Rodenburg R, Stams GJ, Meijer AM, Aldenkamp AP, Deković M. Psychopathology in children with epilepsy: a meta-analysis. J Pediatr Psychol. 2005;30:453–68.
100. Biederman J, Faraone SV. Attention-deficit hyperactivity disorder. Lancet. 2005;366:237–48.
101. Pliszka SR, Crismon ML, Hughes CW, Conners CK, Emslie GJ, Jensen PS, et al. The Texas children's medication algorithm project: revision of the algorithm for pharmacotherapy of attention-deficit/hyperactivity disorder. J Am Acad Child Adolesc Psychiatry. 2006;45: 642–57.
102. Feldman H, Crumine P, Handen BL, Alvin R, Teodori J. Methylphenidate in children with seizures and attention-deficit disorder. Am J Dis Child. 1989;143:1081–6.
103. Gross-Tsur V, Monor O, van der Meere J, Joseph A, Shalev RS. Epilepsy and attention deficit hyperactivity disorder: is methylphenidate safe and effective? J Pediatr. 1997;130: 670–4.
104. Fosi T, Lax-Pericall MT, Scott RC, Neville BG, Aylett SE. Methylphenidate treatment of attention deficit hyperactivity disorder in young people with learning disability and difficult-to-treat epilepsy: evidence of clinical benefit. Epilepsia. 2013;54:2071–81.
105. Santos K, Palmini A, Radziuk AL, Rotert R, Bastos F, Booij L, et al. The impact of methylphenidate on seizure frequency and severity in children with attention-deficit-hyperactivity disorder and difficult-to-treat epilepsies. Dev Med Child Neurol. 2013;55: 654–60.

106. Gonzalez-Heydrich J, Hsin O, Gumlak S, Kimball K, Rober A, Azeem MW, et al. Comparing stimulant effects in youth with ADHD symptoms and epilepsy. Epilepsy Behav. 2014;36:102–7.
107. Gonzalez-Heydrich J, Whitney J, Waber D, Forbes P, Hsin O, Faraone SV, et al. Adaptive phase I study of OROS methylphenidate treatment of attention deficit hyperactivity disorder with epilepsy. Epilepsy Behav. 2010;18:229–37.
108. Wernicke JF, Chilcott KE, Jin L, Edison T, Zhang S, Bangs ME, et al. Seizure risk in patients with attention-deficit-hyperactivity disorder treated with atomoxetine. Dev Med Child Neurol. 2007;49:498–502.
109. Torres A, Whitney J, Rao S, Tilley C, Lobel R, Gonzalez-Heydrich J. Tolerability of atomoxetine for treatment of pediatric attention-deficit/hyperactivity disorder in the context of epilepsy. Epilepsy Behav. 2011;20:95–102.
110. Hernández AJC, Barragán PEJ. Efficacy of atomoxetine treatment in children with ADHD and epilepsy. Epilepsia. 2005;46 Suppl 6:241.
111. Alldredge BK. Seizure risk associated with psychotropic drugs: clinical and pharmacokinetic considerations. Neurology. 1999;53 Suppl 2:S68–75.
112. Torres AR, Whitney J, Gonzalez-Heydrich J. Attention-deficit/hyperactivity disorder in pediatric patients with epilepsy: review of pharmacological treatment. Epilepsy Behav. 2008;12:217–33.
113. The MTA Cooperative Group. A 14-month randomized clinical trial of treatment strategies for attention-deficit/hyperactivity disorder. Arch Gen Psychiatry. 1999;56:1073–86.
114. Engelberts NHJ, Klein M, Adèr HJ, Heimans JJ, Trenité DG, van der Ploeg HM. The effectiveness of cognitive rehabilitation for attention deficits in focal seizures: a randomized controlled study. Epilepsia. 2002;43:587–95.
115. Triplett RL, Velanova K, Luna B, Padmanabhan A, Gaillard WD, Asato MR. Investigating inhibitory control in children with epilepsy: an fMRI study. Epilepsia. 2014;55:1667–76.
116. Williams J, Phillips T, Griebel ML, Sharp GB, Lange B, Edgar T, et al. Factors associated with academic achievement in children with controlled epilepsy. Epilepsy Behav. 2001;2:217–23.
117. Hermann BP, Jones JE, Sheth R, Koehn M, Becker T, Fine J, et al. Growing up with epilepsy: a two-year investigation of cognitive development in children with new onset epilepsy. Epilepsia. 2008;49:1847–58.
118. Fastenau PS, Shen J, Dunn DW, Austin JK. Academic underachievement among children with epilepsy. J Learn Disabil. 2008;41:195–207.
119. Yoo HK, Park S, Wang H-R, Lee JS, Kim K, Paik K-W, et al. Effect of methylphenidate on the quality of life in children with epilepsy and attention deficit hyperactivity disorder. Epileptic Disord. 2009;11:301–8.

Chapter 14
Dementia

Alla Guekht

Abstract Association between epilepsy and dementia has been described centuries ago; still many neurobiological, clinical, and therapeutic issues remain unclear. This comorbidity is currently in the focus of experimental, translational, and clinical research.

There are similarities (as well as differences) between patients with dementias and those with temporal lobe epilepsy (TLE), and between animal models of Alzheimer disease (AD) and TLE. Seizures in the human temporal lobe transiently impair cognition and steadily damage hippocampal circuitry, leading to progressive memory loss; many mechanisms involved in AD influence excitability and cause seizures.

On one hand, there is a multifactorial cognitive deficit in patients with chronic epilepsy; it is driven by the impact of the underlying etiology, the effects of recurrent seizures, adverse effects of antiepileptic drugs (AEDs), and psychosocial issues.

On the other hand, seizures are frequently observed in patients with dementia. The incidence of seizures among patients with dementia varies with the etiology of the dementing illness.

The proper choice of AEDs is essential in symptomatic treatment of seizures in patients with dementia; possible risks and benefits of the drug for the elderly patient should be noted.

Better understanding of the converging neurobiological pathways of epilepsy and dementia could enrich the therapeutic armamentarium and allow improved control of both conditions, ameliorate related abnormalities and potentially modify disease progression.

Keywords Epilepsy • Seizures • Cognitive decline • Alzheimer's disease • Vascular dementia • Apolipoprotein E • β-amyloid • Hippocampal sclerosis • Excitotoxicity • Antiepileptic drugs

A. Guekht, MD, PhD
Department of Neurology, Neurosurgery and Genetics, Russian National Research Medical University and Moscow Research and Clinical Center for Neuropsychiatry, Donskaya, 43, Moscow 115419, Russia
e-mail: guekht@gmail.com

M. Mula (ed.), *Neuropsychiatric Symptoms of Epilepsy*, Neuropsychiatric Symptoms of Neurological Disease, DOI 10.1007/978-3-319-22159-5_14

Introduction

Association between epilepsy and dementia has been described centuries ago [1]. Thomas Willis wrote that dementia could result from the “cruel diseases of the head,” such as epilepsy [2]; the French Encyclopedia [3] also considered “incurable diseases such as epilepsy” one of the causes of dementia.

In fact, neuropsychiatric problems are observed in 30–50 % of patients with chronic epilepsy. Cognitive impairments, especially in memory, concentration, and word finding are well known. Cognitive deficit in patients with chronic epilepsy is multifactorial and includes the impact of the underlying etiology, the effects of recurrent seizures, adverse effects of antiepileptic drugs, and psychosocial issues [4–9]. However, there is an increasing evidence that patients with newly diagnosed epilepsy are cognitively compromised even before the start of antiepileptic drug medication. The cognitive domains most affected are psychomotor speed, higher executive functioning, and memory [10–12].

On the other hand, seizures are frequently observed in patients with dementia. The incidence of seizures among patients with dementia varies with the etiology of the dementing illness [13–17]. Pohlmann-Eden reported that the spectrum of diseases with dementia and associated seizures ranges from more frequent conditions (Alzheimer’s disease) and vascular dementia (VaD), where seizures occur in a small proportion of patients, to rare conditions (Creutzfeldt-Jakob disease) in which seizures are a common reflection of the underlying epileptogenic neurobiological process [18]. The incidence of epilepsy in persons with Down syndrome (DS) is 1.4–17 % and varies with age [19–23].

According to McVicker et al., seizures are quite prevalent at certain phases of DS, and could be seen in about half of patients over age 50 [24].

There are a number of relatively rare conditions that are associated with early-onset dementia, myoclonus, and epilepsy: sialidosis, GM2 gangliosidosis, Lafora disease, ceroidlipofuscinosis, and mitochondrial encephalomyopathies [25–27].

Dementia, stroke, and epilepsy are three most common neurological disorders in the elderly; incidence rates of over 100 per 100,000 for epilepsy in people over 60 years of age have been reported [28–33]. Epilepsy, cerebral atherosclerosis, and age-related cognitive disorders, including Alzheimer’s disease, share many clinical manifestations, risk factors, and structural and pathological brain abnormalities. Plaque deposits in gray matter were first described by Blocq and Marinesco as the result of the examination of nine deceased epileptic patients in 1892 [34]. They did not, however, relate the plaques to dementia; that was accomplished in 1906 by Alois Alzheimer [34–37].

Alzheimer’s Disease and Epilepsy

Patients with AD have an increased risk of developing seizures and epilepsy. AD and other neurodegenerative conditions represent the presumed etiology of 10 % of new-onset epilepsy in patients older than 65 years [38]. There are some prospective investigations that noted a significantly higher incidence of seizures in Alzheimer's disease patients than in elderly controls without dementia [13, 14]. The incidence of unprovoked seizures is clearly higher in sporadic AD than in the reference population, and the increase appears to be independent of disease stage [16, 39].

In patients with Alzheimer's disease, approximately 10–22 % had at least one unprovoked seizure [40]. Relative risk estimates vary considerably between studies, ranging from a sixfold higher risk in one study [15] to a tenfold higher risk in another study [13], depending on whether patients with AD were recruited from a special care facility or from a population-based setting. Also there is considerable variability in the reported lifetime prevalence rates of 1.5–64 % [41].

Interestingly, Scarmeas et al. [17] even reported that unprovoked seizures are not common in AD, as only about 1.5 % of patients with AD developed seizures over the course of a mean of 3.7 years of follow-up; still seizures do occur more frequently than in the general population.

The associations between seizures and the age of onset/stage/severity of AD are also the matter of controversy.

Advanced Alzheimer's disease is often considered a risk factor for new-onset generalized tonic–clonic seizures in older adults; it is associated with a 10 % prevalence of seizures, particularly late in the illness [14]. Indeed, the increasing age is a common and well-established risk factor for both epilepsy and AD [42]. Mendez and Lim also noted that seizures usually occur in later stages of Alzheimer's disease, on average ≥6 years of the disease [40]. In the huge follow-up study with a nested case–control analysis using the United Kingdom–based General Practice Research Database (GPRD), Imfeld et al. demonstrated that the patients with longer standing (more than 3 years) AD had a higher risk of developing seizures or epilepsy than those with a shorter duration of disease, although this difference was not statistically significant [43].

However, a number of studies reported higher incidence of seizures in early AD [44]. In these studies, the highest risk was detected among younger persons with early-onset dementia (50–60 years), an age when their general incidence in the population remains low. It was demonstrated that the relative risk of unprovoked seizures markedly increases in patients with early-onset AD, reaching 3-, 20-, and 87-fold with dementia onset when aged 70–79, 60–69, or 50–59 years, respectively [16]. Also it has been noted that more than 80 % pedigrees of patients with very early onset of dementia (<40 years of age) show overt seizures or epilepsy (mostly generalized convulsive seizures and myoclonic seizures). It is much higher compared to patients with late-onset AD – in this group 5–20 % suffer from convulsive seizures [16, 39, 45–47].

In fact, younger patients with AD may have more aggressive disease or may be more likely to have a clinical episode recognized; also the younger brain may be more susceptible to seizure manifestation [16, 17, 48, 49].

The risk factors of seizures in AD, including the association with the age at AD onset, EEG findings, and apolipoprotein E (ApoE) status, are still being debated in the literature. Younger individuals, African Americans, males, and those with more severe disease and/or focal epileptiform findings on electroencephalogram (EEG) were considered to be prone to have unprovoked seizures [50–52]. However, in some studies no association between age at AD onset, as well as prior EEG findings, or ApoE status was confirmed [16, 17]. Race, when analyzed as a whole, and separately as African-American and Hispanic race, did not alter the relationship between AD and seizures [53].

Overall, AD is associated with high risk of seizures and epilepsy. Further studies on risk factors are needed in order to identify the most vulnerable patient populations.

Vascular Dementia and Epilepsy

Cerebrovascular diseases are the leading cause of symptomatic epilepsies in the elderly [30, 32, 54]. Patients with VaD, like the patients with AD, are at higher risk of developing seizures or epilepsy than dementia-free patients. Indeed, there are numerous risk factors of seizures that are common in patients in stroke, VaD, and epilepsy [42, 53, 55–57].

Many papers during the last decades have been focusing on CADASIL (cerebral autosomal dominant arteriopathy with subcortical infarcts and leukoencephalopathy), which appears to be the most common genetic form of VaD [58–61]. This autosomal dominant disorder of cerebral small vessels maps to chromosome 19 and is caused by Notch3 gene mutations [62]. The underlying vascular lesion is a unique nonamyloid nonatherosclerotic microangiopathy involving arterioles and capillaries, primarily in the brain but also in other organs. Recurrent transient ischemic attacks, migraine and dementia represent the principal symptoms in this systemic vascular disease. During the course of the disease, about 10 % of patients may experience focal or generalized epileptic seizures, mainly related to ischemic stroke. Rarely, seizures may precede the ischemic events and the cognitive impairment [63–66]. Valko et al. described the nonconvulsive status epilepticus in CADASIL patient [67].

The bidirectional association between seizures and epilepsy, on one hand, and VaD, on the other hand, has been reported. In fact, preexisting dementia (present in 12–16 % of stroke patients) was independently associated with the occurrence of late seizures after stroke, and early seizures are independent predictors of new-onset dementia within 3 years after stroke. Besides, preexisting vascular pathologies that may predispose to both seizures and new-onset dementia could be white matter changes, silent infarcts, or microbleeds [56, 68, 69]. De Reuck and Van Maele suggested that seizure occurrence in patients with a lacunar infarct is not related to the severity of the stroke, but rather to the degree of cognitive impairment and is probably the expression of an underlying neurodegenerative process that is also responsible for the mental deterioration [70].

In the elderly patients with epilepsy hyperhomocysteinemia (Hcy) [71], hypercholesterolemia/dyslipidemia, abnormal glucose metabolism and insulin resistance (IR), obesity, and subclinical hypothyroidism may increase the risk of age-accelerated vascular disease, cognitive decline, and cognitive disorders.

An age-accelerated atherosclerosis with increased carotid artery intima media thickness is discussed as an independent risk factor in patients with epilepsy [70]. In fact, the following risk factors are shared between epilepsy and age-related cognitive disorders: increased carotid artery intima media thickness (CA-IMT), Hcy, lipid abnormalities, weight gain and obesity, IR, high levels of inflammatory and oxidative stresses, as well as the brain structural and pathological abnormalities including decreased volume of the hippocampus, increased cortical thinning of the frontal lobe, ventricular expansion and increased white matter ischemic disease, total brain atrophy, and β-amyloid protein deposition in the brain [42, 72, 73].

Depression and hypertension have been also identified as the risk factors for unprovoked seizures [15, 16, 74], which constitute an additional risk in patients with VaD. Some other investigators report that cholinesterase inhibitors itself may increase risk of seizures in dementias of different etiology [52].

Interestingly, Imfeld et al. found out that the role of disease duration as a risk factor for seizures/epilepsy seems to differ between AD and VaD [43]. Patients with longer than 3 years standing AD had a higher risk of developing seizures than those with a shorter disease duration; whereas in patients with VaD the contrary was observed.

The association between vascular dementia and epilepsy, especially risk factors for seizures, requires further investigations, as there are many controversies in the literature. For instance, Conrad et al. reported that no patients with dementia developed seizures in his study [75], in contrast to the study by Cordonnier et al. who found dementia to be an independent risk factor for seizures [68].

Mechanisms

There are several hypotheses of co-occurrence of dementia and seizures epilepsy.

Some authors view dementia and seizures as on two fundamentally independent disorders, with the unfortunate co-occurrence of two disease genes or acquired encephalopathies; this hypothesis is supported by relatively low occurrence of seizures in dementia, compared to some other neurological disorders [17, 41, 76].

However, the vast majority of authors [53, 76–78] tend to explain comorbidity of epilepsy and dementia by the number of mechanisms underlying both conditions.

As many risk factors are shared between VaD and AD, and the importance of mixed vascular-degenerative dementia has been recognized [79–81], the mechanisms of their association with seizures and epilepsy will be discussed together.

There are a number of studies looking at the association between amnestic episodes in patients with AD; in these patients epileptiform EEG discharges such as spikes and sharp waves [82, 83] were found. It was confirmed by the fact that both conditions (specific cognitive disturbances and the associated epileptiform EEG discharges) could be prevented by antiepileptic treatment. On the other hand, epileptiform discharges in patients with temporal lobe epilepsy can also lead to transient amnesia and even simulate similar to AD memory disturbances [46, 84]. Palop et al. reported that transgenic mouse model of Alzheimer's disease was found to have spontaneous nonconvulsive seizures accompanied by electroencephalographic changes, similar to those in human TLE [85].

Most authors agree that neuronal cell loss in mesial temporal lobe structures play key role both in epilepsy and dementia [42, 86–90]. The histopathologic finding of hippocampal sclerosis (HS) can be seen in association with dementia, TLE, and hippocampal ischemic injury [87]; Alzheimer disease is usually associated with some loss of hippocampal pyramidal neurons [91–93]. Korf et al. suggested that atrophy of hippocampus along with entorhinal cortex might be a reliable marker for cognitive impairment and supposed that medial temporal lobe atrophy is one of the most significant predictors of progression mild cognitive impairment (MCI) to dementia [94].

Velez-Pardo et al. found out two distinct patterns of neuronal loss in the CA1 field of familial AD (FAD) patients: (a) diffuse-patchy neuronal loss (in FAD non-epilepsy patients) characterized by both a general decrease of neurons and the presence of multiple, small regions devoid of neurons, and (b) sclerotic-like neuronal loss (FAD epilepsy patients, bearing the PS1[E280A] mutation) similar to that found typically in the CA1 field of epilepsy patients with hippocampal sclerosis [86].

Indeed, decreased volumes of hippocampal formations are a common finding in patients with dementia and TLE.

A huge number of magnetic resonance imaging (MRI) studies, including those with results of the voxel-based morphometry, documented abnormalities in hippocampal, extrahippocampal temporal lobe, and extratemporal lobe in TLE. Within the temporal lobe, they have been observed in entorhinal cortex, parahippocampal regions, amygdala, individual temporal lobe gyrus, and temporal lobe white matter, alongside, or independent of hippocampal sclerosis [95–101].

Pauli et al. (2006) found out that decreased neuronal density in the dentate gyrus evidenced by histology correlates positively with memory impairment in patients with TLE [73].

Excitotoxicity is largely involved in pathogenesis of hippocampal neuronal death in epilepsy, as well as in dementia [102, 103]. Autoradiography study of receptors in the human hippocampus shows the highest binding for glutamate, N-Methyl-D-aspartic acid, or N-Methyl-D-aspartate (NMDA), and α-Amino-3-hydroxy-5-methyl-4-isoxazolepropionic acid (AMPA) receptors in the molecular layer of the dentate gyrus were demonstrated in experimental models of both conditions [104–107].

Koeller et al. suggested that basal cyclin D1 expression may render hippocampal circuits more susceptible to particular epileptogenic agents and excitotoxic cell death, though cD1 is not a direct precipitant in apoptosis [108]. Several studies reported new expression of cell cycle proteins in apoptotic, postmitotic neurons in various neurodegenerative mouse models and in pathological samples from patients having neurodegenerative conditions including AD [109, 110].

Seizures could result from highly specific neuronal excitability changes related to the molecular pathogenesis of certain subtypes of dementia that give rise to both phenotypes.

Dementia phenotypes accompanied by epilepsy may be produced by new mutations in PS1, the most common gene for AD [111]. Importantly, epilepsy is a prevalent comorbid phenotype in probands and affected family members with familial AD; mutations in the gamma-secretase modulatory genes presenilin 1 (PS1) or presenilin 2 (PS2) or amyloid precursor protein (APP) are linked to FAD [76, 112–114]. The tight genetic association between Aβ over-expression and epilepsy has been explained by the fact that the seizures arise exclusively from the presence of any particular Aβ peptide fragment, since mutant AD genes may give rise to cleavage patterns in intracellular and extracellular peptides of alternative lengths and toxicity, or exert other deleterious effects [115]. Exaggerated intracellular Ca2 signaling is a robust phenotype observed in cells expressing FAD-causing mutant presenilins [116].

There is an evidence now that high levels of β-amyloid in the brain destabilizes neuronal activity at the circuit and network levels. The pathological accumulation of oligomeric Aβ assemblies depresses excitatory transmission at the synaptic level, but also triggers aberrant patterns of neuronal circuit activity and epileptiform discharges at the network level. Aβ-induced dysfunction of inhibitory interneurons likely increases synchrony among excitatory principal cells and contributes to the destabilization of neuronal networks [46, 47, 84, 112].

It was demonstrated that elevation of Aβ elicits epileptiform activity, including spikes and sharp waves in EEG recording from cortical and hippocampal networks in human amyloid precursor protein (hAPP) transgenic mice [85].

According to this hypothesis of Aβ-induced cognitive dysfunction [85, 117, 118], high Aβ leads to aberrant excitatory network activity and compensatory inhibitory responses involving learning and memory circuits, which is associated with epileptiform activity and contribute to cognitive decline (Fig. 14.1).

One of the most important genetic risk factor for Alzheimer's disease and vascular dementia is apolipoprotein [119, 120]. It is interesting that ApoE4 carriers without dementia show signs of epileptiform activity and sharp waves on their EEGs after hyperventilation, although their EEGs were normal under resting conditions [51]. ApoE4 also exacerbates epilepsy and promotes memory impairment in patients with long-standing intractable TLE [121].

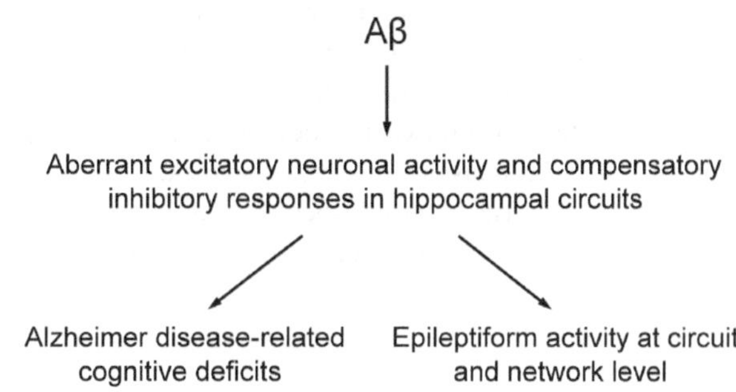

Fig. 14.1 β-Amyloid induces hippocampal remodeling

Hyperhomocysteinemia is another one mechanism that may be involved in the development of seizures in patients with dementing diseases. Elevated plasma levels of homocysteine can be caused by deficiency of vitamin B12 or folate. Genetic factor involved is the C667T substitution of the gene encoding methylenetetrahydrofolate reductase [71]. Kado et al. demonstrated that elevated plasma levels of Hcy (eHcy) is an independent risk factor for facilitating medial temporal lobe atrophy and the evolution from MCI into AD [122]. Hyperhomocysteinemia acts like an excitatory neurotransmitter by competing with inhibitory neurotransmitters such as gamma-aminobutyric acid. Another effect of elevated plasma levels of homocysteine is inducing microvascular permeability by attenuating the γ-aminobutyric acid (GABA)-A/B receptors that may cause disruption of the matrix in the blood–brain barrier. Gorgone et al. (2009) found out that the rate of brain atrophy was higher in epilepsy patients with eHcy [71, 123].

Differential Diagnosis

Persistent cognitive impairment as well as impairment of memory, disturbances of attention, abstract thinking, judgment, calculation, language, and executive function are the common clinical features of different types of dementia.

Dyscognitive epileptic seizures that are not evolving to generalized convulsive episodes also produce impairment of perception, attention, emotions, memory, and represent substantial differential diagnostic challenges, especially in the elderly [124, 125].

Dementia with Lewy bodies (DLB) may cause diagnostic difficulties due to its similarity with many psychiatric, neurologic, and medical conditions in elderly people [126]. Epileptic seizure may cause symptoms that mimic DLB too, so clinicians should consider an epileptic condition as a differential diagnosis for elderly patients with psychiatric symptoms and fluctuating cognition. Definitive diagnosis is based on detection of specific for DLB so called Levy bodies [127]. EEG study and detection of rapid eye movement (REM) sleep behavior disorder that includes vivid dreaming, with persistent dreams, purposeful or violent movements, and falling out of bed can help clinician to identify DLB on early stages of the disease [128]. Nonconvulsive epileptiform activities underlie some of the cognitive impairments observed in AD [46]; EEG monitoring is essential in these cases.

Ictal paresis may be the manifestation of nonconvulsive status epilepticus in elderly people with preexisting dementia. It can be as severe as complete flaccid hemiplegia and can last as long as for a week. EEG study usually reveals continuous epileptiform patterns in parieto-occipital areas and occasionally evolving to the central area, indicative of focal nonconvulsive status epilepticus [129].

Treatment

Comorbidity between dementia and epilepsy has important treatment implications. Population of patients with dementia is aged and rather vulnerable because of multiple other somatic comorbidities. There is a decline in renal and hepatic function with increasing age and weight loss is common, especially in people with AD. Standard doses of drugs may not be appropriate. Doses of drugs for chronic conditions such as hypertension or AEDs that were previously satisfactory may be excessive for an older, frailer person with dementia. All drugs should be reviewed regularly particularly for older people in care homes who are known to take more medications than older people in the wider community [130–132].

Safety and tolerability of all the medications, including those for dementia treatment, is the key issue in the elderly epilepsy patients. Accordingly, lifestyle modification, which is safe and has been proved effective in cognitive decline, especially vascular-related [133, 134], is a reasonable option for these patients. Antiplatelet, antihypertensive, and lipid lowering agents are important for prevention of the recurrent stroke in VaD that might be associated by the further increase of seizure risk.

The well-accepted therapeutic algorithm for the treatment of dementia (AD or VaD) includes acetylcholinesterase inhibitors and/or the N-methyl-D-aspartate (NMDA)–receptor antagonist memantine [135–137]. Fisher et al. reported that donepezil prescribed to improve memory in patients with epilepsy caused a slight increase in frequency of generalized tonic–clonic seizures [138]. On the other hand, Imfeld et al. (2013) did not confirm higher risk of seizures or epilepsy among patients with AD receiving treatment with antidementia drugs compared to patients without it [43].

Emerging therapeutic strategies in dementia have not been substantially studied in terms of safety (and their capacity to provoke seizures), especially in the clinical settings.

It was widely discussed whether the vitamin supplementation can confer additional benefit for treating cognitive decline [139–142]. Low folate levels are risk factors for cognitive decline in adults with concomitant eHcy [143, 144]. Some investigators report that administration of folate with vitamin-B-complex exerts a protective effect on the brain atrophy associated with eHcy [145, 146]. However, supplementation with high doses of folate was reported to worsen long-term episodic memory, total episodic memory and global cognition [71, 147]. Folic acid was initially suspected to be epileptogenic, but that concern has been resolved, as research has demonstrated that folic acid in therapeutic concentrations does not promote seizures. Folic acid level may be too low in persons with epilepsy taking some antiepileptic drugs [148] that might aggravate cognitive decline [149–151].

Low doses of the GABA A receptor antagonist picrotoxin prevented long-term potentiation deficits in the dentate gyrus [152], which may contribute to cognitive impairments, but blocking inhibition with GABA A receptor antagonists can also exacerbate or precipitate seizures, as proved by Palop in animal studies [46].

Some authors offer new avenues of dementia treatment aimed on enhancing of neurogenesis. Importantly, development of strategies that enhance hippocampal neurogenesis such as administration of distinct neurotrophic factors, physical exercise, exposure to enriched environment, antidepressant therapy, and grafting of neural stem cells (NSCs) are proposed for easing various impairments associated with chronic epilepsy [153]. Administration of neurotrophic factors (such as FGF-2, IGF-1 and BDNF) is based on their ability to enhance neurogenesis in both intact and injured aged hippocampus [153–155].

The emerging therapy – grafting of neural stem cells or glial progenitors into the chronically epileptic hippocampus – increases neurogenesis, and might also induce other beneficial effects such as seizure control through generation of new GABAergic interneurons [153, 154, 156] and improved cognitive function through the release of neurotrophic factors by the grafted NSCs.

The alternative strategy to increase neurogenesis could be the administration of antidepressants, especially selective serotonin reuptake inhibitors (SSRI), known by their capacity to enhance neurogenesis by increasing the concentrations of serotonin, norepinephrine, CREB, and multiple neurotrophic factors [157, 158]. In fact, in epilepsy patients with coexisting cognitive impairments and depression, administration of antidepressants may be a useful and clinically safe option [159–161].

Converging pathways between epilepsy and dementia are associated with the causal relationship between Aβ-induced aberrant excitatory neuronal activity and cognitive decline in humans. Accordingly, decreasing of the β-amyloid level and combating other mechanisms related to amyloid pathology could be regarded as important therapeutic targets for the treatment of patients with seizures and dementia, especially AD. Human and amyloid precursor protein (hAPP) transgenic mice simulate key aspects of AD, including pathologically elevated levels of amyloid-β peptides in brain, aberrant neural network activity, remodeling of hippocampal circuits, synaptic deficits, and behavioral abnormalities [85, 118]. It was shown recently that levetiracetam (LEV) can ameliorate hAPP/Aβ-induced network, synaptic, cognitive, and behavioral dysfunctions in experimental setting [162]. Clinical studies demonstrated that in patients with amnestic MCI, low dose of levetiracetam, which attenuated dentate gyrus/CA3 activation, significantly improved performance in some memory tasks [163].

As LEV has been used has been widely used in epilepsy and proved to be effective with good tolerability and few drug interactions [164–167], it might be considered a valuable therapeutic instrument in patients with epilepsy and cognitive decline/dementia.

The proper choice of AEDs is essential in symptomatic treatment of seizures in patients with dementia; possible risks and benefits of the drug for the elderly patient should be noted. In principle, all the AEDs, approved for focal seizures, could be used; however, the key issues are safety in terms of drug-related adverse effect, especially cognitive and favorable pharmacokinetic profile. Frequent comorbidities of dementia such as psychiatric (depression, anxiety, etc.) and numerous somatic (diabetes, hypertension, low bone density, etc.) should be carefully taken in consideration. Patients who have been maintained on long-term enzyme-inducers AEDs as

CBZ, PHT, PB may be at risk of age-accelerated vascular disease that may contribute to the risk of progressive cognitive, brain, and behavioral changes. Accordingly, priority might be given to the new AED [168–171].

The importance of adequate seizure control in patients with comorbid epilepsy and dementia is highlighted by the notion that seizures act as predictors of hippocampal atrophy in Alzheimer's disease [172, 173].

Known for centuries association between epilepsy and dementia is in the focus of experimental, translational, and clinical research during the last decades. There are similarities (as well as differences) between patients with dementias, especially AD and those with temporal lobe epilepsy, and between animal models of AD and TLE. Seizures in the human temporal lobe transiently impair cognition and steadily damage hippocampal circuitry, leading to progressive memory loss; many mechanisms involved in AD influence excitability and cause seizures [46, 76, 118]. Better understanding of the converging neurobiological pathways of epilepsy and dementia could enrich our therapeutic armamentarium and allow to improve control of both conditions, ameliorate related abnormalities, and potentially modify disease progression.

Acknowledgments The author is sincerely grateful to Prof. Natalia Gulyaeva and Drs. Oxana Danilenko and Mikhail Zinchuk for their invaluable assistance in preparation of this chapter.

References

1. Berrios G. Dementia: historical overview. In: Burns A, O'Brien J, Ames D, editors. Dementia. 3rd ed. London: Hodder Arnold; 2005. p. 3–15. doi:10.1201/b13239-3.
2. Willis T. Practice of physick. London: T. Dring, C. Harper, and J. Leigh; 1684. p. 209–14.
3. Diderot D, d'Alembert J. Encyclopédie ou dictionnaire raisonné des sciences, des arts et des métiers [Encyclopedia or systematic dictionary of the sciences, arts and crafts]. Paris: Briasson, David, Le Breton, Durand; 1765. p. 807–8.
4. Fisher RS. Epilepsy from the patient's perspective: review of results of a community-based survey. Epilepsy Behav. 2000;1:9–14. doi:10.1006/ebeh.2000.0107.
5. Brooks-Kayal A. Molecular mechanisms of cognitive and behavioral comorbidities of epilepsy in children. Epilepsia. 2011;52 Suppl 1:13–20. doi:10.1111/j.1528-1167.2010.02906.x.
6. Carreño M, Donaire A, Sánchez-Carpintero R. Cognitive disorders associated with epilepsy: diagnosis and treatment. Neurologist. 2008;14 Suppl 1:26–34. doi:10.1097/01.nrl.0000340789.15295.8f.
7. Aldenkamp AP. Antiepileptic drug treatment and epileptic seizures – effects on cognitive function. In: Trimble M, Schmitz B, editors. The neuropsychiatry of epilepsy. New York: Cambridge University Press; 2002. p. 256–67. doi:10.1017/cbo9780511544354.017.
8. Lin JJ, Mula M, Hermann BP. Uncovering the neurobehavioural comorbidities of epilepsy over the lifespan. Lancet. 2012;380(9848):1180–92. doi:10.1016/S0140-6736(12)61455-X.
9. Korczyn AD, Schachter SC, Brodie MJ, Dalal SS, Engel JJ, Guekht A, et al. Epilepsy, cognition, and neuropsychiatry (Epilepsy, Brain, and Mind, part 2). Epilepsy Behav. 2013;28:283–302. doi:10.1016/j.yebeh.2013.03.012.
10. Taylor J, Kolamunnage-Dona R, Marson AG, Smith PE, Aldenkamp AP, Baker GA. Patients with epilepsy: cognitively compromised before the start of antiepileptic drug treatment? Epilepsia. 2010;51:48–56. doi:10.1111/j.1528-1167.2009.02195.x.

11. Helmstaedter C, Fritz NE, Hoffmann J, Elger CE. Impact of newly diagnosed and untreated symptomatic/cryptogenic epilepsy on cognition. Epilepsia. 2005;46:152.
12. Aniol VA, Ivanova-Dyatlova AY, Keren O, Guekht AB, Sarne Y, Gulyaeva NV. A single pentylenetetrazole-induced clonic-tonic seizure episode is accompanied by a slowly developing cognitive decline in rats. Epilepsy Behav. 2013;26:196–202. doi:10.1016/j.yebeh.2012.12.006.
13. Hauser WA, Morris ML, Heston LL, Anderson VE. Seizures and myoclonus in patients with Alzheimer's disease. Neurology. 1986;36:1226–30. doi:10.1212/wnl.36.9.1226.
14. Romanelli MF, Morris JC, Ashkin K, Coben LA. Advanced Alzheimer's disease is a risk factor for late-onset seizures. Arch Neurol. 1990;47:847–50. doi:10.1001/archneur.1990.00530080029006.
15. Hesdorffer D, Hauser WA, Annegers JF, et al. Dementia and adult-onset unprovoked seizures. Neurology. 1996;46:727–30. doi:10.1212/wnl.46.3.727.
16. Amatniek JC, Hauser WA, DelCastillo-Castaneda C, Jacobs DM, Marder K, Bell K, Albert M, Brandt J, Stern Y. Incidence and predictors of seizures in patients with Alzheimer's disease. Epilepsia. 2006;47:867–72. doi:10.1111/j.1528-1167.2006.00554.x.
17. Scarmeas N, Honig LS, Choi H, Cantero J, Brandt J, Blacker D, Albert M, Amatniek JC, Marder K, Bell K, Hauser WA, Stern Y. Seizures in Alzheimer disease: who, when, and how common? Arch Neurol. 2009;66:992–7. doi:10.1001/archneurol.2009.130.
18. Pohlmann-Eden B, Eden MA. Dementia and epilepsy. In: Trimble MR, Schmitz B, editors. The neuropsychiatry of epilepsy. New York: Kenbridge University Press; 2011. p. 46–56. doi:10.1017/cbo9780511977145.006.
19. Bull MJ, the Committee on Genetics. Health supervision for children with Down syndrome. Pediatrics. 2011;128:393–406. doi:10.1542/peds.2011-1605.
20. Thiel RJ, Fowkes SW. Down syndrome and epilepsy: a nutritional connection? Med Hypotheses. 2004;62:35–44. doi:10.1016/s0306-9877(03)00294-9.
21. Sangani M, Shahid A, Amina S, Koubeissi M. Improvement of myoclonic epilepsy in Down syndrome treated with levetiracetam. Epileptic Disord. 2010;12:151–4. doi:10.1684/epd.2010.0306.
22. Ferlazzo E, Adjien CK, Guerrini R, Calarese T, Crespel A, Elia M, et al. Lennox-Gastaut syndrome with late- onset and prominent reflex seizures in trisomy 21 patients. Epilepsia. 2009;50:1587–95. doi:10.1111/j.1528-1167.2008.01944.x.
23. Barca D, Tarta-Arsene O, Dica A, Iliescu C, Budisteanu M, Motoescu C, Butoianu N, et al. Intellectual disability and epilepsy in Down syndrome. Maedica (Buchar). 2014;9:344–50.
24. McVicker RW, Shanks OE, McClelland RJ. Prevalence and associated features of epilepsy in adults with Down's syndrome. Br J Psychiatry. 1994;164:528–32. doi:10.1192/bjp.164.4.528.
25. Frey LC, Ringel SP, Filley CM. The natural history of cognitive dysfunction in late-onset GM2 gangliosidosis. Arch Neurol. 2005;62:989–94. doi:10.1001/archneur.62.6.989.
26. Shahwan A, Farrell M, Delanty N. Progressive myoclonic epilepsies: a review of genetic and therapeutic aspects. Lancet Neurol. 2005;4:239–48. doi:10.1016/s1474-4422(05)70043-0.
27. Camicioli R. Differentiation from non-Alzheimer dementia. In: Gauthier S, editor. Clinical diagnosis and management of Alzheimer's disease. 3rd ed. Abingdon: Informa Healthcare; 2006. p. 53–66. doi:10.3109/9780203931714-8.
28. Hendrie HC. Epidemiology of Dementia and Alzheimers Disease. J Geriatr Psychiatry. 1998;6 Suppl 1:3–18.
29. Luhdorf K, Jensen LK, Plesner AM. Etiology of seizures in the elderly. Epilepsia. 1986;27:458–63. doi:10.1111/j.1528-1157.1986.tb03567.x.
30. Hauser WA, Annegers JF, Kurland LT. Incidence of epilepsy and unprovoked seizures in Rochester,Minnesota:1935–1984.Epilepsia.1993;34:453–68.doi:10.1111/j.1528-1157.1993.tb02586.x.
31. Annegers JF, Hauser WA, Lee JR, Rocca WA. Secular trends and birth cohort effects in unprovoked seizures: Rochester, Minnesota 1935–1984. Epilepsia. 1995;36:575–9. doi:10.1111/j.1528-1157.1995.tb02570.x.

32. Hussain SA, Haut SR, Lipton RB, Derby C, Markowitz SY, Shinnar S. Incidence of epilepsy in a racially diverse, community-dwelling, elderly cohort: results from the Einstein aging study. Epilepsy Res. 2006;71:195–205. doi:10.1016/j.eplepsyres.2006.06.018.
33. Pugh MJ, Knoefel JE, Mortensen EM, Amuan ME, Berlowitz DR, Van Cott AC. New-onset epilepsy risk factors in older veterans. J Am Geriatr Soc. 2009;57:237–42. doi:10.1111/j.1532-5415.2008.02124.x.
34. Blocq P, Marinesco G. Sur les lésions et la pathogénie de l'épilepsie dite essentielle. La Semaine médicale. 1892;12:445–6.
35. Alzheimer A. Über eine eigenartige. Erkrankung der Hirnrinde. Allgemeine. Zeitschrift fűr Psychiatrie. 1907;64:146–8.
36. Buda O, Arsene D, Ceausu M, Dermengiu D, Curca GC. Georges Marinesco and the early research in neuropathology. Neurology. 2009;72:88–91. doi:10.1212/01.wnl.0000338626.93425.74.
37. Mandell AM, Green RC. Alzheimer' s disease. In: Budson AE, Kowall NW, editors. The handbook of Alzheimer's disease and other dementias. 1st ed. Oxford: Blackwell Publishing Ltd; 2011. p. 1–91. doi:10.1002/9781444344110.ch1.
38. Pandis D, Scarmeas N. Seizures in Alzheimer disease: clinical and epidemiological data. Epilepsy Curr. 2012;12:184–7. doi:10.5698/1535-7511-12.5.184.
39. Larner AJ. Epileptic seizures in AD patients. Neuromolecular Med. 2010;12:71–7. doi:10.1007/s12017-009-8076-z.
40. Mendez M, Lim G. Seizures in elderly patients with dementia: epidemiology and management. Drugs Aging. 2003;20:791–803. doi:10.2165/00002512-200320110-00001.
41. Friedman D, Honig LS, Scarmeas N. Seizures and epilepsy in Alzheimer's disease. CNS Neurosci Ther. 2012;18:285–94. doi:10.1111/j.1755-5949.2011.00251.x.
42. Hamed SA. Atherosclerosis in epilepsy: its causes and implications. Epilepsy Behav. 2014;41:290–6. doi:10.1016/j.yebeh.2014.07.003.
43. Imfeld P, Bodmer M, Schuerch M, Jick SS, Meier CR. Seizures in patients with Alzheimer's disease or vascular dementia: a population-based nested case–control analysis. Epilepsia. 2013;54:700–7. doi:10.1111/epi.12045.
44. Hommet C, Mondon K, Camus V, De Toffol B, Constans T. Epilepsy and dementia in the elderly. Dement Geriatr Cogn Disord. 2008;25:293–300. doi:10.1159/000119103.
45. Doran M, Harvie AK, Larner AJ. Antisocial behaviour orders: the need to consider underlying neuropsychiatric disease. Int J Clin Pract. 2006;60:861–2. doi:10.1111/j.1742-1241.2006.01008.x.
46. Palop JJ, Mucke L. Epilepsy and cognitive impairments in Alzheimer disease. Arch Neurol. 2009;66:435. doi:10.1001/archneurol.2009.15.
47. Palop JJ, Mucke L. Amyloid-β induced neuronal dysfunction in Alzheimer's disease: from synapses toward neural networks. Nat Neurosci. 2010;13:812–8. doi:10.1038/nn.2583.
48. Waldemar G, Dubois B, Emre M, Georges J, McKeith IG, Rossor M, et al. Alzheimer's disease and other disorders associated with dementia. In: Hughes R, Brainin M, Gilhus NE, editors. European handbook of neurological management. Oxford: Blackwell Publishing; 2006. p. 266–98. doi:10.1002/9780470753279.ch19.
49. Jacobs D, Sano M, Marder K, Bell K, Bylsma F, Lafleche G, et al. Age at onset of Alzheimer's disease: relation to pattern of cognitive dysfunction and rate of decline. Neurology. 1994;44:1215–20. doi:10.1212/wnl.44.7.1215.
50. Tunde-Ayinmode MF, Abiodun OA, Ajiboye PO, Buhari OI, Sanya EO. Prevalence and clinical implications of psychopathology in adults with epileps seen in an outpatient clinic in Nigeria. Gen Hosp Psychiatry. 2014;36:703–8. doi:10.1016/j.genhosppsych.2014.08.009.
51. Ponomareva NV, Korovaitseva GI, Rogaev EI. EEG alterations in non-demented individuals related to apolipoprotein E genotype and to risk of Alzheimer disease. Neurobiol Aging. 2008;29:819–27. doi:10.1016/j.neurobiolaging.2006.12.019.

52. Bernardi S, Scaldaferri N, Vanacore N, Trebbastoni A, Francia A, D'Amico A, Prencipe M. Seizures in Alzheimer's disease: a retrospective study of a cohort of outpatients. Epileptic Disord. 2010;12:16–21.
53. Sherzai D, Losey T, Vega S, Sherzai A. Seizures and dementia in the elderly: Nationwide Inpatient Sample 1999–2008. Epilepsy Behav. 2014;36:53–6. doi:10.1016/j.yebeh.2014.04.015.
54. Annegers JF, Hauser WA, Lee JR, Rocca WA. Incidence of acute symptomatic seizures in Rochester, Minnesota, 1935–1984. Epilepsia. 1995;36:327–33. doi:10.1111/j.1528-1157.1995.tb01005.x.
55. Cleary P, Shorvon S, Tallis R. Late-onset seizures as a predictor of subsequent stroke. Lancet. 2004;363:1184–6. doi:10.1016/s0140-6736(04)15946-1.
56. Pendlebury ST. Stroke-related dementia: rates, risk factors and implications for future research. Maturitas. 2009;64:165–71. doi:10.1016/j.maturitas.2009.09.010.
57. Chang CS, Liao CH, Lin CC, Lane HY, Sung FC, Kao CH. Patients with epilepsy are at an increased risk of subsequent stroke: a population-based cohort study. Seizure. 2014;23:377–81. doi:10.1016/j.seizure.2014.02.007.
58. Chabriat H, Vahedi K, Iba-Zizen MT, et al. Clinical spectrum of CADASIL: a study of 7 families. Cerebral autosomal dominant arteriopathy with subcortical infarcts and leukoencephalopathy. Lancet. 1995;346:934–9.
59. Dichgans M. CADASIL: a monogenic condition causing stroke and subcortical vascular dementia. Cerebrovasc Dis. 2002;13 Suppl 2:37–41. doi:10.1159/000049148.
60. Kalimo H, Ruchoux MM, Viitanen M, Kalaria RN. CADASIL: a common form of hereditary arteriopathy causing brain infarcts and dementia. Brain Pathol. 2002;12:371–84. doi:10.1111/j.1750-3639.2002.tb00451.x.
61. Román G. Therapeutic strategies for vascular dementia. In: Burns A, O'Brien J, Ames D, editors. Dementia. 3rd ed. London: CRC Press; 2005. p. 574–600. doi:10.1201/b13239-83.
62. Joutel A, Corpechot C, Ducros A, Vahedi K, Chabriat H, Mouton P, et al. Notch3 mutations in CADASIL, a hereditary adult onset condition causing stroke and dementia. Nature. 1996;383:707–10. doi:10.1038/383707a0.
63. Dichgans M, Mayer M, Uttner I, Brüning R, Müller-Höcker J, Rungger G, et al. The phenotypic spectrum of CADASIL: clinical findings in 102 cases. Ann Neurol. 1998;44:731–9. doi:10.1002/ana.410440506.
64. Desmond DW, Moroney JT, Lynch T, Chan SS, Chin S, Mohr JP. The natural history of CADASIL: a pooled analysis of previously published cases. Stroke. 1999;30:1230–3. doi:10.1161/01.str.30.6.1230.
65. Haan J, Lesnik Oberstein SAJ, Ferrari MD. Epilepsy in cerebral autosomal dominant arteriopathy with subcortical infarcts and leukoencephalopathy. Cerebrovasc Dis. 2007;24:316–7. doi:10.1159/000106518.
66. Velizarova R, Mourand I, Serafini A, Crespel A, Gelisse P. Focal epilepsy as first symptom in CADASIL. Seizure. 2011;20:502–4. doi:10.1016/j.seizure.2011.02.006.
67. Valko PO, Siccoli MM, Schiller A, Wieser HG, Jung HH. Non-convulsive status epilepticus causing focal neurological deficits in CADASIL. BMJ Case Rep. 2009. doi:10.1136/bcr.07.2008.0529.
68. Cordonnier C, Henon H, Derambure P, Pasquier F, Leys D. Influence of pre-existing dementia on the risk of post-stroke epileptic seizures. J Neurol Neurosurg Psychiatry. 2005;76:1649–53. doi:10.1136/jnnp.2005.064535.
69. Cordonnier C, Henon H, Derambure P, Pasquier F, Leys D. Early epileptic seizures after stroke are associated with increased risk of new-onset dementia. J Neurol Neurosurg Psychiatry. 2007;78:514–6. doi:10.1136/jnnp.2006.105080.
70. De Reuck J, Van Maele G. Cognitive impairment and seizures in patients with lacunar strokes. Eur Neurol. 2009;61:159–63. doi:10.1159/000186507.
71. Ansari R, Mahta A, Mallack E, Luo JJ. Hyperhomocysteinemia and neurologic disorders: a review. J Clin Neurol. 2014;10:281–8. doi:10.3988/jcn.2014.10.4.281.

72. Golarai G, Greenwood AC, Feeney DM, Connor JA. Physiological and structural evidence for hippocampal involvement in persistent seizure susceptibility after traumatic brain injury. J Neurosci. 2001;21:8523–37.
73. Pauli E, Hildebrandt M, Romstöck J, Stefan H, Blümcke I. Deficient memory acquisition in temporal lobe epilepsy is predicted by hippocampal granule cell loss. Neurology. 2006;67:1383–9. doi:10.1212/01.wnl.0000239828.36651.73.
74. Ng SK, Hauser WA, Brust J, Susser M. Hypertension and the risk of new-onset unprovoked seizures. Neurology. 1993;43:425–8. doi:10.1212/wnl.43.2.425.
75. Conrad J, Pawlowski M, Dogan MJ, Kovac S, Ritter MA, Evers S. Seizures after cerebrovascular events: risk factors and clinical features. Seizure. 2013;22:275–82. doi:10.1016/j.seizure.2013.01.014.
76. Noebels J. A perfect storm: converging paths of epilepsy and Alzheimer's dementia intersect in the hippocampal formation. Epilepsia. 2011;52 Suppl 1:39–46. doi:10.1111/j.1528-1167.2010.02909.x.
77. Prevett M, Enevoldson TP, Duncan JS. Adult onset acid maltase deficiency associated with epilepsy and dementia: a case report. J Neurol Neurosurg Psychiatry. 1992;55:509. doi:10.1136/jnnp.55.6.509.
78. Larner AJ. Presenilin-1 mutation Alzheimer's disease: a genetic epilepsy syndrome? Epilepsy Behav. 2011;21:20–2. doi:10.1016/j.yebeh.2011.03.022.
79. Kalaria RN, Maestre GE, Arizaga R, Friedland RP, Galasko D, Hall K, et al. Alzheimer's disease and vascular dementia in developing countries: prevalence, management, and risk factors. Lancet Neurol. 2008;7:812–26. doi:10.1016/S1474-4422(08)70169-8.
80. Korczyn AD. Mixed dementia--the most common cause of dementia. Ann N Y Acad Sci. 2002;977:129–34. doi:10.1111/j.1749-6632.2002.tb04807.x.
81. Zekry D, Duyckaerts C, Hauw JJ. Mixed dementia: a neuropathologic point od view. Psychol Neuropsychiatr Vieil. 2005;3:251–9.
82. Vossel KA, Beagle AJ, Rabinovici GD, Shu H, Lee SE, Naasan G, et al. Seizures and epileptiform activity in the early stages of Alzheimer disease. JAMA Neurol. 2013;70:1158–66. doi:10.1001/jamaneurol.2013.136.
83. Rabinowicz AL, Starkstein SE, Leiguarda RC, Coleman AE. Transient epileptic amnesia in dementia: a treatable unrecognized cause of episodic amnestic wandering. Alzheimer Dis Assoc Disord. 2000;14:231–3. doi:10.1097/00002093-200010000-00008.
84. Sinforiani E, Manni R, Bernasconi L, Banchieri LM, Zucchella C. Memory disturbances and temporal lobe epilepsy simulating Alzheimer's disease: a case report. Funct Neurol. 2003;8:39–41.
85. Palop JJ, Chin J, Roberson ED, Wang J, Thwin MT, Bien-Ly N, et al. Aberrant excitatory neuronal activity and compensatory remodeling of inhibitory hippocampal circuits in mouse models of Alzheimer's disease. Neuron. 2007;55:697–711. doi:10.1016/j.neuron.2007.07.025.
86. Velez-Pardo C, Arellano JI, Cardona-Gomez P, Jimenez Del Rio M, Lopera F, De Felipe J. CA1 hippocampal neuronal loss in familial Alzheimer's disease presenilin-1 E280 Amutation is related to epilepsy. Epilepsia. 2004;45:751–6. doi:10.1111/j.0013-9580.2004.55403.x.
87. Hatanpaa KJ, Raisanen JM, Herndon E, Burns DK, Foong C, Habib AA, et al. Hippocampal sclerosis in dementia, epilepsy, and ischemic injury: differential vulnerability of hippocampal subfields. J Neuropathol Exp Neurol. 2014;73:136–42. doi:10.1097/OPX.0000000000000170.
88. Timsit S, Rivera S, Ouaghi P, Guischard F, Tremblay E, Ben-Ari Y, Khrestchatisky M. Increased cyclin D1 in vulnerable neurons in the hippocampus after ischaemia and epilepsy: a modulator of in vivo programmed cell death? Eur J Neurosci. 1999;11:263–78. doi:10.1046/j.1460-9568.1999.00434.x.
89. Szabo K, Förster A, Gass A. Conventional and diffusion-weighted MRI of the hippocampus. Front Neurol Neurosci. 2014;34:71–84. doi:10.1159/000357925.

90. Bandopadhyay R, Liu JY, Sisodiya SM, Thom M. A comparative study of the dentate gyrus in hippocampal sclerosis in epilepsy and dementia. Neuropathol Appl Neurobiol. 2014;40:177–90. doi:10.1111/nan.12087.
91. Counts SE, Alldred MJ, Che S, Ginsberg SD, Mufson EJ. Synaptic gene dysregulation within hippocampal CA1 pyramidal neurons in mild cognitive impairment. Neuropharmacology. 2014;79:172–9. doi:10.1016/j.neuropharm.2013.10.018.
92. Merino-Serrais P, Benavides-Piccione R, Blazquez-Llorca L, Kastanauskaite A, Rábano A, Avila J, et al. The influence of phospho-τ on dendritic spines of cortical pyramidal neurons in patients with Alzheimer's disease. Brain. 2013;136:1913–28. doi:10.1093/brain/awt088.
93. Kerchner GA, Holbrook K. Novel presenilin-1 Y159F sequence variant associated with early-onset alzheimer's disease. Neurosci Lett. 2012;531:142–4. doi:10.1016/j.neulet.2012.10.037.
94. Korf ES, Wahlund LO, Visser PJ, Scheltens P. Medial temporal lobe atrophy on MRI predicts dementia in patients with mild cognitive impairment. Neurology. 2004;63:94–100. doi:10.1212/01.wnl.0000133114.92694.93.
95. Bernasconi N, Bernasconi A, Andermann F, Dubeau F, Feindel W, Reutens DC. Entorhinal cortex in temporal lobe epilepsy: a quantitative MRI study. Neurology. 1999;52:1870–6. doi:10.1212/wnl.52.9.1870.
96. Bernhardt BC, Hong SJ, Bernasconi A, Bernasconi N. Magnetic resonance imaging pattern learning in temporal lobe epilepsy: classification and prognostics. Ann Neurol. 2015;77:436–46. doi:10.1002/ana.24341.
97. Peng B, Wu L, Zhang L, Chen Y. The relationship between hippocampal volumes and non-verbal memory in patients with medial temporal lobe epilepsy. Epilepsy Res. 2014;108:1839–44. doi:10.1016/j.eplepsyres.2014.09.007.
98. Barron DS, Tandon N, Lancaster JL, Fox PT. Thalamic structural connectivity in medial temporal lobe epilepsy. Epilepsia. 2014;55:50–5. doi:10.1111/epi.12637.
99. Paterson A, Winder J, Bell KE, McKinstry CS. An evaluation of how MRI is used as a pre-operative screening investigation in patients with temporal lobe epilepsy. Clin Radiol. 1998;53:353–6. doi:10.1016/s0009-9260(98)80008-1.
100. Salmenperä T, Kälviäinen R, Partanen K, Pitkänen A. Quantitative MRI volumetry of the entorhinal cortex in temporal lobe epilepsy. Seizure. 2000;9:208–15. doi:10.1053/seiz.1999.0373.
101. Keller SS, Roberts N. Voxel-based morphometry of temporal lobe epilepsy: an introduction andreviewoftheliterature.Epilepsia.2008;49:741–57.doi:10.1111/j.1528-1167.2007.01485.x.
102. Yang Y, Kinney GA, Spain WJ, Breitner JC, Cook DG. Presenilin-1 and intracellular calcium stores regulate neuronal glutamate uptake. J Neurochem. 2004;88:1361–72. doi:10.1046/j.1471-4159.2003.02279.x.
103. Eid T, Behar K, Dhaher R, Bumanglag AV, Lee TSW. Roles of glutamine synthetase inhibition in epilepsy. Neurochem Res. 2012;37:2339–50. doi:10.1007/s11064-012-0766-5.
104. Traynelis SF, Dingledine R, McNamara JO, Butler L, Rigsbee L. Effect of kindling on potassium-induced electrographic seizures in vitro. Neurosci Lett. 1989;105:326–32. doi:10.1016/0304-3940(89)90642-3.
105. Tamminga CA, Southcott S, Sacco C, Wagner AD, Ghose S. Glutamate dysfunction in hippocampus: relevance of dentate gyrus and CA3 signaling. Schizophr Bull. 2012;38:927–35. doi:10.1093/schbul/sbs062.
106. Fujita S, Toyoda I, Thamattoor AK, Buckmaster PS. Preictal activity of subicular, CA1, and dentate gyrus principal neurons in the dorsal hippocampus before spontaneous seizures in a rat model of temporal lobe epilepsy. J Neurosci. 2014;34:16671–87. doi:10.1523/JNEUROSCI.0584-14.2014.
107. Wan P, Wang S, Zhang Y, Lv J, Jin QH. Involvement of dopamine D1 receptors of the hippocampal dentate gyrus in spatial learning and memory deficits in a rat model of vascular dementia. Pharmazie. 2014;69:709–10.

108. Koeller HB, Ross ME, Glickstein SB. Cyclin D1 in excitatory neurons of the adult brain enhances kainate-induced neurotoxicity. Neurobiol Dis. 2008;31:230–41. doi:10.1016/j.nbd.2008.04.010.
109. Freeman RS, Estus S, Johnson Jr EM. Analysis of cell cycle-related gene expression in postmitotic neurons: selective induction of Cyclin D1 during programmed cell death. Neuron. 1994;12:343–55. doi:10.1016/0896-6273(94)90276-3.
110. Yang Y, Mufson EJ, Herrup K. Neuronal cell death is preceded by cell cycle events at all stages of Alzheimer's disease. J Neurosci. 2003;23:2557–63.
111. Alberici A, Bonato C, Borroni B, Cotelli M, Mattioli F, Binetti G, et al. Dementia, delusions and seizures: storage disease or genetic AD? Eur J Neurol. 2007;14:1057–9. doi:10.1111/j.1468-1331.2007.01664.x.
112. Minkeviciene R, Rheims S, Dobszay MB, Zilberter M, Hartikainen J, Fülöp L, et al. Amyloid beta-induced neuronal hyperexcitability triggers progressive epilepsy. J Neurosci. 2009;29:3453–62. doi:10.1523/JNEUROSCI.5215-08.2009.
113. Minkeviciene R, Ihalainen J, Malm T, Matilainen O, Keksa-Goldsteine V, Goldsteins G, et al. Age-related decrease in stimulated glutamate release and vesicular glutamate transporters in APP/PS1 transgenic and wild-type mice. J Neurochem. 2008;105:584–94. doi:10.1111/j.1471-4159.2007.05147.x.
114. Palop JJ, Mucke L. Synaptic depression and aberrant excitatory network activity in Alzheimer's disease: two faces of the same coin? Neuromolecular Med. 2010;12:48–55. doi:10.1007/s12017-009-8097-7.
115. LaFerla FM, Green KN, Oddo S. Intracellular amyloid-beta in Alzheimer's disease. Nat Rev Neurosci. 2007;8:499–509. doi:10.1038/nrn2168.
116. Shilling D, Müller M, Takano H, Mak DO, Abel T, Coulter DA, et al. Suppression of InsP3 receptor-mediated Ca2+ signaling alleviates mutant presenilin-linked familial Alzheimer's disease pathogenesis. J Neurosci. 2014;34:6910–23. doi:10.1523/JNEUROSCI.5441-13.2014.
117. Leonard AS, McNamara JO. Does epileptiform activity contribute to cognitive impairment in Alzheimer's disease? Neuron. 2007;55:677–8. doi:10.1016/j.neuron.2007.08.014.
118. Scharfman HE. Alzheimer's disease and epilepsy: insight from animal models. Future Neurol. 2012;7:177–92. doi:10.2217/fnl.12.8.
119. Karlsson IK, Bennet AM, Ploner A, Andersson TM, Reynolds CA, Gatz M, et al. Apolipoprotein E ε4 genotype and the temporal relationship between depression and dementia. Neurobiol Aging. 2015. doi:10.1016/j.neurobiolaging.2015.01.008.
120. Rohn TT. Is apolipoprotein E4 an important risk factor for vascular dementia? Int J Clin Exp Pathol. 2014;7:3504–11.
121. Busch RM, Lineweaver TT, Naugle RI, Kim KH, Gong Y, Tilelli CQ, et al. ApoE-epsilon4 is associated with reduced memory in long-standing intractable temporal lobe epilepsy. Neurology. 2007;68:409–14. doi:10.1212/01.wnl.0000253021.60887.db.
122. Kado DM, Karlamangla AS, Huang MH, Troen A, Rowe JW, Selhub J, et al. Homocysteine versus the vitamins folate, B6, and B12 as predictors of cognitive function and decline in older high-functioning adults: MacArthur Studies of Successful Aging. Am J Med. 2005;118:161–7. doi:10.1016/j.amjmed.2004.08.019.
123. Gorgone G, Caccamo D, Pisani LR, Currò M, Parisi G, Oteri G, et al. Hyperhomocysteinemia in patients with epilepsy: does it play a role in the pathogenesis of brain atrophy? A preliminary report. Epilepsia. 2009;50 Suppl 1:33–6. doi:10.1111/j.1528-1167.2008.01967.x.
124. Licht EA, Fujikawa DG. Nonconvulsive status epilepticus with frontal features: quantitating severity of subclinical epileptiform discharges provides a marker for treatment efficacy, recurrence and outcome. Epilepsy Res. 2002;51:13–21. doi:10.1016/s0920-1211(02)00107-9.
125. Pacagnella D, Lopes TM, Morita ME, Yasuda CL, Cappabianco FA, Bergo F, et al. Memory impairment is not necessarily related to seizure frequency in mesial temporal lobe epilepsy with hippocampal sclerosis. Epilepsia. 2014;55:1197–204. doi:10.1111/epi.12691.

126. Park IS, Yoo SW, Lee KS, Kim JS. Epileptic seizure presenting as dementia with Lewy bodies. Gen Hosp Psychiatry. 2014;36:3–5. doi:10.1016/j.genhosppsych.2013.10.015.
127. Mrak RE, Griffin WT. Dementia with Lewy bodies: definition, diagnosis, and pathogenic relationship to Alzheimer's disease. Neuropsychiatr Dis Treat. 2007;3:619–25.
128. Vyas U, Franco R. Rem behavior disorder (RBD) as an early marker for development of neurodegenerative diseases. BJMP. 2012;5:506.
129. Oono M, Uno H, Umesaki A, Nagatsuka K, Kinoshita M, Naritomi H. Severe and prolonged ictal paresis in an elderly patient. Epilepsy Behav Case Rep. 2014;2:105–7. doi:10.1016/j.ebcr.2014.03.009.
130. Jones R. Co-existent medical problems and concomitant diseases. In: Gauthier S, editor. Clinical diagnosis and management of Alzheimer's disease. Abingdon: Taylor & Francis Group, LLC; 2007. p. 257–65. doi:10.3109/9780203931714-26.
131. Leppik IE. The place of levetiracetam in the treatment of epilepsy. Epilepsia. 2001;42:44–5. doi:10.1111/j.1528-1167.2001.00010.x.
132. Krämer G. Epileptic seizures and epilepsy in the elderly]. Ther Umsch. 2001;58:684–90.
133. Brainin M, Matz K, Nemec M, Teuschl Y, Dachenhausen A, Asenbaum-Nan S, et al. Prevention of poststroke cognitive decline: ASPIS – a multicenter, randomized, observer-blind, parallel group clinical trial to evaluate multiple lifestyle interventions - study design and baseline characteristics. Int J Stroke. 2013. doi:10.1111/ijs.12188.
134. Teuschl Y, Matz K, Brainin M. Prevention of post-stroke cognitive decline: a review focusing onlifestyleinterventions.EurJNeurol.2013;20:35–49.doi:10.1111/j.1468-1331.2012.03757.x.
135. Danysz W, Parsons CG. Alzheimer's disease, β-amyloid, glutamate, NMDA receptors and memantine--searching for the connections. Br J Pharmacol. 2012;167:324–52. doi:10.1111/j.1476-5381.2012.02057.x.
136. Thomas SJ, Grossberg GT. Memantine: a review of studies into its safety and efficacy in treating Alzheimer's disease and other dementias. Clin Interv Aging. 2009;4:367–77. doi:10.2147/cia.s6666.
137. Parsons CG, Danysz W, Dekundy A, Pulte I. Memantine and cholinesterase inhibitors: complementary mechanisms in the treatment of Alzheimer's disease. Neurotox Res. 2013;24:358–69. doi:10.1007/s12640-013-9398-z.
138. Fisher RS, Bortz JJ, Blum DE, Duncan B, Burke H. A pilot study of donepezil for memory problems in epilepsy. Epilepsy Behav. 2001;2:330–4. doi:10.1006/ebeh.2001.0221.
139. Kim H, Kim G, Jang W, Kim SY, Chang N. Association between intake of B vitamins and cognitive function in elderly Koreans with cognitive impairment. Nutr J. 2014;13:118. doi:10.1186/1475-2891-13-118.
140. Li MM, Yu JT, Wang HF, Jiang T, Wang J, Meng XF, et al. Efficacy of vitamins B supplementation on mild cognitive impairment and Alzheimer's disease: a systematic review and meta-analysis. Curr Alzheimer Res. 2014;11:844–52.
141. Agnew-Blais JC, Wassertheil-Smoller S, Kang JH, Hogan PE, Coker LH, Snetselaar LG, et al. Folate, vitamin B-6, and vitamin B-12 intake and mild cognitive impairment and probable dementia in the Women's Health Initiative Memory study. J Acad Nutr Diet. 2015;115:231–41. doi:10.1016/j.jand.2014.07.006.
142. Annweiler C, Dursun E, Féron F, Gezen-Ak D, Kalueff AV, Littlejohns T, et al. 'Vitamin D and cognition in older adults': updated international recommendations. J Intern Med. 2015;277:45–57. doi:10.1111/joim.12279.
143. Song JH, Park MH, Han C, Jo SA, Ahn K. Serum homocysteine and folate levels are associated with late-life dementia in a Korean population. Osong Public Health Res Perspect. 2010;1:17–22. doi:10.1016/j.phrp.2010.12.006.
144. Loria-Kohen V, Gómez-Candela C, Palma-Milla S, Amador-Sastre B, Hernanz A, Bermejo LM. A pilot study of folic acid supplementation for improving homocysteine levels, cognitive and depressive status in eating disorders. Nutr Hosp. 2013;28:807–15. doi:10.3305/nh.2013.28.3.6335.

145. Ford AH, Flicker L, Alfonso H, Thomas J, Clarnette R, Martins R, et al. Vitamins B(12), B(6), and folic acid for cognition in older men. Neurology. 2010;75:1540–7. doi:10.1212/wnl.0b013e3181f962c4.
146. Blasko I, Hinterberger M, Kemmler G, Jungwirth S, Krampla W, Leitha T, Heinz Tragl K, Fischer P. Conversion from mild cognitive impairment to dementia: influence of folic acid and vitamin B12 use in the VITA cohort. J Nutr Health Aging. 2012;16:687–94. doi:10.1007/s12603-012-0051-y.
147. Singleton AB, Farrer MJ, Bonifati V. The genetics of Parkinson's disease: progress and therapeutic implications. Mov Disord. 2013;28:14–23. doi:10.1002/mds.25249.
148. Morrell MJ, Sarto GE, Shafer PO, Borda EA, Herzog A, Callanan M. Health issues for women with epilepsy: a descriptive survey to assess knowledge and awareness among healthcare providers. J Womens Health Gend Based Med. 2000;9:959–65. doi:10.1089/15246090050199982.
149. Hernández R, Fernández Mde L, Miranda G, Suástegui R. Decrease of folic acid and cognitive alterations in patients with epilepsy treated with phenytoin or carbamazepine, pilot study. Rev Invest Clin. 2005;57:522–31.
150. Sener U, Zorlu Y, Karaguzel O, Ozdamar O, Coker I, Topbas M. Effects of common antiepileptic drug monotherapy on serum levels of homocysteine, vitamin B12, folic acid and vitamin B6. Seizure. 2006;2:79–85. doi:10.1016/j.seizure.2005.11.002.
151. Ogawa Y, Kaneko S, Otani K, Fukushima Y. Serum folic acid levels in epileptic mothers and their relationship to congenital malformations. Epilepsy Res. 1991;8:75–8. doi:10.1016/0920-1211(91)90039-i.
152. Yoshiike Y, Kimura T, Yamashita S, Furudate H, Mizoroki T, Murayama M, et al. GABAA receptor-mediated acceleration of aging-associated memory decline in APP/PS1 mice and its pharmacological treatment by picrotoxin. PLoS One. 2008;3:3029. doi:10.1371/journal.pone.0003029.
153. Kuruba R, Hattiangady B, Shetty AK. Hippocampal neurogenesis and neural stem cells in temporal lobe epilepsy. Epilepsy Behav. 2009;14 Suppl 1:65–73. doi:10.1016/j.yebeh.2008.08.020.
154. Hattiangady B, Shetty AK. Subcutaneous administration of BDNF dramatically enhances dentate neurogenesis in the injured aged hippocampus. Soc Neurosci Abstr. 2007;562:12.
155. Jin K, Sun Y, Xie L, Batteur S, Mao XO, Smelick C, et al. Neurogenesis and aging: FGF-2 and HB-EGF restore neurogenesis in hippocampus and subventricular zone of aged mice. Aging Cell. 2003;2:175–83. doi:10.1046/j.1474-9728.2003.00046.x.
156. Shetty AK, Hattiangady B. Prospects of stem cell therapy for temporal lobe epilepsy. Stem Cells. 2007;25:2396–407. doi:10.1634/stemcells.2007-0313.
157. Kohl Z, Winner B, Ubhi K, Rockenstein E, Mante M, Münch M, et al. Fluoxetine rescues impaired hippocampal neurogenesis in a transgenic A53T synuclein mouse model. Eur J Neurosci. 2012;35:10–9. doi:10.1111/j.1460-9568.2011.07933.x.
158. Peters ME, Vaidya V, Drye LT, Rosenberg PB, Martin BK, Porsteinsson AP, et al. Sertraline for the treatment of depression in Alzheimer disease: genetic influences. J Geriatr Psychiatry Neurol. 2011;24(4):222–8. doi:10.1177/0891988711422527.
159. Mula M, Schmitz B, Sander JW. The pharmacological treatment of depression in adults with epilepsy. Expert Opin Pharmacother. 2008;9:3159–68. doi:10.1517/14656560802587024.
160. Pisani F, Spina E, Oteri G. Antidepressant drugs and seizure susceptibility: from in vitro data to clinical practice. Epilepsia. 1999;40 Suppl 10:S48–56. doi:10.1111/j.1528-1157.1999.tb00885.x.
161. Harden CL, Goldstein MA. Mood disorders in patients with epilepsy: epidemiology and management. CNS Drugs. 2002;16:291–302. doi:10.2165/00023210-200216050-00002.
162. Sanchez PE, Zhu L, Verret L, Vossel KA, Orr AG, Cirrito JR, et al. Levetiracetam suppresses neuronal network dysfunction and reverses synaptic and cognitive deficits in an Alzheimer's disease model. Proc Natl Acad Sci U S A. 2012;109:2895–903. doi:10.1073/pnas.1121081109.

163. Bakker A, Krauss GL, Albert MS, Speck CL, Jones LR, Stark CE, et al. Reduction of hippocampal hyperactivity improves cognition in amnestic mild cognitive impairment. Neuron. 2012;74:467–74. doi:10.1016/j.neuron.2012.03.023.
164. Ben-Menachem E, Gilland E. Efficacy and tolerability of levetiracetam during 1-year follow-up in patients with refractory epilepsy. Seizure. 2003;12:131–5. doi:10.1016/s1059-1311(02)00251-0.
165. Cereghino JJ, Biton V, Abou-Khalil B, Dreifuss F, Gauer LJ, Leppik I. Levetiracetam for partial seizures: results of a double-blind, randomized clinical trial. Neurology. 2000;55(2):236–42. doi:10.1212/wnl.55.2.236.
166. Brodie MJ, Perucca E, Ryvlin P, Ben-Menachem E, Meencke HJ. Levetiracetam Monotherapy Study Group. Comparison of levetiracetam and controlled-release carbamazepine in newly diagnosed epilepsy. Neurology. 2007;68:402–8. doi:10.1212/01.wnl.0000252941.50833.4a.
167. Shorvon SD, Löwenthal A, Janz D, Bielen E, Loiseau P. Multicenter double-blind, randomized, placebo-controlled trial of levetiracetam as add-on therapy in patients with refractory partial seizures. European Levetiracetam Study Group. Epilepsia. 2000;41:1179–86. doi:10.1111/j.1528-1157.2000.tb00323.x.
168. Patsalos PN. Antiepileptic drug interactions. London: Springer; 2013. doi:10.1007/978-1-4471-2434-4.
169. Perucca E, French J, Bialer M. Development of new antiepileptic drugs: challenges, incentives, and recent advances. Lancet Neurol. 2007;6:793–804. doi:10.1016/s1474-4422(07)70215-6.
170. French JA, Gazzola DM. New generation antiepileptic drugs: what do they offer in terms of improved tolerability and safety? Ther Adv Drug Saf. 2011;2:141–58. doi:10.1177/2042098611411127.
171. Johannessen Landmark C, Patsalos PN. Drug interactions involving the new second- and third-generation antiepileptic drugs. Expert Rev Neurother. 2010;10:119–40. doi:10.1586/ern.09.136.
172. Dhikav V, Anand K. Potential predictors of hippocampal atrophy in Alzheimer's disease. Drugs Aging. 2011;28:1–11. doi:10.2165/11586390-000000000-00000.
173. Dhikav V, Anand K. Hippocampal atrophy may be a predictor of seizures in Alzheimer's disease. Med Hypotheses. 2007;69:234–5. doi:10.1016/j.mehy.2006.11.031.

Chapter 15
Stress and Epilepsy

Clare M. Galtrey and Hannah R. Cock

Abstract The notion that stress, the physiological and/or behavioral response to event(s) interpreted as threatening to well-being, plays a role in triggering seizures or even causing epilepsy has been extensively studied in both experimental and clinical contexts. People with epilepsy consistently report stress as one of the most common triggers, although disentangling from confounders such as sleep deprivation, mood, and alcohol, and cause from effect has proved challenging. A great deal of effort (and money) has gone into pre-clinical and clinical research, including more recently functional imaging studies, such that we now have a good understanding of pathways and potential mechanisms. Similarly, there has been considerable work looking at ways to reduce stress, which can undoubtedly be of benefit in terms of psychological well-being, though may not improve seizure control. There has been very little consideration of cost-effectiveness or cost-utility thus far, which is of particular importance when there are inevitable limitations on resources. Thus beyond heightened awareness about the potential for stress and epilepsy to interact, little of this work has as yet translated into meaningful changes for clinical practice. Hopefully, further carefully directed preclinical and especially clinical research will lead to greater understanding of the interaction and benefit to patients.

Keywords Epilepsy • Seizures • Stress • Mechanisms • Treatment • Epileptogenesis • Prenatal • Delayed Effects

---

C.M. Galtrey, MA, PhD, MB BChir, MRCP
Epilepsy Group, Atkinson Morley Regional Neuroscience Centre,
St. George's University Hospitals NHS Foundation Trust,
Blackshaw Road, London SW17 0QT, UK
e-mail: clare.galtrey@gmail.com

H.R. Cock, BSc, MD, MBBS, FRCP (✉)
Epilepsy Group, Atkinson Morley Regional Neuroscience Centre,
St. George's University Hospitals NHS Foundation Trust,
Blackshaw Road, London SW17 0QT, UK

Institute of Biomedical and Medical Education, St. George's University of London,
Cranmer Terrace, London SW17 0RE, UK
e-mail: hannahrc@sgul.ac.uk

M. Mula (ed.), *Neuropsychiatric Symptoms of Epilepsy*, Neuropsychiatric Symptoms of Neurological Disease, DOI 10.1007/978-3-319-22159-5_15

Introduction

Stress and epilepsy interact on many levels: many patients with epilepsy report that stress influences the frequency and severity of their seizures; recent or past stressors might be the cause of their epilepsy, and for most the occurrence of a seizure, or a diagnosis of epilepsy per se is a stressful event both at the time, and for some more chronically. As a result patients may be resistant to evidence-based treatment changes, or expend considerable efforts on seeking explanations or attempting to exclude stress from day to day life, often without clear benefit. On rare occasions beliefs may be held so firmly the individual struggles to accept the diagnosis of epilepsy at all, as illustrated by Box 15.1.

Box 15.1. Stress and Epilepsy: Illustrative Case Summaries

1. A 35-year-old nurse presented with witnessed generalized tonic–clonic seizures occurring from sleep with lateral tongue biting on two consecutive nights while staying with a friend who called an ambulance on both occasions. Attending paramedics noted post-ictal drowsiness and obvious tongue injury. She also reported waking on 3–4 occasions in the preceding year with a bitten tongue and feeling unwell, but had not sought medical attention. She had a history of viral encephalitis aged 18 from which she had made a full recovery. She also disclosed having had particularly stressful life events in the days leading up to the recent cluster, and prior to events over the preceding year. MRI was normal and EEG showed frequent left temporal inter-ictal discharges. A diagnosis of epilepsy was made independently by two neurologists specializing in epilepsy – one on presentation to hospital with her second witnessed seizure, and a second at a later clinic appointment. At the time of writing, the patient remains adamantly of the view that her attacks were caused by stress for which she has now sought counseling, and against advice has not started treatment with any antiepileptic drug.
2. An otherwise well man underwent a left amygdalohippocampectomy for refractory temporal lobe epilepsy at the age of 33 years, and was found to have hippocampal sclerosis together with a dysplastic amygdala on histology. Pre-operatively he experienced infrequent convulsions, but clusters of focal seizures with altered awareness and automatisms every 3–4 weeks since the age of 15 despite antiepileptic medication. Post-operatively he remains seizure free (14 months) on stable doses of two drugs, other than a single episode at 10 months when he had been increasingly stressed by a change in work-hours (shifts) over 1–2 weeks and forgot several doses of his medication over consecutive days.
3. A woman, aged 33 at the time, had been very distressed following an episode towards the end of her second pregnancy when she awoke to find an

intruder in her home. Sometime after this she presented to her general practitioner with daily episodes of sudden fear and panic, which were attributed to stress. Despite counseling the attacks worsened, and by age 36 were interrupting activities with brief periods of amnesia, described by her husband as associated with episodes of being fidgety and pacing around over 20–30 s, sometimes with injuries. Citalopram had been added, without benefit and aged 39 she sought a private neurology opinion – a diagnosis of temporal lobe epilepsy, supported by left temporal abnormalities on MRI and EEG. However, despite witnessing a typical attack, the neurologist felt she also had post-traumatic panic attacks and continued to reinforce stress management approaches. As there was only marginal benefit with the levetiracetam, she was referred for a specialist epilepsy opinion aged 40, where pre-surgical evaluation was commenced in addition to switching her levetiracetam to lamotrigine, and withdrawing the citalopram. Video EEG subsequently confirmed all of her attacks were focal seizures. On Lamotrigine she has at the time of writing had no daytime attacks for over 2 years, and only infrequent attacks from sleep so has deferred further investigation.

A considerable body of work in this area, both pre-clinical and clinical, illustrates that although potential mechanisms have been well elucidated, the association between stress and epilepsy is complex. This chapter will explore what evidence there is from both clinical and basic scientific research to support any causal association between stress, the occurrence of seizures and epilepsy, with a view to informing both future research and clinical practice.

Stress is defined as the physiological and/or behavioral response to an event or events that are interpreted as threatening to the well-being of the individual response [1]. Stress is a widely used term in lay, physiological, and psychological contexts, each with a different perspective. Precipitating events can be physical, environmental, psychological, and pharmacological. Most stress now is not life threatening but psychosocial, with both interpersonal and environmental contributors that are perceived as straining or exceeding the individuals' adaptive capacities. The element of perception is key, and reflects individual differences in personality, as well as physical or health differences. Nonetheless, however defined, stress is present to a greater or lesser extent for all of us at times throughout life.

Many known triggers for seizures (in some cases also leading to epilepsy) are of themselves stressful, for example traumatic brain injury, alcohol withdrawal, acute stroke, which we will not be discussing other than where stress has been considered as a specific contributor. Similarly it is self-evident that for most the occurrence of a seizure, or a diagnosis of epilepsy per se, is a stressful event both at the time, and for some more chronically. It is also well recognized that there is a high prevalence of anxiety and depression in patients with epilepsy. These topics are covered in detail in Chaps. 2 and 4 and will not be further discussed here, other than in relation to the potential interaction with stress and seizure control. Finally, it is important to recognize that a major confounder in this area is the high rate of misdiagnosis with dissociative non-epileptic attacks (Chap. 9), where previous or current life stressors have an established role, often being labeled and managed as epilepsy which again we do not intend to cover in this chapter.

The key clinical issues we will address in this chapter are to whether stress can precipitate seizures or contribute to deterioration in seizure control in an individual with epilepsy, and whether stress may increase the likelihood of an individual developing epilepsy in the first place. We will start by summarizing the clinical evidence that stress and seizures are linked, as this is the context for then reviewing definitions and the neurobiology of stress. We will end by considering possible treatments and future research.

Clinical Association of Stress and Seizures

The idea that stress precipitates seizures dates back centuries, as reviewed by Shorvon [2], including: Gowers in 1881 (mental anxiety, frights, excitement, emotion); Turner in 1907 (shock, emotional excitement, fear, anxiety, and overwork); and Lennox in 1960 (emotional disturbances are considered a contributor to the epileptic threshold). More recently still, some have proposed stress-induced seizures might be a specific type of reflex epilepsy [3], or perhaps more controversially that all seizures in temporal lobe epilepsy are provoked, usually by stress [4]. But what evidence is there to really support this?

In retrospective studies, stress is consistently identified as the most common seizure trigger (Table 15.1). However such studies are inherently dependent on patient perception and memory, and often have inherent selection biases, so methodologically unreliable. Loss of self-control is the most disturbing psychosocial consequence of epilepsy and trying to find connections between their seizures and external or internal events that give a feeling of predictability is a natural likely coping mechanism [5]. However, if nothing else such studies illustrate that irrespective of evidence, this is something that concerns patients, so should be of interest to clinicians.

Others have tried to minimize selection bias by studying seizure and epilepsy following traumatic events affecting whole populations. For example, 30 patients evacuated due to flooding in the Netherlands had significantly more seizures during or shortly after the evacuation period ($p<0.05$) compared to matched control patients from a non-flooded area [19]. Similarly, a survey of children with epilepsy during and after the 1991–1992 Croatian War [20] showed that those from directly affected areas ($n=52$) had more seizures than before the war ($p<0.001$), and then those from unaffected areas ($n=34$; $p<0.009$), who were mostly stable throughout. The actual numbers however are still small, the studies retrospective, and stress is inferred rather than confirmed/measured. Furthermore disasters on this scale are very prone to confounding factors such as non-adherence with medication and sleep deprivation as was found during a study in Persian Gulf War [21], although medication

Table 15.1 Retrospective, self-report studies linking seizures and stress [6–18]

Ref.	No	Country	Epilepsy type	Setting	Method	% patients reporting stress as seizure trigger
[6]	177	USA	Mixed	Neurology clinics	Self-report questionnaire	58
[7]	517	Australia	Mixed	Neurology clinics	Self-report questionnaire	41.2 % (trigger); 59 % (plays a role in frequency)
[8]	1628	UK	Mixed, (mostly focal)	Community	Self-report questionnaire	28 %
[9]	79	UK	Mixed	Specialist residential schools	Interview of patients, carer questionnaire	38.5 % by patients; 58.7 % by carers
[10]	400	USA	Mixed	Tertiary care epilepsy center	Self-report questionnaire	30 %
[11]	100	UK	Mixed, refractory	Neurology/neuropsychiatry epilepsy clinics	Semistructured interview	53 % (open questions); 66 % (closed questions)
[12]	89	USA	Mixed	Epilepsy clinic	Self-report Questionnaire	64 %
[13]	1677	Norway and Denmark	Mixed	Twins and family members from registry	Self-report questionnaire	20.9 %
[14]	40	Singapore	Mixed	Epilepsy patients hospitalized for seizures	Structured interview	10 %
[15]	75	Brazil	Juvenile myoclonic epilepsy	Epilepsy clinic	Semistructured interview	83 %
[16]	200	USA	Mixed	Inpatient epilepsy monitoring or outpatient epilepsy clinic	Questionnaire	49.5 %

(continued)

Table 15.1 (continued)

Ref.	No	Country	Epilepsy type	Setting	Method	% patients reporting stress as seizure trigger
[a][17]	433	UK	Mixed	Community longitudinal cohort study	Self-report postal questionnaires, two time points 5 months apart. Modeling based on results	Neither perceived stress nor anxiety independently influence seizure frequency when depression controlled for
[18]	2112	USA	Refractory Focal, + auras	epilepsy clinic 17 %	Self-report questionnaire	67 %

Abbreviations: *UK* United Kingdom, *USA* United States of America, *N/A* not available, *TLE* temporal lobe epilepsy, *IGE* idiopathic generalized epilepsy

[a]Indicates studies where patients were prospectively identified, although the data was then historical/retrospective

adherence was reported as similar between groups in the Croatian study. That said, larger population-based studies also support an association. A Danish national registry study, examining the influence of losing a child on the subsequent risk of epilepsy in either parent, demonstrated a significant 50 % increased risk overall in bereaved versus non-bereaved parents, particularly in fathers within the first 3 years. This could not be explained by sociodemographic factors, and is truly population based, though the effects of potential lifestyle confounders such as alcohol and substance abuse, and misdiagnoses could not be excluded [22]. A retrospective analysis of medical information and duty assignments (combat, maintenance, or administrative) from over 300,000 compulsorily drafted Israeli Defense Forces males followed for 30 months gave conflicting results [23]: The risk of new onset seizures was slightly (RR 1.29, 95 % CI 1.03–1.62), but significantly ($p=0.03$) higher in the "high stress" combat than other units. However, in those with previous or current epilepsy (some of whom if seizure free, and off treatment with normal EEGs were assigned to combat), there was no identifiable effect on risk of recurrence.

There are a smaller number of prospective studies though hampered by a lack of clear definitions and standardized assessment tools. Stressful verbal stimuli presented to healthy controls have been shown to produce subtle EEG changes (narrowing of the bandwidth and regional changes in frequency) of sufficient magnitude that a blinded reviewer could correctly identify 92 % of stress stimuli on EEG alone [24]. Similarly in people with a variety of epilepsies, stressful interviews induced changes (exaggerated spiking, paroxysmal activity, or epileptiform complexes) in the majority [25] and there are case series of stress inducing audio/video recordings inducing seizures in patients with temporal lobe epilepsy in particular [26]. There are few larger or longer term truly prospective studies (Table 15.2). These broadly support an association, but have struggled to separate the effects of stress per se from confounders such as sleep deprivation, alcohol, and missing medication, or to separate cause from effect. However, as highlighted by one of the most recent prospective studies, the relationship between, and difficulties distinguishing stress from premonitory sensations and mood is particularly challenging to disentangle [27]. Thus changes in the brain preceding a seizure might increase patient perceptions of stress and anxiety rather than the converse. Nonetheless, overall there is reasonable support from clinical studies that stress might lower seizure thresholds, on which basis we now proceed to look more closely at putative mechanisms.

Mechanisms and Consequences of Stress

The definition of stress depends on the context. In lay usage, stress is defined in the Oxford English Dictionary as "A state of mental or emotional strain or tension resulting from adverse or very demanding circumstances." In the historical scientific study of stress, as reviewed by [31], Claude Bernard (1865) noted that the maintenance of life is critically dependent on keeping our internal milieu constant

Table 15.2 Prospective studies examining seizures and stress [6, 28–30]

Ref	No	Country	Epilepsy type	Setting	Method	Results
[28]	12	USA	Mixed, refractory ≥4 seizures per month, with carer >10 h/week	Epilepsy clinic	Prospective diaries for 3 months, events, seizures, tension, blinded to purpose of study	Significantly fewer seizures associated with low vs. high stress days ($p=0.005$); 7/12 (58 %) individuals with significant stress association (not possible to determine cause v effect)
[6]	6	USA	Mixed, refractory, selected from 177 surveyed as reporting highest stress-seizure association	Neurology clinic	Detailed in patient ratings and EEG assessments to explore mechanisms, including hypothesis testing individual challenges	Main mechanism sleep deprivation in 1/6, hyperventilation 4/6; no exacerbation (EEG or seizures) in 4/4 given cortisol injections
[29]	46 (37 analyzed)	USA	Mixed, refractory, average 3.3 seizures/week	Neurology clinics	Prospective diaries for 10–36 weeks, seizures and life events	No significant association when controlled for confounders (sleep deprivation, alcohol, missing medication)
[30]	71	USA	Localization-related epilepsy	Epilepsy centre and referring practices	Prospective paper diary, collected over >30 days (15,635 diary days)	1 unit increased stress (on 10 point scale) associated with an increased risk of seizure the following day (OR 1.06, 95 % CI 1.01–1.12 multivariate model; $p=0.03$)

in the face of a changing environment. Cannon (1929) called this "homeostasis." Selye (1956) used the term "stress" to represent the effects of anything that seriously threatens homeostasis. The actual or perceived threat to an organism is referred to as the "stressor" and the response to the stressor is called the "stress response." Although stress responses evolved as adaptive processes, Selye observed that severe, prolonged stress responses might lead to tissue damage and disease. Lazarus and Folkman (1984) described a model of psychological stress where the environmental event or "stressor" initially undergoes primary appraisal of the stimulus as threatening followed by secondary appraisal when the individual coping resources are appraised as insufficient, with both psychological and behavioral consequences [31]. McEwen and Lasley [32] extended the definition of the stress response with the term allostasis which is the process by which bodily functions change in response to environmental challenges. When allostasis is moderate, it has beneficial effects that aid adaption to change, but when it is excessive or prolonged, it has adverse effects known as the "allostatic load" that result in chronic disease mainly affecting the cardiovascular system, the immune system, and the brain.

Stressors can be physical (e.g., sleep deprivation, hyperventilation, excessive exercise, fever, illness, menstrual cycle), psychological (e.g., fear, sadness, anger), environmental (e.g., temperature, noise, lighting, smells), or pharmacological (e.g., substances of abuse such as cocaine or amphetamines, medication withdrawal such as benzodiazepines, withdrawal of caffeine or alcohol). Many of these stressors are well-known triggers for seizures which we will not be discussing. Most of the stress reported by patients is psychosocial, with both interpersonal and environmental contributors that are perceived as straining or exceeding the individual's adaptive capacities.

Extensive experimental and functional imaging studies comprehensively reviewed elsewhere [33, 34] means we now have a good understanding of the neuroanatomy and neurobiology of stress. Broadly speaking physiological stressors (e.g., pain) are appraised by brainstem and hypothalamus (Fig. 15.1), whereas complex emotional and experiential stressors are appraised in multiple limbic forebrain structures (amygdala, hippocampus, and prefrontal cortex with inputs from higher order sensory processing e.g., olfactory nuclei, preform cortex, and insular cortex) and memory (medial septum, entorhinal cortex, and cingulate cortex). Together with inputs from attention and arousal (e.g., locus coeruleus and raphe nucleus) these converge on subcortical structures to stimulate medial parvocellular paraventricular nucleus of the hypothalamus. The acute response involves both fast (seconds–minutes), and slower components (minutes–hours; Fig. 15.2 [35]) vital for adaption and recovery. However all also have the potential to cause harm, particularly where there are repeated or chronic stressors. The considerable and varied impact of stress on brain function is also being increasingly recognized, with "hot spots" of receptors for key stress mediators in key strategic hubs for networks involved in learning and memory, decision-making, hormonal, autonomic, and emotional responses [36].

The fast initiation response rapidly releases corticotropin-releasing hormone (CRH) that acts via the CRH1 receptor to activate the sympathetic nervous system. The medulla releases noradrenaline that stimulates the preganglionic neurons in intermediolateral cell column of the spinal cord to produce sympathetic response leading to the release of noradrenaline and adrenaline from the adrenal medulla. Resultant behavioral changes include the largely protective fight or flight reactions, but can become maladaptive including increased eating, smoking, drug use, and increased vigilance leading to anxiety and worrying. CRHI also activates the hypothalamic–pituitary–adrenal (HPA) axis. Neurons in medial parvocellular paraventricular nucleus

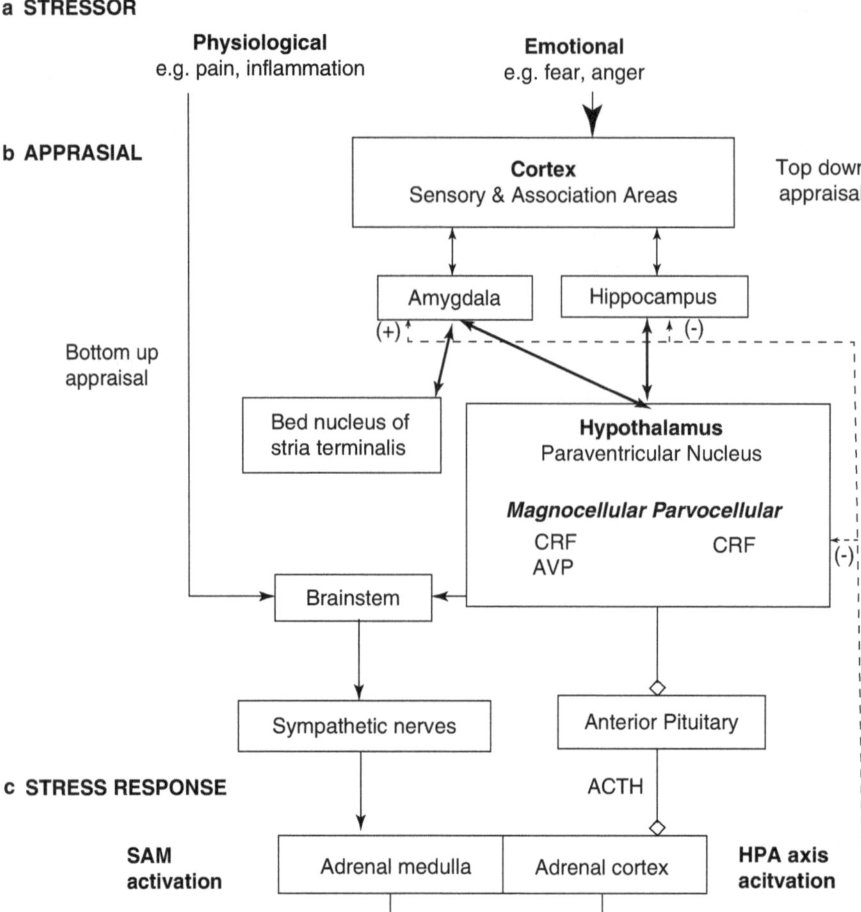

Fig. 15.1 Anatomy and pathways involved in stress. Stress is the non-specific response of the body to any demand for change, and has multiple components. (**a**) Stressor: Stressors can be physiological, e.g., pain or emotional, e.g., fear. (**b**) Appraisal: Physiological stressors activate the brainstem and hypothalamus. Emotional stressors activate limbic structures. Both systems activate the paraventricular nucleus (*PVN*) of the hypothalamus and the brainstem via direct projections and the limbic system indirectly. (**c**) Stress Response: The PVN of hypothalamus releases corticotropin-releasing hormone (*CRH*). This activates both the sympathetic adrenergic pathway (*SAM*) of the autonomic nervous system (*ANS*) and the HPA (hypothalamic–pituitary–adrenal) axis. The PVN neurons secrete CRH and vasopressin (*AVP*) into the portal system to the anterior pituitary to produce adrenocorticotropic hormone (*ACTH*). ACTH stimulates the adrenal cortex to release cortisol

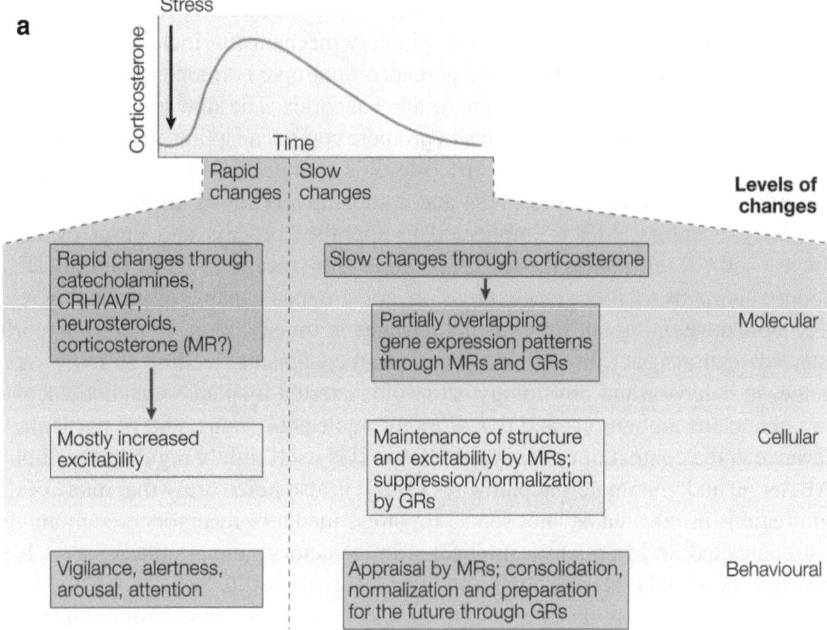
a
Stress
Corticosterone
Time
Rapid changes
Slow changes
Levels of changes
Rapid changes through catecholamines, CRH/AVP, neurosteroids, corticosterone (MR?)
Slow changes through corticosterone
Partially overlapping gene expression patterns through MRs and GRs
Molecular
Mostly increased excitability
Maintenance of structure and excitability by MRs; suppression/normalization by GRs
Cellular
Vigilance, alertness, arousal, attention
Appraisal by MRs; consolidation, normalization and preparation for the future through GRs
Behavioural

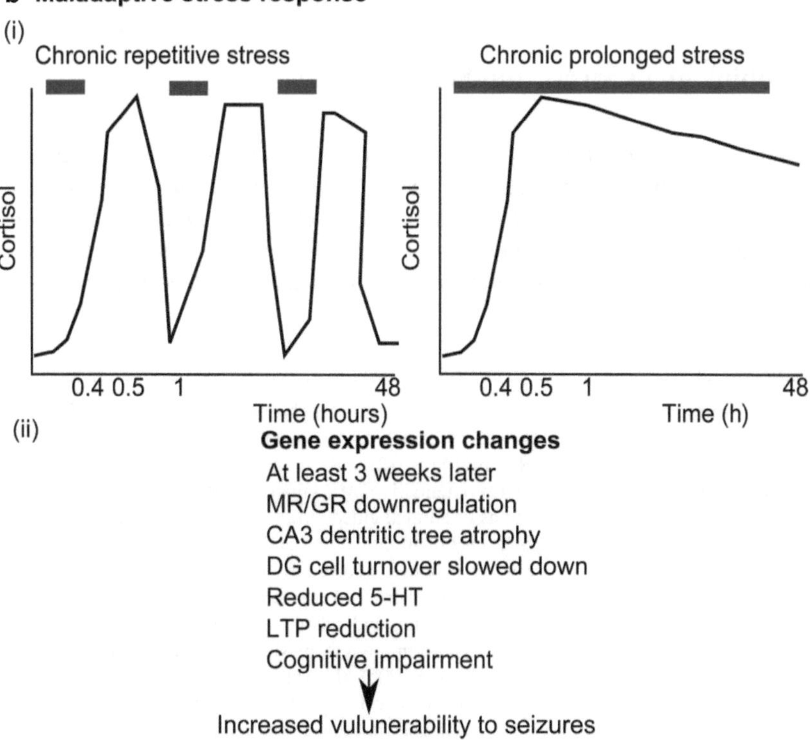
b Maladaptive stress response
(i)
Chronic repetitive stress
Chronic prolonged stress
Cortisol
0.4 0.5 1 48
Time (hours)
Time (h)
(ii)
Gene expression changes
At least 3 weeks later
MR/GR downregulation
CA3 dentritic tree atrophy
DG cell turnover slowed down
Reduced 5-HT
LTP reduction
Cognitive impairment
Increased vulunerability to seizures

of the hypothalamus release corticotropin-releasing hormone (CRH) and arginine vasopressin (AVP) which in turn activate pituitary mechanisms, including the release of opioids, melanocortin peptides, and adrenocorticotropic hormone (ACTH). ACTH stimulates glucocorticoid release from the adrenal cortex. The slow termination phase acts via CRH2 receptor and urocortins to promote coping, adaption, and recovery.

In an effective stress response, corticosteroids operate in both stress systems via high-affinity mineralocorticoid (MR) and comparatively lower affinity glucocorticoid (GR) receptors. MR is implicated in appraisal process and onset of stress response and GR terminates the stress reactions. Both receptors act by binding DNA response elements to alter gene expression, and are thus capable of producing relatively slow developing but long-lasting changes in transcription. In addition, corticosteroids can also act through non-genomic mechanisms, leading to more rapid changes in behavior and physiology. Control is exerted by parasympathetic activation via nucleus ambiguous and dorsal motor nucleus of vagus, and of particularly relevance in the context of epilepsy the HPA axis is itself tightly regulated by limbic GABAergic and glutamatergic pathways [37]. It is also noteworthy that many of the brain regions implicated as "hot spots" for stress mediator receptors are among the most connected and frequently implicated in refractory human epilepsies such as the cortex, amygdala, hippocampus, and locus coeruleus [36, 38].

So what evidence is there to support a direct role for stress in the context of seizures?

Neurobiology of Stress and Seizures

The time course of the stress is crucial in determining both its biological effects and effects on health including seizures. Selye (1956) observed that acute stress responses evolved as adaptive processes but severe, prolonged stress responses might lead to tissue damage and disease [31]. McEwen again extended this stating when allostasis is moderate, it has beneficial effects that aid adaption to change, but

Fig. 15.2 Normal and maladaptive responses to acute and chronic stress [35]. *5-HT* 5-hydroxytryptomine, *AVP* arginine vasopressin, *CA3* Cornu ammonus (of the hippocampus), *CRH* cortisol-releasing hormone, *CRHR1(2)* CRH receptor 1(2), *DG* dentate granule (hippocampus), *GR* glucocorticoid receptors, *LTP* long-term potentiation, *MR* mineralocorticoid receptors. (**a**) Acute stress response: (i) Blood concentrations of adrenal glucocorticoids rise to peak levels 15–30 min and then decline slowly to pre-stress levels 60–90 min later. (ii) Fast activation changes happen in seconds–minutes. The cortisol released acts via MR involved in the appraisal process and the onset of the stress response. Slow coping and recovery occur over minutes to hours in response to acute events. The slower response is vital for adaption and recovery and CRH also activates CRH2 receptor to produce urocortins (Reprinted by permission from Macmillan Publishers Ltd: de Kloet et al. [35] Figure 1 © Nature Publishing Group 2005). (**b**) Maladaptive mechanisms in the stress response over time: (i) Normal processes can become deranged where there are repeated or chronic stressors with abnormal elevations of cortisol, and (ii) later downstream consequences

when it is excessive or prolonged the cost of reinstating homeostasis becomes too high leading to "allosteric load" [39]. This inappropriate stress response produces a vulnerable phenotype and leaves genetically predisposed individuals and increased risk of chronic disease affecting the cardiovascular system, the immune system, and the brain [32]. This general model also appears broadly true for stress and seizures, though as we shall go on to outline in animal models the effect of acute stress on seizures depends on type of stressors and circuits involved.

Acute Stress and Seizures

Even in one brain region, in a single model, the consequences of an acute stress reaction can vary. For example acute stress, via CRH and ACTH initially has a largely pro-convulsant effect on CA1/CA3 excitation in the hippocampus. However, enhanced calcium influx several hours later protects against further excessive activity but is associated with a higher risk of neuronal injury if activation does occur. In contrast, increased corticosteroid levels in the dentate gyrus have less effect on activity, or calcium influx, but can enhance inhibition via effects on GABA receptors and be mostly anticonvulsant at least in the short term [40]. This complexity, together huge variation in the species, seizure triggers, stressors, and outcome studied in the basic science literature probably accounts for similarly varied results and conclusions, as reviewed by [41]. As they detail, the largest group of experiments is in rodent models exposed to swim stress creating both physical and psychological stress. If the seizures were induced by a GABA-A antagonist (e.g., picrotoxin, bicuculline, pentylenetetrazol) acute stress was anticonvulsive, but exacerbated electroconvulsive shock seizures, and had no effect on different various other models (e.g., kainite, strychnine, glycine, and acetylcholine antagonist or 4-aminopyridine-induced seizures). The anticonvulsant effects are most likely mediated via neuroactive steroids acting at GABA-A receptors increasing inhibition and decreasing seizure activity [42, 43]. Supporting this, changes in GABA-A subunit expression have been demonstrated following acute stress [44]. Thus overall in terms of acute stress, such studies demonstrate a range of putative pro- and anticonvulsant mechanisms, but are of little use beyond that in terms of understanding the interaction between stress and seizures in man. As Sawyer and Escayg [41] point out however, the increasing availability of genetically modified mice carrying human epilepsy mutations, or mutations in stress pathway genes provide an opportunity to examine this relationship in a more direct manner in the future.

Chronic Stress and Seizures

The results of animal models of chronic stress consistently demonstrate that chronic stress increases seizures [40]. Studies in different rodent models consistently show that increasing corticosterone (equivalent to cortisol in man) by exogenous administration lowers the threshold for provoked seizures in kindling [45–47] and chemiconvulsant models [48, 49]. Similarly, exogenous corticosterone enhances spike-wave discharges in a genetic model of absence epilepsy [50], and increased spontaneous inter-ictal epileptiform discharges in a post-pilocarpine status epilepticus rat epilepsy model [50, 51], though neither study was able to demonstrate changes in seizure frequency perhaps due to relatively short time scales. Conversely, removal of corticosterone by removal of adrenal gland or pituitary decreases seizures in kindling [52–54] and chemiconvulsant models [49, 55].

Other stress studies tell the same story including: polygenic gerbils with spontaneous seizures exposed to chronic novelty stress [56]; genetic model of absence epilepsy in rats show that spike and wave discharges do not increase after a single foot shock stressor but increases over 3 days of repeated stressor [57, 58]; worsened seizures in rodents with GABA-A antagonist induced seizures exposure to the chronic stress of social isolation [59, 60]. Heightened stress reactions are also postulated, with reasonable evidence, to be the primary mechanism underpinning one well characterized mouse strain with reflex focal epilepsy (El mice) [61].

Possible mechanisms are that corticotropin-releasing hormone that is released in the brain as first response to stress causes increase in neuronal discharge and modulates glutamatergic transmission, [62] and that glucocorticoid increases excitatory glutamate [63]. Conversely a decrease in GABAergic inhibition is seen in chronic stress [64–66], likely mediated via a change in neurosteroids [43].

Putative Roles of Stress in Epilepsy

The distinction between acute symptomatic seizures in a "normal brain," and epilepsy, characterized by an enduring predisposition to recurrent unprovoked seizures (Fig. 15.3a) is not as clear cut as current definitions imply (nor for that matter is the definition of "normal"), but having a conceptualization of the process that generates chronic seizures, epileptogenesis is nonetheless useful. Epilepsy is most commonly conceptualized as a spectrum in which a potentially (in the case of, e.g., genetic malformations) or previously normal brain is functionally altered and biased towards the generation of the abnormal electrical activity subserving recurrent unprovoked seizures. There may be a initial predisposing brain insult (e.g., genetic, neurodevelopmental, trauma, infection, stroke), sometimes itself involving seizures (e.g., febrile convulsions, status epilepticus), followed by a latent period during which the brain is altered by progressive cellular and network changes to create an epileptic brain that is prone to spontaneous unprovoked seizures (epilepsy) [67] (Fig. 15.3b), although in some instances it may be that the proposed insult and latent period are indistinguishable.

There are several potential mechanisms by which stress might enhance this process (Fig. 15.3a–d). While it is likely these mechanisms interact, each will be discussed separately.

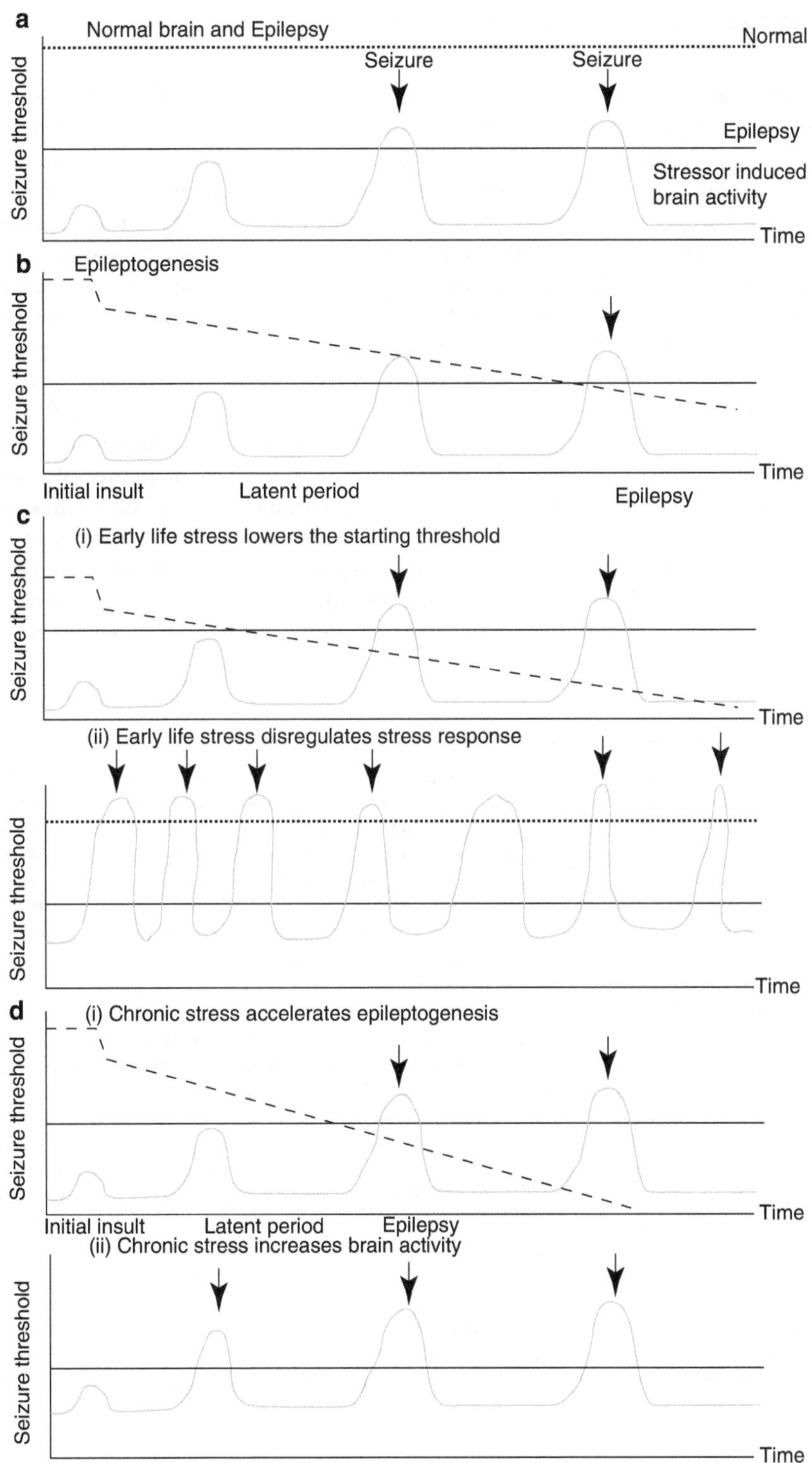
a
Normal brain and Epilepsy
Normal
Seizure
Seizure
Epilepsy
Stressor induced brain activity
Seizure threshold
Time
b
Epileptogenesis
Seizure threshold
Time
Initial insult
Latent period
Epilepsy
c
(i) Early life stress lowers the starting threshold
Seizure threshold
Time
(ii) Early life stress disregulates stress response
Seizure threshold
Time
d
(i) Chronic stress accelerates epileptogenesis
Seizure threshold
Time
Initial insult
Latent period
Epilepsy
(ii) Chronic stress increases brain activity
Seizure threshold
Time

Stress Increases the Excitability of Brain Activity

As discussed previously, stress may act as an insult of itself, and lower the seizure threshold and promote hyperexcitability via a range of mechanisms, rendering the brain more susceptible to unprovoked seizures, or at risk of more severe or frequent seizures (and their consequences) in the event of an additional insult (see Fig. 15.3a,b). There is evidence of HPA axis dysfunction with epilepsy in rodent models with acutely provoked (kindled) seizures [61, 68–71] as well as in clinical studies of status epilepticus [72–74], although antiepileptic drug treatment is a potential confounder in all the clinical studies. What is less clear, there is something inherently different about the HPA axis regulation in people who go on to develop epilepsy, or if having seizures and epilepsy is stressful leading to secondary HPA axis dysfunction, or both. It is possible the hippocampus normally acts to shut off the HPA axis but excessive exposure to glucocorticoids can cause the hippocampus to shrink, disinhibiting the HPA axis and resulting in a vicious cycle of unopposed allostatic load. Functional imaging studies in humans are starting to try unlock the link and causality between the cortical and physiologic responses to acute stress and the relationship between seizure control in epilepsy and both the HPA axis and fMRI signal reactivity [75], though, have a long way to go. Stress has been postulated to be of particular importance in patients with temporal lobe epilepsy, in which context

Fig. 15.3 Putative mechanisms underlying relationship between stress and epilepsy. *Dashed black line* seizure threshold in "normal" brain, *Solid black line* seizure threshold in brain with epilepsy, *gray line* brain activity fluctuations, *arrows* seizures occur. (**a**) Normal brain and stable epilepsy: It is possible to trigger seizures in a "normal" brain only with extreme physiological challenge (e.g., hypoxia, hypoglycemia, mechanical insults; acute symptomatic seizures, not shown). In a person with epilepsy, seizures occur at a lower threshold and are by definition unprovoked, though may be triggered at this lower threshold by lesser events, which may include stress. (**b**) Epileptogenesis: After brain insult (e.g., neurodevelopmental, genetic, traumatic, stroke, infectious, or prolonged seizures) a process of epileptogenesis begins by which the previously normal brain is functionally altered and biased towards the generation of the abnormal electrical activity. This can take a variable period of time from days to years. At some point an individual's seizure threshold reaches the level at which unprovoked (± triggers) spontaneous recurrent seizures occur, i.e., the threshold defining epilepsy. The individual seizure threshold may continue to decrease after the onset of epilepsy, as shown, or may stabilize, which may vary between individuals. (**c**) (i) Early life stress lowers the starting threshold: Early life stress may create a vulnerable phenotype, meaning they start with a lower than normal seizure threshold, such that on a subsequent epileptogenic insult it will reach the epileptic threshold, with unprovoked seizures sooner. (ii) Early life stress disregulates stress response: Early life stress has minimal effect on the background threshold, but alters the HPA axis so that background and/or stress responses, and their effects on brain activity are exaggerated resulting in seizures. (**d**) (i) Chronic stress accelerates epileptogenesis: Chronic stress accelerates the process of epileptogenesis so that following an epileptogenic insult the epilepsy threshold is reached sooner in the time course and earlier seizures occur. (ii) Chronic stress increases brain activity: Increases in background brain activity during periods of chronic stress result in seizures being triggered more readily, including by fluctuations that would not previously have been ictogenic

that decreased functional connectivity this patient group [76] might reflect underlying network abnormalities resulting in epilepsy, but that also affect their response to acute stress. In support, one recent case control study ($n=23$ each group) in left-sided temporal lobe epilepsy has shown a significant relationship between seizure control and both the hypothalamic–pituitary–adrenal axis and fMRI signal reactivity to acute psychosocial stress [75].

Early Life Stress Creates a Vulnerable Phenotype

The idea that insults in prenatal or early life might prime the developing brain for seizures and epileptogenesis is attractive, given the recognized association between for example cerebral palsy and epilepsy, and febrile convulsions and later epilepsy. In this context, stress has been much studied in animal models as we will go on to summarize (see Fig. 15.3c). To explore this in humans would have huge methodological challenges, which is likely why there is very limited clinical data on the effect of early life stress on seizures. One population-based cohort study involved children born to women who had lost a close relative during pregnancy or 1 year before pregnancy, with hospitalization due to epilepsy as the outcome measure. There was no association between this particular form of prenatal stress and risk of epilepsy [77]. However, despite that this was a national registry study, involving over 1.5 million children, of whom almost 40,000 were in the exposed group, there were no direct measures with respect to the timing and duration of stress, nor either of which might be important, and/or modified by individual coping mechanisms and circumstances, although this too has been little studied, though not yet demonstrated where this issue is addressed [78]. More recently, a case control study of 120 children under 30 months of age consecutively seen at a child care center in China with infantile spasms ($n=60$), other epilepsy ($n=30$), or healthy children ($n=30$) reported a significant association with prenatal maternal stress in the infantile spasm group [79]. Maternal stress was assessed retrospectively, though using a scale validated for this population (Pregnant Woman Life Event Scale), and that scores were similar in the other epilepsy and healthy group, but more than doubled in the infantile spasm group argues against this all being recall bias. Pre-clinical data however is strong that early life stress predisposes the brain to provoked seizures and to later epilepsy. For example, as covered in recent reviews [80, 81] if pregnant female rodents are stressed (e.g., by restraint, bright lights, or injections) several groups have shown it is easier to induce seizures up to several weeks later in the pups in response to kindling [82], audiogenic stimuli [83], and chemoconvulsants [84]. Similarly, postnatal stress induced by separation of pups from their mother (typically for brief periods aged 2–9 or 14 days) renders the pups more susceptible to later seizures with kindling [85–88] and chemoconvulsants [89–91]. Attempts to explore the effect of more subtle early life stressors, specifically quality of parenting on seizure risk by cross-fostering experiments between strains of seizure-prone and seizure-resistant rodents have given opposing results [92, 93], and are confounded by the likely stress of maternal separation per se in the pups. Clinical studies looking at the interaction between family environment and epilepsy have mostly focused on psychosocial outcomes rather than seizures, or on the consequences of epilepsy on the family [94], and would be difficult methodologically. There is however preliminary data emerging from functional imaging in humans that show associations between white matter integrity of various limbic regions of the brain and early cortisol reactivity to stress may be moderated by parenting [95], which is also of potential relevance to epileptogenesis.

There are several possible mechanisms underlying the link between early life stress and epilepsy including (1) hyperactivity of the HPA axis that leads the adults with an impaired stress response to aversive stimuli including increase in stress hormone release and impairment of HPA negative feedback [96, 97]; (2) changes in hippocampal structure and function, mediated by early CRH elevation [98]; (3) hyper excitable neurotransmission in the limbic system due to decreased GABA inhibition [99]; (4) induction of immune and inflammatory pathways [100] which are implicated in neural damage in epilepsy [101]; (5) decreased brain derived neurotrophic factor (BDNF) in the adult brain which, considered a critical mediator of neuroprotection in epilepsy [102]; (6) delayed development of white matter in the brain [103], commonly associated with a broad range of epilepsy phenotypes.

Chronic Stress Accelerates the Process of Epileptogenesis

The same mechanisms, proposed to enhance vulnerability in the developing brain, may also play a role in epileptogenesis at a later stage in the mature brain, though again this is largely speculative in clinical terms (see Fig. 15.3d). A very broad range of mechanisms have been proposed to play a role in epileptogenesis, including at a molecular level microglia and astrocyte activation, oxidative stress and reactive oxygen species production, mitochondria and damage of blood–brain barrier [104], which others have proposed converge at the level of circuit dysfunction [67]. Chronic stress has been shown to influence many of these mechanisms. Thus chronic stress may potentiate the process of epileptogenesis via increased microglia and astrocyte activation with an increase in inflammatory mediators NF-B, TNF alpha, IL1, prostaglandins and free radicals such as nitric oxide [105], as well as causing abnormal neurogenesis in the hippocampus [106], with demonstrable lasting changes in brain structure and function [107]. Stress also alters dentate granule cell proliferation and regulates dendritic and synaptic plasticity [108, 109]. Two types of plasticity occur: remodeling of dendrites of hippocampal pyramidal neurons in response to repeated stress and chronic elevation of glucocorticoids and inhibition of neurogenesis of granule cells in the dentate gyrus, each contributing to hippocampal network hyperexcitability and increased seizure susceptibility.

Association Between Seizures, Stress, Anxiety, and Depression

Depression and anxiety are common comorbidities of epilepsy and there are complex bidirectional relationships between both, and with stress. Stressful events can undoubtedly precipitate depression and anxiety, postulated to involve changes in corticotropin releasing factor (CRFR1) and serotonin (5-HT2R) receptors [110]. This is altered by genetic determinants and environmental factors, particularly stressor experiences encountered early in life [111].

Several studies have tried to dissect the causal relationships between stress, anxiety, depression, and other confounding factors such as sleep deprivation. A longitudinal cohort study of over 400 community recruited patients using a range of validated scales applied retrospectively at two time points looked in detail at the interaction of anxiety, depression, and perceived stress on seizure frequency and concluded that depression underpinned the relationship [17]. In contrast cross-sectional studies, both of over 200 patients attending an epilepsy center [16, 112], 50–80 % respectively of whom reported stress as a seizure trigger, concluded that anxiety was the most important factor. Others have shown a high correlation between stress, sleep deprivation, and fatigue [10], though others [12] including a more methodologically robust multivariate analysis of prospective paper diaries collected over up to 1 year [30], albeit in smaller numbers ($n=71$), concluded that sleep deprivation, anxiety, and stress were all independent predictors of seizure occurrence.

It is also important to recognize in this context that conditions, previously thought of as psychiatric comorbidities or consequences of epilepsy, may be in fact manifestations of genetic disturbances in the same pathways and that there may be overlapping or common mechanisms between epilepsy, mood, and the stress response [2]. For example: there is HPA axis dysfunction in anxiety and depression [113]; people with epilepsy who report experiencing emotional seizure triggers show attentional biases toward threat [114]; people with epilepsy may have a lower stress threshold and a chronic state of heightened arousal, with autonomic nervous system connections to the amygdala, then hippocampus, hypothalamus, and cortex, involved in both stress perception and stress responses [115].

Stress Management in the Treatment of Epilepsy

Just as has been found in other chronic diseases [116], irrespective of the exact mechanisms, and despite the difficulties separating cause from effect with respect to seizures and epilepsy, there is little doubt that stress is important to people with epilepsy, will impact on quality of life, and may directly or indirectly also influence seizure control. Thus as well as for research purposes, there is arguably a strong incentive for us to more proactively identify stress in our patients, and more importantly provide support and treatment. Psychoeducational approaches are the most well studied, but we also briefly discuss the potential roles of pharmacological and electrical stimulation.

Psychoeducational Approaches

It could be argued that stress management should be dealt with by mental health services, rather as part of epilepsy management; however, evidence from other chronic diseases including cardiac [117], diabetes [118], and multiple sclerosis [119] suggests that this is best achieved through an integrated clinic, with improvements both in disease control and quality of life. With respect to epilepsy, at least some consensus and guidance documents already include statements that argue in support of a similar approach. For example, UK guidance highlights the importance of ensuring people feel supported to manage their condition, and improved functional abilities as key areas for enhancing quality of life [120], specifically include stress as a topic that patients should receive information on [121], and recommend that both psychologists and psychiatrists are part of a multidisciplinary epilepsy team at least at tertiary centers, although there are no psychiatric/psychological outcomes in proposed US standards for epilepsy care [122].

There are several types of interventions that have been explored to reduce stress in epilepsy, and have been comprehensively reviewed elsewhere [123, 124]. All the suggested therapies aim to increase the individual's ability to prevent the build-up of seizure activity and reduce both nonspecific seizure precipitants (e.g., stress, sleep deprivation) and specific internal (e.g., emotional distress) and/or external (e.g., sensory and environmental) contextual seizure precipitants. Proposed mechanisms of action include (1) stress reduction techniques to increase the parasympathetic response, thereby decreasing stress and seizures; (2) improving psychiatric comorbidity to improve seizures; (3) understanding that seizures are triggered and therefore potentially controllable is motivating for many patients; (4) learning a new response to pre-ictal and early ictal phenomena that engage neurons adjacent or contralateral to the area of hyperexcitable neurons, in order to prevent further recruitment and, hence, the spread of seizure activity and (5) a recognition that adjustment to having seizures can be difficult and can be enhanced by providing educational materials, introducing adaptive coping, communication skills, general problem-solving skills, and nonjudgmental awareness.

Cognitive–behavioral therapy, mind–body approaches, and multimodel educative interventions have consistently demonstrated significant effects on improving psychological well-being, and enhancing epilepsy knowledge and adjustment as compared with controls. However, the effects on seizure control remain inconsistent across studies (Table 15.3), and a Cochrane review concluded there was no reliable evidence for stress management therapies in terms of seizure control [125].

One clinical trial [142], "Stress Management Intervention for Living With Epilepsy" (SMILE, NCT01444183), has just ended recruitment and should be reported in 2015, though was halted early due to slow recruitment and funding limitations (n=66, personal communication, Privitera 2015). Although there is clearly potential for future larger studies, as illustrated in Table 15.3, many interventions are resource intensive, and neither cost-effectiveness nor cost-utility have been considered in previous studies to our knowledge but are clearly of substantial importance.

Table 15.3 Evidence for psychobehavioral treatments including strategies for stress in epilepsy [126–141]

Ref	No	Country	Epilepsy type and setting	Intervention	Design, primary endpoint	Results
Behavioral/cognitive behavioral approaches						
[126]	8 vs. 10 vs. 9	Canada	Mixed (including 2 each group with NES), all with significant psychosocial problems; epilepsy clinics	8 × 2-h sessions of group CBT vs. 8 2-h sessions of vs. supportive counseling or wait list control	Single blind RCT; daily seizure diaries, patient and physician standard scales, 4 month follow-up	No change in any group on seizures or psychosocial difficulties
[127]	6 vs. 6 vs. 6	Sweden	Mixed, refractory; neurology clinics	6-week contingent relaxation vs. 6-week attention control vs. no treatment	Open RCT (10 weeks baseline and post-treatment follow-up), and open follow-up (all active) up to 72 weeks total	Median seizure frequency 66 %↓ post-treatment vs. 2 %↓ wait list, 68 %↑ attention control ($p<0.05$ all pairs); all improved 30 weeks post treatment (open; $p=.001$)
[128]	16	Germany	Mixed, refractory; neurology clinics	Therapist guided psychological intervention (“self-control training”) over 3–30 months	Prospective case series, 6 months – 3 years follow-up, no predefined endpoint	68 % improved (50 % by >80 %, 18 % by 50–79 %)
[129]	18 vs. 19	Australia	Mixed, >60 years old; community and clinics	6× weekly 2 h-sessions group CBT vs. 6× 1 h relaxation sessions	Open RCT Mood and psychosocial functioning scales, seizure frequency, 3 month follow-up vs. baseline	Significant improvements mood and functioning and seizure frequency both groups, significantly more with CBT time point

(continued)

Table 15.3 (continued)

Ref	No	Country	Epilepsy type and setting	Intervention	Design, primary endpoint	Results
[130]	40 vs. 40	USA	Mixed epilepsy, with depression/dysthymia; epilepsy center and referring neurology clinics	× 50-min sessions of home-based sessions vs. usual care ("PEARLS" for depression)	Open RCT, up to 18 months follow-up; Depression related scores: retrospective recall of seizures/month	No change in seizure frequency, despite improvement in depression
[131]	60	Germany, Switzerland, and USA	Mixed, 57 % refractory; neurology clinics	Therapist guided behavioral intervention ("Andrews/Reiter," self-control/trigger focused)	Retrospective case series, patient self-reports; Changes in seizure frequency at end of program vs. baseline with stable/reduced Medication	>50 % reduction in seizures in 50 % of patients (not statistically evaluated)
Mind-body approaches						
[132]	10 vs. 10 vs. 12	India	Mixed, refractory; neurology clinics	Yoga (20–30 min/day, 1 month daily training, *X*2/week thereafter) vs. mimic exercises (same) vs. no treatment	Open RCT; weekly seizure diaries 6 month follow-up	Mean seizure/month 85 % ↓ yoga vs. 14 % mimic vs. 6 % control ($p<0.001$) including 4/10 yoga but none of mimic or controls seizure free
[133]	14 vs. 13	South Africa	Mixed, refractory; residents or day workers at Centre for Epilepsy	4 sessions of ACT vs. 4 sessions of supportive Therapy, boosters at 6 and 12 months	Open RCT, Seizure Index (frequency/month × duration in seconds) and monthly frequency	Seizure Index vs. 23–55 in ACT group vs. >2000 in control ($p<0.001$); frequency/month @12 months 0.62±o0.86 vs. 5.8±53.51 ($p<0.001$)

[134]	10 vs. 8	India	Mixed, refractory; epilepsy clinic	4 sessions of ACT vs. 4 sessions of yoga, boosters at 6 and 12 months	Open RCT, 12 months follow-up; Change score (baseline vs. 12 months, seizure index frequency/month × duration in seconds for each group)	CT Seizure Index 395 ± 351 pre, 62 +/104 post ($p < 0.05$); Yoga 75 ± 54 Pre, 15 ±423 post ($p < 0.05$) vs. decreased seizure index
Education interventions						
[135]	20 vs. 18	USA	Mixed, epilepsy centers	2-day Sepulveda educational program "SEE" to patient/family vs. wait list control	Open RCT, 4 months follow-up, multiple outcomes including seizure index, mood, coping, knowledge, drug levels	Increased knowledge vs. no change; Increased knowledge and medication adherence; No change seizures or other measures
[136]	113 vs. 129	Germany, Austria, Switzerland	Epilepsy centers	9 units of MOSES (Modular Service Package Epilepsy) educational treatment program on epilepsy knowledge, self-confidence, and illness management vs. wait list control	Open RCT, multiple outcomes including seizure frequency, coping and mental health, 6-month follow-up. Univariate analysis	Significant improvements in coping with epilepsy, Improved satisfaction with therapy, drug tolerability. No other changes
[137]	96 vs. 96	USA	Mixed; online, community and Clinics weeks vs. waitlist control	W internet-based self-management program "WebEase" for 6 weeks vs. waitlist control	Open RCT, multiple outcomes including stress scales, QoL, self-control measures (no seizure outcomes)	No significant change any stress measures. Only medication adherence and self-efficacy improved

(continued)

Table 15.3 (continued)

Ref	No	Country	Epilepsy type and setting	Intervention	Design, primary endpoint	Results
[a]*Biofeedback interventions review* [138]						
[139]	25	Germany	Mixed refractory, at least 1 seizure/week; Epilepsy center	28 × 1 h training sessions for self-regulation vertex EEG surface-negative SCP	UCase series, 8 week baseline vs. up to 1-year follow-up; SCP control (all), seizure frequency ($n = 18$)	Achieved significant SCP control; 17 at least some; Significant improvements seizure frequency ($p < 0.01$; 6 seizure free; 7 reduced).
[140]	10 vs. 8	UK	Mixed refractory; epilepsy clinics	12 × 30 min Galvanic skin response biofeedback training to modulate arousal state vs. sham control	Single blind RCT, 3 months baseline, 1 month treatment, 3 month follow-up; % change baseline seizure frequency/week	–49.26 ± 441.64 % improvement in treatment group ($p = 0.017$; 6/10 > 50 % seizure reduction including 1 seizure free)
[141]	87 (10 studies)	USA and Europe	Mixed refractory; epilepsy clinics and centers	EEG biofeedback training sessions, varied methodologies/durations	Meta-analysis prospective, peer reviewed studies that evaluated sensorimotor rhythm (SMR) uptraining or SCP control; weekly seizure frequency	Significant intervention effect ($p < 0.001$; 74 % subjects improved seizure frequency)

ACT acceptance and commitment therapy, *CBT* cognitive behavioral therapy, *NES* non-epileptic seizures, *RCT* randomized controlled trial, *SCP* slow cortical potentials

[a]There are over 60 such studies in the review mentioned, only selected included here

Vagal Nerve Stimulation, Stress, and Epilepsy

Vagal nerve stimulation (VNS) is now an established treatment for epilepsy, and known to both decrease seizure frequency and improve mood [143], with known effects on the autonomic nervous system [144] likely to also influence stress, which might thus be one of its modes of action. In support of this, non-invasive transcutaneous vagus nerve stimulation in healthy individuals during fMRI has been shown to cause widespread decreased activation to high threshold stimulation in emotional/stress related regions of the limbic system, associated with significant improvements in well-being afterwards compared to sham stimulation [145].

Pharmacological Strategies to Alter Stress

The interaction between stress and epilepsy is being explored with respect to existing and new drug treatments in a number of ways including:

1. Many of our current AEDs, believed to act by increasing inhibitory (GABAergic) activity reduce excitatory activity, are also widely used in the in treatment of mood disorders, for example valproate, carbamazepine, and lamotrigine as mood stabilizers, and pregabalin for anxiety, though further research is needed to prove if mechanisms involved in stress, such as HPA axis modulation, are directly or indirectly relevant to efficacy.
2. Neurosteroids themselves are also being explored as potential antiepileptic drugs. Fluctuations in endogenous levels might account for seizure frequency variations in for example pregnancy and menstruation [146], and exogenous administration has been shown to alter limbic system connectivity in functional imaging studies in humans [147], of potential relevance to the treatment of mood disorders and of epilepsy. For one such neurosteroid, Ganaxolone, a synthetic analogue of allopregnanolone and a potent allosteric modulator of $GABA_A$ receptors, there are promising results from Phase II clinical trials including for partial onset seizures and infantile spasms, with phase 3 studies are still on-going [148].
3. Steroids and ACTH are of course already widely used in some pediatric epilepsies [149], with established benefits for seizures albeit with also well-established side effects, though the effects on stress have not been explored and would be difficult to disentangle. While there is enthusiasm in theory for blocking stress hormones as a treatment for epilepsy and its comorbidities, that stress hormones also play an essential role in the immune system and metabolic functions, as well as compensatory rises in hormone levels where antagonists are used, are substantial barriers. Ideally a glucocorticoid antagonist would only affect the glucocorticoid release in response to stress, without impacting on basal levels or the diurnal rhythm of glucocorticoid secretion [150], but this work still has a long way to go.

Conclusions

Stress, however defined and whatever you believe about its role in susceptibility to seizures and epileptogenesis, is a topic that we hope you are now convinced it would be foolish to ignore in epilepsy-related research or clinical practice. People with epilepsy report this as a trigger more commonly than any other factor, and there are both pre-clinical and clinical studies to support this association, together with an increasing understanding about potential mechanisms. There is also good pre-clinical evidence that prenatal/early life stress may create a vulnerability although we may never know how relevant this is for human epilepsy.

Future animal studies, if continuing to dissect the mechanisms is considered important, should we suggest move away from seizure provocation studies, and focus on more clinically relevant models of chronic epilepsy, perhaps taking advantage of increasingly available transgenic models in relation to epilepsy and stress mechanisms, as well as recognizing that for the most part it is prolonged psychological stressors which have the greatest effect on patients. Emerging functional imaging technologies also provide methods which can start to examine mechanisms and treatment effects less subjectively in both healthy controls, and those with epilepsy.

Any clinical studies exploring cause and effect are inevitably likely to be compromised by the numerous confounders, varied definitions, and overlap with mood and other psychosocial variables so are if of dubious benefit. Prospective studies are at least less liable to recall biases, but logistically challenging and resource intensive. There is already good clinical trial evidence to support that psychoeducational stress management strategies improve quality of life and enhance well-being, on which basis this should surely anyway be available as part of any epilepsy care package. The role of such interventions in improving seizure control, and which approach is most effective requires further study, but must surely include cost-effectiveness and cost-utility analysis. Pharmacological and electrical manipulation of stress pathways might already play a role in some current antiepileptic treatments, though developing this in terms of a new target for drug development in epilepsy has substantial obstacles.

Throughout this chapter we have largely referred to epilepsy as though it were a single condition, whereas the reality is of course very different. As well as considering the many separate identified electroclinical syndromes, it may be that people with epilepsy who report stress as a seizure precipitant are an additional subset, perhaps because of functional brain connectivity which may be secondary to underlying mood disorders – early life stress or genetics? If this is the case it is possible that treatment effects may differ for those in whom stress is contributory compared to others, and that these differences may not align with specific electroclinical syndromes, suggesting we have yet more work to do in terms of developing individualized treatment plans in the future.

References

1. McEwen BS. The neurobiology of stress: from serendipity to clinical relevance. Brain Res. 2000;886(1–2):172–89.
2. Shorvon SD. The causes of epilepsy: changing concepts of etiology of epilepsy over the past 150 years. Epilepsia. 2011;52(6):1033–44.
3. Gilboa T. Emotional stress-induced seizures: another reflex epilepsy? Epilepsia. 2012;53(2):e29–32.
4. Eggers AE. Temporal lobe epilepsy is a disease of faulty neuronal resonators rather than oscillators, and all seizures are provoked, usually by stress. Med Hypotheses. 2007;69(6):1284–9.
5. Spatt J, Langbauer G, Mamoli B. Subjective perception of seizure precipitants: results of a questionnaire study. Seizure. 1998;7(5):391–5.
6. Mattson RH. Emotional effects on seizure occurrence. Adv Neurol. 1991;55:453–60.
7. Hayden M, Penna C, Buchanan N. Epilepsy: patient perceptions of their condition. Seizure. 1992;1(3):191–7.
8. Hart YM, Shorvon SD. The nature of epilepsy in the general population. I. Characteristics of patients receiving medication for epilepsy. Epilepsy Res. 1995;21(1):43–9.
9. Cull CA, Fowler M, Brown SW. Perceived self-control of seizures in young people with epilepsy. Seizure. 1996;5(2):131–8.
10. Frucht MM, Quigg M, Schwaner C, Fountain NB. Distribution of seizure precipitants among epilepsy syndromes. Epilepsia. 2000;41(12):1534–9.
11. Spector S, Cull C, Goldstein LH. Seizure precipitants and perceived self-control of seizures in adults with poorly-controlled epilepsy. Epilepsy Res. 2000;38(2–3):207–16.
12. Haut SR, Vouyiouklis M, Shinnar S. Stress and epilepsy: a patient perception survey. Epilepsy Behav. 2003;4(5):511–4.
13. Nakken KO, Solaas MH, Kjeldsen MJ, Friis ML, Pellock JM, Corey LA. Which seizure-precipitating factors do patients with epilepsy most frequently report? Epilepsy Behav. 2005;6(1):85–9.
14. Tan JH, Wilder-Smith E, Lim EC, Ong BK. Frequency of provocative factors in epileptic patients admitted for seizures: a prospective study in Singapore. Seizure. 2005;14(7):464–9.
15. da Silva SP, Lin K, Garzon E, Sakamoto AC, Yacubian EM. Self-perception of factors that precipitate or inhibit seizures in juvenile myoclonic epilepsy. Seizure. 2005;14(5):340–6.
16. Sperling MR, Schilling CA, Glosser D, Tracy JI, Asadi-Pooya AA. Self-perception of seizure precipitants and their relation to anxiety level, depression, and health locus of control in epilepsy. Seizure. 2008;17(4):302–7.
17. Thapar A, Kerr M, Harold G. Stress, anxiety, depression, and epilepsy: investigating the relationship between psychological factors and seizures. Epilepsy Behav. 2009;14(1):134–40.
18. Dionisio J, Tatum WO. Triggers and techniques in termination of partial seizures. Epilepsy Behav. 2010;17(2):210–4.
19. Swinkels WA, Engelsman M, Kasteleijn-Nolst Trenite DG, Baal MG, de Haan GJ, Oosting J. Influence of an evacuation in February 1995 in The Netherlands on the seizure frequency in patients with epilepsy: a controlled study. Epilepsia. 1998;39(11):1203–7.
20. Bosnjak J, Vukovic-Bobic M, Mejaski-Bosnjak V. Effect of war on the occurrence of epileptic seizures in children. Epilepsy Behav. 2002;3(6):502–9.
21. Neufeld MY, Sadeh M, Cohn DF, Korczyn AD. Stress and epilepsy: the Gulf war experience. Seizure. 1994;3(2):135–9.
22. Christensen J, Li J, Vestergaard M, Olsen J. Stress and epilepsy: a population-based cohort study of epilepsy in parents who lost a child. Epilepsy Behav. 2007;11(3):324–8.
23. Moshe S, Shilo M, Chodick G, Yagev Y, Blatt I, Korczyn AD, et al. Occurrence of seizures in association with work-related stress in young male army recruits. Epilepsia. 2008;49(8):1451–6.

24. Berkhout J, Walter DO, Adey WR. Alterations of the human electroencephalogram induced by stressful verbal activity. Electroencephalogr Clin Neurophysiol. 1969;27(5):457–69.
25. Stevens JR. Emotional activation of the electroencephalogram in patients with convulsive disorders. J Nerv Ment Dis. 1959;128(4):339–51.
26. Feldman RG, Paul NL. Identity of emotional triggers in epilepsy. J Nerv Ment Dis. 1976;162(5):345–53.
27. Haut SR, Hall CB, Borkowski T, Tennen H, Lipton RB. Modeling seizure self-prediction: an e-diary study. Epilepsia. 2013;54(11):1960–7.
28. Temkin NR, Davis GR. Stress as a risk factor for seizures among adults with epilepsy. Epilepsia. 1984;25(4):450–6.
29. Neugebauer R, Paik M, Hauser WA, Nadel E, Leppik I, Susser M. Stressful life events and seizure frequency in patients with epilepsy. Epilepsia. 1994;35(2):336–43.
30. Haut SR, Hall CB, Masur J, Lipton RB. Seizure occurrence: precipitants and prediction. Neurology. 2007;69(20):1905–10.
31. Lovallo WR. Stress and health: biological and psychological interactions (behavioral medicine & health psychology). 2nd ed. Thousand Oaks: SAGE Publications, Inc; London, UK. 2004.
32. McEwen BS, Lasley EN. The end of stress as we know it. 1st ed. Washington: Joseph Henry Press; 2002. 262 p.
33. Ulrich-Lai YM, Herman JP. Neural regulation of endocrine and autonomic stress responses. Nat Rev Neurosci. 2009;10(6):397–409.
34. Allendorfer JB, Szaflarski JP. Contributions of fMRI towards our understanding of the response to psychosocial stress in epilepsy and psychogenic nonepileptic seizures. Epilepsy Behav. 2014;35:19–25.
35. de Kloet ER, Joels M, Holsboer F. Stress and the brain: from adaptation to disease. Nat Rev Neurosci. 2005;6(6):463–75.
36. Joels M, Baram TZ. The neuro-symphony of stress. Nat Rev Neurosci. 2009;10(6):459–66.
37. Herman JP, Ostrander MM, Mueller NK, Figueiredo H. Limbic system mechanisms of stress regulation: hypothalamo-pituitary-adrenocortical axis. Prog Neuropsychopharmacol Biol Psychiatry. 2005;29(8):1201–13.
38. Joels M, Sarabdjitsingh RA, Karst H. Unraveling the time domains of corticosteroid hormone influences on brain activity: rapid, slow, and chronic modes. Pharmacol Rev. 2012;64(4):901–38.
39. McEwen BS. Allostasis and allostatic load: implications for neuropsychopharmacology. Neuropsychopharmacology. 2000;22(2):108–24.
40. Joels M. Stress, the hippocampus, and epilepsy. Epilepsia. 2009;50(4):586–97.
41. Sawyer NT, Escayg A. Stress and epilepsy: multiple models, multiple outcomes. J Clin Neurophysiol. 2010;27(6):445–52.
42. Reddy DS. Is there a physiological role for the neurosteroid THDOC in stress-sensitive conditions? Trends Pharmacol Sci. 2003;24(3):103–6.
43. Reddy DS. Role of hormones and neurosteroids in epileptogenesis. Front Cell Neurosci. 2013;7.
44. Mitchell EA, Herd MB, Gunn BG, Lambert JJ, Belelli D. Neurosteroid modulation of GABAA receptors: molecular determinants and significance in health and disease. Neurochem Int. 2008;52(4–5):588–95.
45. Weiss GK, Castillo N, Fernandez M. Amygdala kindling rate is altered in rats with a deficit in the responsiveness of the hypothalamo-pituitary-adrenal axis. Neurosci Lett. 1993;157(1):91–4.
46. Karst H, de Kloet ER, Joels M. Episodic corticosterone treatment accelerates kindling epileptogenesis and triggers long-term changes in hippocampal CA1 cells, in the fully kindled state. Eur J Neurosci. 1999;11(3):889–98.
47. Taher TR, Salzberg M, Morris MJ, Rees S, O'Brien TJ. Chronic low-dose corticosterone supplementation enhances acquired epileptogenesis in the rat amygdala kindling model of TLE. Neuropsychopharmacology. 2005;30(9):1610–6.

48. Roberts AJ, Keith LD. Mineralocorticoid receptors mediate the enhancing effects of corticosterone on convulsion susceptibility in mice. J Pharmacol Exp Ther. 1994;270(2):505–11.
49. Bowers BJ, Bosy TZ, Wehner JM. Adrenalectomy increases bicuculline-induced seizure sensitivity in long-sleep and short-sleep mice. Pharmacol Biochem Behav. 1991;38(3):593–600.
50. Schridde U, van Luijtelaar G. Corticosterone increases spike-wave discharges in a dose- and time-dependent manner in WAG/Rij rats. Pharmacol Biochem Behav. 2004;78(2):369–75.
51. Castro OW, Santos VR, Pun RY, McKlveen JM, Batie M, Holland KD, et al. Impact of corticosterone treatment on spontaneous seizure frequency and epileptiform activity in mice with chronic epilepsy. PLoS One. 2012;7(9), e46044.
52. Rose RP, Bridger WH. Hormonal influences on seizure kindling: the effects of post-stimulation ACTH or cortisone injections. Brain Res. 1982;231(1):75–84.
53. Rose RP, Morell F, Hoeppner TJ. Influences of pituitary-adrenal hormones on kindling. Brain Res. 1979;169(2):303–15.
54. Cottrell GA, Nyakas C, de Kloet ER, Bohus B. Hippocampal kindling: corticosterone modulation of induced seizures. Brain Res. 1984;309(2):373–6.
55. Lee PH, Grimes L, Hong JS. Glucocorticoids potentiate kainic acid-induced seizures and wet dog shakes. Brain Res. 1989;480(1–2):322–5.
56. Scotti AL, Bollag O, Nitsch C. Seizure patterns of Mongolian gerbils subjected to a prolonged weekly test schedule: evidence for a kindling-like phenomenon in the adult population. Epilepsia. 1998;39(6):567–76.
57. Tolmacheva EA, Oitzl MS, van Luijtelaar G. Stress, glucocorticoids and absences in a genetic epilepsy model. Horm Behav. 2012;61(5):706–10.
58. Tolmacheva EA, van Luijtelaar G. The role of ovarian steroid hormones in the regulation of basal and stress induced absence seizures. J Steroid Biochem Mol Biol. 2007;104(3–5):281–8.
59. Matsumoto K, Nomura H, Murakami Y, Taki K, Takahata H, Watanabe H. Long-term social isolation enhances picrotoxin seizure susceptibility in mice: up-regulatory role of endogenous brain allopregnanolone in GABAergic systems. Pharmacol Biochem Behav. 2003;75(4):831–5.
60. Chadda R, Devaud LL. Sex differences in effects of mild chronic stress on seizure risk and GABAA receptors in rats. Pharmacol Biochem Behav. 2004;78(3):495–504.
61. Forcelli PA, Orefice LL, Heinrichs SC. Neural, endocrine and electroencephalographic hyperreactivity to human contact: a diathesis-stress model of seizure susceptibility in El mice. Brain Res. 2007;1144:248–56.
62. Hollrigel GS, Chen K, Baram TZ, Soltesz I. The pro-convulsant actions of corticotropin-releasing hormone in the hippocampus of infant rats. Neuroscience. 1998;84(1):71–9.
63. Moghaddam B, Bolinao ML, Stein-Behrens B, Sapolsky R. Glucocorticoids mediate the stress-induced extracellular accumulation of glutamate. Brain Res. 1994;655(1–2):251–4.
64. Serra M, Pisu MG, Mostallino MC, Sanna E, Biggio G. Changes in neuroactive steroid content during social isolation stress modulate GABAA receptor plasticity and function. Brain Res Rev. 2008;57(2):520–30.
65. Dong E, Matsumoto K, Uzunova V, Sugaya I, Takahata H, Nomura H, et al. Brain 5alpha-dihydroprogesterone and allopregnanolone synthesis in a mouse model of protracted social isolation. Proc Natl Acad Sci U S A. 2001;98(5):2849–54.
66. MacKenzie G, Maguire J. Chronic stress shifts the GABA reversal potential in the hippocampus and increases seizure susceptibility. Epilepsy Res. 2015;109:13–27.
67. Goldberg EM, Coulter DA. Mechanisms of epileptogenesis: a convergence on neural circuit dysfunction. Nat Rev Neurosci. 2013;14(5):337–49.
68. Szafarczyk A, Caracchini M, Rondouin G, Ixart G, Malaval F, Assenmacher I. Plasma ACTH and corticosterone responses to limbic kindling in the rat. Exp Neurol. 1986;92(3):583–90.
69. Karst H, Bosma A, Hendriksen E, Kamphuis W, de Kloet ER, Joels M. Effect of adrenalectomy in kindled rats. Neuroendocrinology. 1997;66(5):348–59.

70. Mazarati AM, Shin D, Kwon YS, Bragin A, Pineda E, Tio D, et al. Elevated plasma corticosterone level and depressive behavior in experimental temporal lobe epilepsy. Neurobiol Dis. 2009;34(3):457–61.
71. An SJ, Park SK, Hwang IK, Kim HS, Seo MO, Suh JG, et al. Altered corticotropin-releasing factor (CRF) receptor immunoreactivity in the gerbil hippocampal complex following spontaneous seizure. Neurochem Int. 2003;43(1):39–45.
72. Zobel A, Wellmer J, Schulze-Rauschenbach S, Pfeiffer U, Schnell S, Elger C, et al. Impairment of inhibitory control of the hypothalamic pituitary adrenocortical system in epilepsy. Eur Arch Psychiatry Clin Neurosci. 2004;254(5):303–11.
73. Galimberti CA, Magri F, Copello F, Arbasino C, Cravello L, Casu M, et al. Seizure frequency and cortisol and dehydroepiandrosterone sulfate (DHEAS) levels in women with epilepsy receiving antiepileptic drug treatment. Epilepsia. 2005;46(4):517–23.
74. Calabrese VP, Gruemer HD, Tripathi HL, Dewey W, Fortner CA, DeLorenzo RJ. Serum cortisol and cerebrospinal fluid beta-endorphins in status epilepticus. Their possible relation to prognosis. Arch Neurol. 1993;50(7):689–93.
75. Allendorfer JB, Heyse H, Mendoza L, Nelson EB, Eliassen JC, Storrs JM, et al. Physiologic and cortical response to acute psychosocial stress in left temporal lobe epilepsy - a pilot cross-sectional fMRI study. Epilepsy Behav. 2014;36:115–23.
76. Bernhardt BC, Hong S, Bernasconi A, Bernasconi N. Imaging structural and functional brain networks in temporal lobe epilepsy. Front Hum Neurosci. 2013;7:624.
77. Li J, Vestergaard M, Obel C, Precht DH, Christensen J, Lu M, et al. Prenatal stress and epilepsy in later life: a nationwide follow-up study in Denmark. Epilepsy Res. 2008;81(1):52–7.
78. Donnelly KM, Schefft BK, Howe SR, Szaflarski JP, Yeh HS, Privitera MD. Moderating effect of optimism on emotional distress and seizure control in adults with temporal lobe epilepsy. Epilepsy Behav. 2010;18(4):374–80.
79. Shang N-X, Zou L-P, Zhao J-B, Zhang F, Li H. Association between prenatal stress and infantile spasms: a case–control study in China. Pediatr Neurol. 2010;42(3):181–6.
80. Haung L-T. Early-life stress impacts the developing hippocampus and primes seizure occurrence: cellular, molecular, and epigenetic mechanisms. Front Mol Neurosci. 2014;7(Article 8):1–15.
81. Jones NC, O'Brien TJ, Carmant L. Interaction between sex and early-life stress: influence on epileptogenesis and epilepsy comorbidities. Neurobiol Dis. 2014;72 Pt B:233–41.
82. Edwards HE, Dortok D, Tam J, Won D, Burnham WM. Prenatal stress alters seizure thresholds and the development of kindled seizures in infant and adult rats. Horm Behav. 2002;42(4):437–47.
83. Beck SL, Gavin DL. Susceptibility of mice to audiogenic seizures is increased by handling their dams during gestation. Science. 1976;193(4251):427–8.
84. Frye CA, Bayon LE. Prenatal stress reduces the effectiveness of the neurosteroid 3 alpha,5 alpha-THP to block kainic-acid-induced seizures. Dev Psychobiol. 1999;34(3):227–34.
85. Salzberg M, Kumar G, Supit L, Jones NC, Morris MJ, Rees S, et al. Early postnatal stress confers enduring vulnerability to limbic epileptogenesis. Epilepsia. 2007;48(11):2079–85.
86. Jones NC, Kumar G, O'Brien TJ, Morris MJ, Rees SM, Salzberg MR. Anxiolytic effects of rapid amygdala kindling, and the influence of early life experience in rats. Behav Brain Res. 2009;203(1):81–7.
87. Kumar G, Jones NC, Morris MJ, Rees S, O'Brien TJ, Salzberg MR. Early life stress enhancement of limbic epileptogenesis in adult rats: mechanistic insights. PLoS One. 2011;6(9), e24033.
88. Koe AS, Salzberg MR, Morris MJ, O'Brien TJ, Jones NC. Early life maternal separation stress augmentation of limbic epileptogenesis: the role of corticosterone and HPA axis programming. Psychoneuroendocrinology. 2014;42:124–33.
89. Huang LT, Holmes GL, Lai MC, Hung PL, Wang CL, Wang TJ, et al. Maternal deprivation stress exacerbates cognitive deficits in immature rats with recurrent seizures. Epilepsia. 2002;43(10):1141–8.

90. Lai MC, Lui CC, Yang SN, Wang JY, Huang LT. Epileptogenesis is increased in rats with neonatal isolation and early-life seizure and ameliorated by MK-801: a long-term MRI and histological study. Pediatr Res. 2009;66(4):441–7.
91. Ozlem A, Moshe SL, Galanopoulou AS. Early life status epilepticus and stress have distinct and sex-specific effects on learning, subsequent seizure outcomes, including anticonvulsant response to phenobarbital. CNS Neurosci Ther. 2014;21(2):181–92.
92. Leussis MP, Heinrichs SC. Quality of rearing guides expression of behavioral and neural seizure phenotypes in EL mice. Brain Res. 2009;1260:84–93.
93. Gilby KL, Sydserff S, Patey AM, Thorne V, St-Onge V, Jans J, et al. Postnatal epigenetic influences on seizure susceptibility in seizure-prone versus seizure-resistant rat strains. Behav Neurosci. 2009;123(2):337–46.
94. Ellis N, Upton D, Thompson P. Epilepsy and the family: a review of current literature. Seizure Europ J Epilepsy. 2000;9(1):22–30.
95. Sheikh HI, Joanisse MF, Mackrell SM, Kryski KR, Smith HJ, Singh SM, et al. Links between white matter microstructure and cortisol reactivity to stress in early childhood: Evidence for moderation by parenting. Neuro Image Clin. 2014;6:77–85.
96. Maccari S, Morley-Fletcher S. Effects of prenatal restraint stress on the hypothalamus-pituitary-adrenal axis and related behavioural and neurobiological alterations. Psychoneuroendocrinology. 2007;32 Suppl 1:S10–5.
97. McEwen BS. Sex, stress and the brain: interactive actions of hormones on the developing and adult brain. Climacteric. 2014;17(S2):18–25.
98. Brunson KL, Eghbal-Ahmadi M, Bender R, Chen Y, Baram TZ. Long-term, progressive hippocampal cell loss and dysfunction induced by early-life administration of corticotropin-releasing hormone reproduce the effects of early-life stress. Proc Natl Acad Sci U S A. 2001;98(15):8856–61.
99. Hsu FC, Zhang GJ, Raol YS, Valentino RJ, Coulter DA, Brooks-Kayal AR. Repeated neonatal handling with maternal separation permanently alters hippocampal GABAA receptors and behavioral stress responses. Proc Natl Acad Sci U S A. 2003;100(21):12213–8.
100. Knuesel I, Chicha L, Britschgi M, Schobel SA, Bodmer M, Hellings JA, et al. Maternal immune activation and abnormal brain development across CNS disorders. Nat Rev Neurol. 2014;10(11):643–60.
101. Vezzani A, Aronica E, Mazarati A, Pittman QJ. Epilepsy and brain inflammation. Exp Neurol. 2013;244:11–21.
102. Bazak N, Kozlovsky N, Kaplan Z, Matar M, Golan H, Zohar J, et al. Pre-pubertal stress exposure affects adult behavioral response in association with changes in circulating corticosterone and brain-derived neurotrophic factor. Psychoneuroendocrinology. 2009; 34(6):844–58.
103. Howell BR, McCormack KM, Grand AP, Sawyer NT, Zhang X, Maestripieri D, et al. Brain white matter microstructure alterations in adolescent rhesus monkeys exposed to early life stress: associations with high cortisol during infancy. Biol Mood Anxiety Disord. 2013;3(1):1–14.
104. Amini E, Rezaei M, Mohamed Ibrahim N, Golpich M, Ghasemi R, Mohamed Z, et al. A molecular approach to epilepsy management: from current therapeutic methods to preconditioning efforts. Mol Neurobiol. 2015;52(1):492–513.
105. Sorrells SF, Caso JR, Munhoz CD, Sapolsky RM. The stressed CNS: when glucocorticoids aggravate inflammation. Neuron. 2009;64(1):33–9.
106. Danzer SC. Depression, stress, epilepsy and adult neurogenesis. Exp Neurol. 2012;233(1):22–32.
107. McEwen BS, Eiland L, Hunter RG, Miller MM. Stress and anxiety: structural plasticity and epigenetic regulation as a consequence of stress. Neuropharmacology. 2012;62(1):3–12.
108. Schoenfeld TJ, Gould E. Stress, stress hormones, and adult neurogenesis. Exp Neurol. 2012;233(1):12–21.
109. Magarinos AM, Verdugo JM, McEwen BS. Chronic stress alters synaptic terminal structure in hippocampus. Proc Natl Acad Sci U S A. 1997;94(25):14002–8.

110. Magalhaes AC, Holmes KD, Dale LB, Comps-Agrar L, Lee D, Yadav PN, et al. CRF Receptor1 regulates anxiety behaviour via sensitization of 5-HT2 receptor signaling. Nat Neurosci. 2010;13(5):622–9.
111. Anisman H, Merali Z, Stead JD. Experiential and genetic contributions to depressive- and anxiety-like disorders: clinical and experimental studies. Neurosci Biobehav Rev. 2008;32(6):1185–206.
112. Privitera M, Walters M, Lee I, Polak E, Fleck A, Schwieterman D, et al. Characteristics of people with self-reported stress-precipitated seizures. Epilepsy Behav. 2014;41:74–7.
113. Baumeister D, Lightman SL, Pariante CM. The interface of stress and the HPA axis in behavioural phenotypes of mental illness. Curr Top Behav Neurosci. 2014;18:13–24.
114. Lanteaume L, Bartolomei F, Bastien-Toniazzo M. How do cognition, emotion, and epileptogenesis meet? A study of emotional cognitive bias in temporal lobe epilepsy. Epilepsy Behav. 2009;15(2):218–24.
115. Novakova B, Harris PR, Ponnusamy A, Reuber M. The role of stress as a trigger for epileptic seizures: a narrative review of evidence from human and animal studies. Epilepsia. 2013;54(11):1866–76.
116. Byles JE, Robinson I, Banks E, Gibson R, Leigh L, Rodgers B, et al. Psychological distress and comorbid physical conditions: disease or disability? Depress Anxiety. 2014;31(6): 524–32.
117. Child A, Sanders J, Sigel P, Hunter MS. Meeting the psychological needs of cardiac patients: an integrated stepped-care approach within a cardiac rehabilitation setting. Br J Cardiol. 2010;17:175–9.
118. Surwit RS, van Tilburg MA, Zucker N, McCaskill CC, Parekh P, Feinglos MN, et al. Stress management improves long-term glycemic control in type 2 diabetes. Diabetes Care. 2002;25(1):30–4.
119. Moss-Morris R, Dennison L, Landau S, Yardley L, Silber E, Chalder T. A randomized controlled trial of cognitive behavioral therapy (CBT) for adjusting to multiple sclerosis (the saMS trial): does CBT work and for whom does it work? J Consult Clin Psychol. 2013;81(2):251–62.
120. NICE. Quality standard for the epilepsies in adults. Manchester: National Institute of Clinical Excellence; 2013. ISBN 978-1-4731-0048-0.
121. NICE. The epilepsies: the diagnosis and management of the epilepsies in adults and children in primary and secondary care: pharmacological update. London: 2012 1/25/2012. Report No.: Clinical Guideline 20.
122. Fountain NB, Van Ness PC, Swain-Eng R, Tonn S, Bever CT, For the American Academy of Neurology Epilepsy Measure Development Panel and the American Medical Association-Convened Physician Consortium for Performance Improvement Independent Measure Development Process. Quality improvement in neurology: AAN epilepsy quality measures: Report of the Quality Measurement and Reporting Subcommittee of the American Academy of Neurology. Neurology. 2011;76(1):94–9.
123. Muller B. Psychological approaches to the prevention and inhibition of nocturnal epileptic seizures: a meta-analysis of 70 case studies. Seizure. 2001;10(1):13–33.
124. Tang V, Michaelis R, Kwan P. Psychobehavioral therapy for epilepsy. Epilepsy Behav. 2014;32:147–55.
125. Ramaratnam S, Baker GA, Goldstein LH. Psychological treatments for epilepsy. Cochrane Database Syst Rev. 2008;3:1–32.
126. Tan SY, Bruni J. Cognitive-behavior therapy with adult patients with epilepsy: a controlled outcome study. Epilepsia. 1986;27(3):225–33.
127. Dahl J, Melin L, Lund L. Effects of a contingent relaxation treatment program on adults with refractory epileptic seizures. Epilepsia. 1987;28(2):125–32.
128. Schmid-Schonbein C. Improvement of seizure control by psychological methods in patients with intractable epilepsies. Seizure. 1998;7(4):261–70.
129. McLaughlin DP, McFarland K. A randomized trial of a group based cognitive behavior therapy program for older adults with epilepsy: the impact on seizure frequency, depression and psychosocial well-being. J Behav Med. 2011;34(3):201–7.

130. Chaytor N, Ciechanowski P, Miller JW, Fraser R, Russo J, Unutzer J, et al. Long-term outcomes from the PEARLS randomized trial for the treatment of depression in patients with epilepsy. Epilepsy Behav. 2011;20(3):545–9.
131. Michaelis R, Schonfeld W, Elsas SM. Trigger self-control and seizure arrest in the Andrews/Reiter behavioral approach to epilepsy: a retrospective analysis of seizure frequency. Epilepsy Behav. 2012;23(3):266–71.
132. Panjwani U, Selvamurthy W, Singh SH, Gupta HL, Thakur L, Rai UC. Effect of Sahaja yoga practice on seizure control & EEG changes in patients of epilepsy. Indian J Med Res. 1996;103:165–72.
133. Lundgren T, Dahl J, Melin L, Kies B. Evaluation of acceptance and commitment therapy for drug refractory epilepsy: a randomized controlled trial in South Africa--a pilot study. Epilepsia. 2006;47(12):2173–9.
134. Lundgren T, Dahl J, Yardi N, Melin L. Acceptance and Commitment Therapy and yoga for drug-refractory epilepsy: a randomized controlled trial. Epilepsy Behav. 2008;13(1):102–8.
135. Helgeson DC, Mittan R, Tan SY, Chayasirisobhon S. Sepulveda epilepsy education: the efficacy of a psychoeducational treatment program in treating medical and psychosocial aspects of epilepsy. Epilepsia. 1990;31(1):75–82.
136. May TW, Pfafflin M. The efficacy of an educational treatment program for patients with epilepsy (MOSES): results of a controlled, randomized study. Modular service package epilepsy. Epilepsia. 2002;43(5):539–49.
137. DiIorio C, Bamps Y, Walker ER, Escoffery C. Results of a research study evaluating WebEase, an online epilepsy self-management program. Epilepsy Behav. 2011;22(3):469–74.
138. Egner T, Sterman MB. Neurofeedback treatment of epilepsy: from basic rationale to practical application. Expert Rev Neurother. 2006;6(2):247–57.
139. Rockstroh B, Elbert T, Birbaumer N, Wolf P, Duchting-Roth A, Reker M, et al. Cortical self-regulation in patients with epilepsies. Epilepsy Res. 1993;14(1):63–72.
140. Nagai Y, Goldstein LH, Fenwick PB, Trimble MR. Clinical efficacy of galvanic skin response biofeedback training in reducing seizures in adult epilepsy: a preliminary randomized controlled study. Epilepsy Behav. 2004;5(2):216–23.
141. Tan G, Thornby J, Hammond DC, Strehl U, Canady B, Arnemann K, et al. Meta-analysis of EEG biofeedback in treating epilepsy. Clin EEG Neurosci. 2009;40(3):173–9.
142. Polak EL, Privitera MD, Lipton RB, Haut SR. Behavioral intervention as an add-on therapy in epilepsy: designing a clinical trial. Epilepsy Behav. 2012;25(4):505–10.
143. Morris GL, Gloss D, Buchhalter J, Mack KJ, Nickels K, Harden C. Evidence-based guideline update: vagus nerve stimulation for the treatment of epilepsy: report of the Guideline Development Subcommittee of the American Academy of Neurology. Neurology. 2013;81(16):1453–9.
144. Clancy JA, Mary DA, Witte KK, Greenwood JP, Deuchars SA, Deuchars J. Non-invasive vagus nerve stimulation in healthy humans reduces sympathetic nerve activity. Brain Stimul. 2014;7(6):871–7.
145. Kraus T, Hoesl K, Kiess O, Schanze A, Kornhuber J, Forster C. BOLD fMRI deactivation of limbic and temporal brain structures and mood enhancing effect by transcutaneous vagus nerve stimulation. J Neural Transm. 2007;114(11):1485–93.
146. Reddy DS. Neurosteroids: endogenous role in the human brain and therapeutic potentials. Prog Brain Res. 2010;186:113–37.
147. Sripada RK, Welsh RC, Marx CE, Liberzon I. The neurosteroids allopregnanolone and dehydroepiandrosterone modulate resting-state amygdala connectivity. Hum Brain Mapp. 2014;35(7):3249–61.
148. Bialer M, Johannessen SI, Levy RH, Perucca E, Tomson T, White HS. Progress report on new antiepileptic drugs: a summary of the eleventh Eilat conference (EILAT XI). Epilepsy Res. 2013;103(1):2–30.
149. Gupta R, Appleton R. Corticosteroids in the management of the paediatric epilepsies. Arch Dis Child. 2005;90(4):379–84.
150. Maguire J, Salpekar JA. Stress, seizures, and hypothalamic-pituitary-adrenal axis targets for the treatment of epilepsy. Epilepsy Behav. 2013;26(3):352–62.

Chapter 16
Epilepsy in Psychiatric Disorders

Massimiliano Beghi, Ettore Beghi, and Cesare Maria Cornaggia

Abstract Around 20 % of people with intellectual disability (ID) develop epileptic seizures. ID is a risk factor for the development of epileptic seizures also in patients with autism (21.5 % vs 8 % in the general population). In both these conditions generalized seizures are more common than partial seizures. The incidence of epilepsy is four to seven times higher in patients with depression than in the general population. Epilepsy and depression share an unusually high co-occurrence leading to a common etiology. A lifetime history of depression is also associated with a worse seizure outcome even after anterior temporal lobectomy. Patients treated with an antidepressant have a 50 % reduction in the occurrence of seizures. Epilepsy and bipolar disorder also could share a number of biochemical and pathophysiological underpinnings, even though the current literature is scarce. Patients with schizophrenia have an 11-fold increase in the prevalence of comorbid epilepsy. At therapeutic doses, drugs with high epileptogenic potential include clozapine and phenothiazines; drugs with intermediate epileptogenic potential include maprotiline and tricyclic antidepressants, while drugs with low epileptogenic potential include bupropion. The antidepressants with higher seizure potential after overdose are imipramine, desipramine, nortriptyline, maprotiline, and bupropion.

Keywords Epilepsy • Psychiatric Disorders • Comorbidity • Psychotropic Drugs • Neurobiology • Side Effects • Anxiety

---

M. Beghi, MD (✉)
Department of Mental Health, Medicine and Surgery, Department of Psychiatry, G. Salvini Hospital, via Beatrice d'Este 28, Milan 20017- Rho, Italy
e-mail: mbeghi@aogarbagnate.lombardia.it

E. Beghi, MD
Laboratory of Neurological Disorders, Department of Neurosciences, IRCCS-Istituto di Ricerche Farmacologiche Mario Negri, via La Masa 19, Milan 20156, Italy
e-mail: ettore.beghi@marionegri.it

C.M. Cornaggia, MD
Department of Surgery and Interdisciplinary Medicine, University of Milano Bicocca, via Cadore 48, Monza, Italy
e-mail: cesaremaria.cornaggia@unimib.it

M. Mula (ed.), *Neuropsychiatric Symptoms of Epilepsy*, Neuropsychiatric Symptoms of Neurological Disease, DOI 10.1007/978-3-319-22159-5_16

Table 16.1 Age-adjusted odds ratios (ORs) with 95 % confidence intervals (CIs) for development of unprovoked seizures after a first discharge diagnosis of depression, psychosis, bipolar disorder, anxiety disorder, suicide attempt, or psychiatric disorders combined [1]

	Symptomatic		Cryptogenic/idiopathic	
Diagnosis	OR	95 % CI	OR	95 % CI
Depression	1.5	0.8–2.6	3.9	2.4–6.1
Psychosis	2.1	1.2–3.9	2.5	1.4–4.4
Bipolar disorder	2.3	0.9–5.6	3.3	1.4–7.9
Anxiety disorder	1.4	0.6–3.6	4.0	2.1–7.6
Suicide attempt	1.2	0.5–2.8	3.9	2.4–6.2
Psychiatric disorders combined[a]	1.9	1.3–2.9	3.5	2.5–5.0

Reprinted with permission Wolters Kluwer Health, from Adelöw et al. [1], © 2012
Abbreviations: *CI* confidence interval, *OR* odds ratio
[a]The diagnosis psychiatric disorders combined includes all the other diagnoses except suicide attempt, for which each patient can have more than one psychiatric diagnosis

Introduction

Despite an abundant literature exploring psychiatric disorders in epilepsy, little is known on the epidemiology of epilepsy in psychiatric disorders. Some recent studies [1, 2] found an increased rate of psychiatric comorbidity preceding epileptic seizure onset and indicating a bidirectional relationship and common underlying mechanisms lowering seizure threshold and increasing the risk for psychiatric disorders and suicide (Table 16.1). In this chapter we make a summary of the available evidence on this topic, trying to explain the underlying mechanisms.

Neurodevelopmental Disorders and Epilepsy

Intellectual disability (ID), the term used instead of the previous one of mental retardation, might be not properly considered a psychiatric disorder, but it has been always included in the psychiatric disorders category, both in the Diagnostic and Statistical Manual (DSM) [3] and in the International Classification of Diseases (ICD) [4]. The fifth recent edition of DSM [3] uses, in the broader category of "Neurodevelopmental Disorders," the term "intellectual developmental disorders" (IDD), pointing out two substantial concepts: first of all the "IDD" is no longer considered a "disability" but a "disorder"; second, the term strongly links the symptoms to the brain evolution process. About this aspect, cognitive or behavioral disorders are associated and lie under the same etiopathogenic mechanism. This is thus the only condition strongly related to epilepsy in terms of diagnosis, prognosis, and treatment [5]. The comorbidity between IDD and epilepsy is high. Around 20 % of people with IDD develop seizures with a stable prevalence during the last decades [6, 7]. The risk for epilepsy increases with the severity of ID [8]. In patients with ID, generalized seizures are more common than partial seizures (63 % vs 33 %) [9].

Autism Spectrum Disorder and Epilepsy

Although there is a strong correlation between autism spectrum disorder and epilepsy, the prevalence of comorbidity varies widely according to the patient's IQ, with more autistic patients with IDD having epilepsy (Relative Risk [RR] = 0.555; 95 % confidence interval [CI]: 0.42–0.73; $p < 0.001$). The pooled prevalence of epilepsy was 21.5 % in autistic subjects with IDD versus 8 % in autistic subjects without IDD [10]. There is a significant difference in RR according to gender, favoring comorbidity of epilepsy in autistic girls (RR M/F = 0.549; 95 % CI: 0.45–0.66; $p < 0.001$) [10]. The male:female ratio of autism spectrum disorder comorbid with epilepsy was close to 2:1, whereas the male:female ratio of autism spectrum disorder without epilepsy was 3.5:1 [10–12]. Generalized tonic–clonic seizures predominate (88 %). This indicates that the familial liability to autism spectrum disorder can be associated with the risk for epilepsy in the proband [11]. Although the presence of epilepsy in probands was not associated with an increased risk of epilepsy in their relatives, it was associated with the presence of a broader autism spectrum disorder phenotype in other family members [11].

Patients' histories were consistent with generalized tonic-clonic seizures in 88 % of individuals. The possibility of simple or complex partial seizures was increased in eight other individuals but was not confirmed in any of them [11]. Seizure frequency has a great impact on the individuals' lives. Specialist medical care is needed in this severely communication-disabled population [12].

Attention-Deficit Hyperactivity Disorder and Epilepsy

In a study of 148 children with first unprovoked seizure and 89 seizure-free sibling controls, attention problems were 2.4 times more common before identification of the first seizure (8.1 %) than in controls (3.4 %) [13]. In a more recent study [14], a history of attention-deficit hyperactivity disorder (ADHD) was 2.5 times more common among children with newly diagnosed seizures than among control subjects (95 % CI, 1.1–5.5). The association was restricted to ADHD predominantly of the inattentive type (odds ratio [OR], 3.7; 95 % CI, 1.1–12.8), while no association was found in the hyperactive/impulsive type (OR, 1.8; 95 % CI, 0.6–5.7) nor in the combined type (OR, 2.5; 95 % CI, 0.3–18.3). Seizure type, etiology, gender, or seizure frequency at diagnosis (1 or >1) did not affect findings [14].

Depression and Epilepsy

Depression and epilepsy seem strictly correlated. The incidence of depression is 5–20 times higher and epilepsy 4–7 times higher for each group, respectively [15].

Depression itself and antidepressants have been examined as risk factors for developing epilepsy. Individuals with a history of major depression and/or suicide attempts are at increased risk for developing new-onset epilepsy [16–19], raising the possibility that depression and epilepsy share a common pathophysiology. Further evidence for this hypothesis can be found in studies showing that current neuropsychiatric disability and depression are associated with a worse seizure outcome in people with new-onset epilepsy and that a lifetime history of psychiatric disorders, and more specifically of depression, is associated with a worse seizure outcome after anterior temporal lobectomy [20]. Epilepsy and depression share an unusually high co-occurrence leading to a common etiology. Disrupted production of adult-born hippocampal granule cells in both disorders may contribute to this high co-occurrence [21]. Chronic stress and depression are associated with decreased granule cell neurogenesis [21]. Epilepsy is associated with increased production and aberrant integration of new cells early in the disease and decreased production of new cells late in the disease [21]. In both cases, these changes in neurogenesis play important roles. Aberrant integration of adult-generated cells during the development of epilepsy may impair the ability of the dentate gyrus to prevent excess excitatory activity from reaching hippocampal pyramidal cells, which promote seizures [17]. Moreover, studies in mice underline that lack of exercise, very common in depressed patients, causes a reduction in galanine production, with consequent increase in seizure frequency [22].

The mechanism leading to seizures in these individuals may thus be correlated with the pathophysiology of depression, suggesting different treatment strategies. The treatment of depression can improve seizure frequency. In placebo-controlled studies of serotonine selective reuptake inhibitors (SSRIs) or serotonine and norepinephrine reuptake inhibitors (SNRIs) for treating depression, those treated with a drug showed a 50 % reduction in the occurrence of seizures as adverse events, and those on placebo experienced a 19-fold increased risk for developing seizures compared to the general population [20]. These findings may imply serotonergic mechanisms underlying the observed comorbidity [20].

Bipolar Disorder and Epilepsy

Although mood disorders represent a frequent psychiatric comorbidity among patients with epilepsy, data regarding bipolar disorders are still limited. Recent data suggest that mood instability is actually frequent among patients with epilepsy but is phenomenologically different from that described in bipolar disorders [23]. Epilepsy and bipolar disorders are both episodic conditions that can later become chronic. Mania may represent a privileged window into the neurobiology of mood regulation and the neurobiology of epilepsy itself [23]. The kindling paradigm, invoked as a model for understanding seizure disorders, has also been applied to the episodic nature of bipolar disorders [24]. These two conditions apparently share a number of biochemical and pathophysiological underpinnings. Common mechanisms at the level of ion channels might include the anti-kindling and the calcium-antagonistic and potassium outward current-modulating properties of antiepileptic drugs. All these lines of research appear to be converging on a richer understanding of neurobiological underpinnings between bipolar disorders and epilepsy. In bipolar patients, changes in second-messenger systems, such as G-proteins, phosphatidylinositol, protein kinase C, myristoylated alanine-rich C kinase substrate, or calcium activity, have been described along with changes in c-fos expression [23]. Future research on intracellular mechanisms might become decisive for a better understanding of the similarities between these two disorders [24].

Psychosis and Epilepsy

The view of psychosis, and more specifically schizophrenia, as a neuropsychiatric condition contributed to a scientific notion that structural brain abnormalities in these patients could directly contribute to an increased risk of seizures [25]. Patients with schizophrenia have been reported to have an 11-fold increase in the prevalence of comorbid epilepsy [26]. The most recent evidence suggests that there is significant overlap in epidemiological, clinical, neuropathological, and neuroimaging features of the two diseases, which share biological liability. Those include ventricular enlargement in both conditions, the leucine-rich glioma inactivated (LGI) family gene loci overlap in both conditions, and other similarities [25]. Pathological studies of the brains of schizophrenic patients have revealed disorganization of the typical laminar structure of the hippocampus [27]. Pathological abnormalities in the hippocampus might result in the widespread disruption of the corticolimbic structures, such as the prefrontal cortex, with consequent development of schizophrenic symptoms [27]. In 1953, Landolt introduced EEG recordings as a means of better elucidating this peculiar antagonism, and coined the term "paradoxical" or "forced EEG normalization" (FN) [28], stating that "FN is a phenomenon characterized by the fact that, with the occurrence of psychotic states, the EEG becomes less abnormal, or entirely normal, as compared with previous and subsequent EEG findings." Various mechanisms have been proposed as underlying the antagonistic relationship between epileptic activity and psychosis, including an imbalance of inhibition and over-activation, kindling processes, the propagation of epileptic discharges along unusual pathways, and neurotransmitter alterations [29].

Seizures and Psychotropic Drugs

A wide range of substances, including psychotropic drugs, increase the risk of epileptic seizures. In a systematic review, Ruffmann et al. [30] addressed the issue of the epileptogenic potential of marketed drugs given at therapeutic doses. The authors clinically appraised the available reports emphasizing that a correlation between drug exposure and occurrence of seizures does not necessarily lead to a causal association. To be considered a risk factor, the association should meet a temporal sequence, should be strong (the larger the difference of exposure, the greater the strength of association), consistent (reproducible in different populations), with biological gradient (dose-response effect) and plausibility (consistent with a recognized biological mechanism) [30]. According to these criteria, drugs with high epileptogenic potential include clozapine and phenothiazines; drugs with intermediate epileptogenic potential include maprotiline and tricyclic antidepressants (TCA), while drugs with low epileptogenic potential include bupropion.

Alper et al. [31], accessing public domain data from the US Food and Drug Administration (FDA), compared seizure incidence among active drug and placebo groups in psychopharmacological clinical trials and the published rates of unprovoked seizures in the general population, involving a total of 75,873 patients. The authors found that an increased seizure incidence was observed with the antipsychotics clozapine and olanzapine, and chlorimipramine, a TCA indicated for the treatment of obsessive compulsive disorder (OCD) (Table 16.2). Alprazolam, bupropion immediate-release (IR) form, and quetiapine were also associated with higher than expected seizure incidence. However, only antidepressants have been found to be associated with an increased risk of seizures when adjusting for the duration of exposure. There are many chemical pathways that trigger epileptic seizures. Drugs that antagonize adenosine (A1), histamine (H1), and g-aminobutyric acid (GABA) receptors, and substances that stimulate cholinergic and glutamatergic receptors, can trigger seizures [32].

Antidepressants and Risk of Seizure

The incidence of seizures is significantly lower among patients with antidepressants than patients with placebo, as shown in Table 16.2 (standardized incidence ratio 0.48; 95 % CI, 0.36–0.61) [31].

A solid body of evidence now supports the concept that the noradrenergic and serotonergic effects of antidepressants are anticonvulsant at therapeutic doses, whereas higher doses, such as those that occur with supratherapeutic exposure or an intentional overdose, activate other neurochemical pathways that can culminate in seizures [32]. The drugs with higher seizure potential in overdose were imipramine, desipramine, nortriptyline, amoxapine, maprotiline, and bupropion (Table 16.3).

A recent study carried out in Switzerland [33] identified 15,441 single-agent exposures. Seizures occurred in 313 cases. Antidepressants with a high seizure potential were bupropion (31.6 %, seizures in 6 of 19 cases, 95 % CI: 15.4–50.0 %), maprotiline (17.5 %, 10/57, 95 % CI: 9.8–29.4 %), venlafaxine (13.7 %, 23/168, 95 % CI: 9.3–19.7 %), citalopram (13.1 %, 34/259, 95 % CI: 9.5–17.8 %), and mefenamic acid (10.9 %, 51/470, 95 % CI: 8.4–14.0 %).

In adolescents, 23.9 % (95 % CI: 17.6–31.7 %) of cases exposed to mefenamic acid resulted in seizures, but only 5.7 % (95 % CI: 3.3–9.7 %) in adults ($p=0.001$).

Table 16.2 Standardized incidence ratio (SIR) for seizure incidence in active drug arm relative to placebo, for antidepressant, antipsychotic, and over-the-counter (OCD) indication categories [31]

Indication category	Number of patients, active drug arm	Average trial duration[a] years (days, active drug arm	Placebo seizure rate (per 100,000 PEY)	Observed number of seizures	Expected number of seizures[b]	SIR	95 % CI
Antidepressant							
All	33,885	0.319 (116 days)	1166.7	60	126.1	.48[c]	(0.36–0.61)
All, excluding bupropion IR	29,466			34	109.6	.31[c]	(0.21–0.43)
Bupropion IR only	4,419			26	16.4	1.58[c]	(1.03–2.32)
Antipsychotic							
All	20,368	0.470 (172 days)	784.3	154	75.1	2.05[c]	(1.74–2.40)
All, excluding clozapine	18,626			93	68.7	1.35[c]	(1.09–1.66)
All, excluding clozapine and olanzapine	16,126			70	59.5	1.18	(0.92–1.49)
All, excluding clozapine, olanzapine, and quetiapine	13,739			52	50.7	1.03	(0.77–1.35)
Clozapine only	1,742			61	6.4	9.50[c]	(7.27–12.20)
Olanzapine only	2,500			23	9.2	2.50[c]	(1.58–3.74)
Quetiapine only	2,387			18	8.8	2.05[c]	(1.21–3.23)
OCD							
All	8,318	0.402 (146 days)	433.4	37	14.5	2.55[c]	(1.80–3.52)
All, excluding clomipramine	4,799			12	8.4	1.44	(0.74–2.51)
Clomipramine only	3,519			25	6.1	4.08[c]	(2.64–6.02)

Reprinted from Biological Psychiatry, Alper et al. [31], © 2007, with permission from Elsevier

PEY person exposure years, *OCD* obsessive compulsive disorder, *SR* standardized incidence ratio

[a]Average trial duration = (total number of PEY)/(number of subjects), for those trials which provided information on PEY

[b]Expected number of seizures = (number of patients, active drug arm) × (average trial duration, active drug arm) × (placebo seizure rate)

[c]Significant at level of $p<0.05$

Table 16.3 Risk stratification for antidepressant overdose-induced seizures [32]

Risk for antidepressant overdose-induced seizures			
Antidepressant class representative drugs from each class	Low risk <5 % seizure incidence after overdose	Intermediate risk 5–10 % seizure incidence after overdose	High risk >10 % seizure incidence after overdose
MAOIs			
Isocarboxazid[b]	+	–	–
Moclobemide	+	–	–
Phenelzine[b]	+	–	–
Selegiline[b]	+	–	–
Tranylcypromine[b]	+	–	–
CAs			
Tertiary amines			
Amitrtiptyline	–	+	–
Clomipramine	–	+	–
Doxepin	–	+	–
Imipramine	–		+
Trimipramine	–	+	–
Secondary amines			
Desipramine	–	–	+
Nortriptyline	–	–	+
Protriptyline	–	+	–
Other			
Amoxapine	–	–	+
Maprotiline	–	–	+
SSRIs			
Citalopram[c]	–	+	–
Escitalopram	+	–	–
Fluoxetine	+	–	–
Fluvoxamine	+	–	–
Paroxetine	+	–	–
Sertraline	+	–	–
Atypical antidepressants			
Bupropion	–	–	+
Duloxetine	Risk unknown	–	–
Mirtazapine	+	–	–
Reboxetine	Risk unknown	–	–
Trazodone	+	–	–
Venlafaxine[d]	–	+	–

[a]Data compiled from multiple sources referenced throughout the article. The table was constructed solely by the authors

[b]Seizure risk with overdose presumed to be low based on lack of convincing clinical evidence and/or the drug shares a similar structure and/or pharmacologic mechanism to drugs within its class that have been determined to be low risk

[c]Seizure risk with overdose should be considered high with ingestions exceeding 600 mg

[d]Seizure risk may be high with large ingestions

For citalopram these numbers were 22.0 % (95 % CI: 12.8–35.2 %) and 10.9 % (95 % CI: 7.1–16.4 %), respectively ($p=0.058$). The probability of seizures with mefenamic acid, citalopram, trimipramine, and venlafaxine increased as the ingested dose increased [33].

From a clinical point of view, current data show that a treatment should be given despite its epileptogenic risk.

Tricyclic Agents (TCA)

The incidence of seizures in patients treated with therapeutic doses (150–300 mg) of TCA is 1–2 % and time to seizures ranges between 3 days and 12 months [30]. The incidence of seizures with cyclic agents (CA) toxicity is varied, ranging from 3 % to more than 20 % and is directly correlated to TCA blood concentration, that is the best predictor of seizures, if compared to EEG findings [34]. Toxicity associated with CAs is caused by antagonism against a1-adrenergic, H1 histamine, and muscarinic receptors; blockade of cardiac ion channels (Na1 and K1); and interference with chloride conductance through GABA Cl ionophores. Each drug within this class shows variability in these pharmacologic mechanisms of action and their toxic effects [32].

Maprotiline

At therapeutic doses, seizures are recorded in 0.4 % of patients in clinical trials and in 0.025 % of patients in post marketing surveillance [30]. One retrospective study found a seizure rate of 15.6 % in patients taking between 75 and 300 mg daily [35]. Although it is uncertain what mechanisms are responsible for maprotiline-induced seizures, two possibilities include the inhibitory effect that maprotiline exerts on G-protein- activated inwardly rectifying K (GIRK) channels and antagonism of H1 receptors [32].

Selective Serotonin Reuptake Inhibitors (SSRIs) and Serotonin and Norepinephrine Reuptake Inhibitors (SNRIs)

Despite their relative receptor selectivity, SSRIs can be proconvulsant in the setting of an overdose. How this occurs is still not known [36]. A review of SSRI poisoning admissions to an Australian toxicology unit reported a seizure incidence of 2 % for citalopram, 1 % for fluoxetine, 4 % for fluvoxamine, 2 % for paroxetine, and 2 % for sertraline [37]. Venlafaxine (SNRI) seems more correlated with seizures than SSRI [36].

SSRI overdose can cause serotonin syndrome that increases the risk for seizures, but not all SSRI overdose-induced seizures result from serotonin syndrome. Inhibition of glycine receptors and hyponatremia can also play a role in SSRI overdose-induced seizures. Seizures induced by citalopram may occur from QTc prolongation or inhibition of GIRK channels [36].

Bupropion

The drug is available in immediate-release (IR), sustained-release (SR), and extended-release (XL) formulations. The risk for seizures in therapeutic doses (150–600 mg) is relatively low (0.2 % in prospective studies and 0.4 % in retrospective studies) [30]. In randomized clinical trials the prevalence increased to 0.8 % but half cases had other risk factors [30]. On the other hand, seizure activity occurred in 21 % of patients with overdose involving the IR formulation, 11 % of patients who primarily overdosed on the SR formulation, and 32 % of patients who overdosed on the XL formulation [32]. Seizures induced by overdose of bupropion are problematic because they can be repeated and can progress to status epilepticus. Another problem with bupropion overdose-induced seizures is the delayed onset with which they can occur. Seizure activity has been reported to occur up to 8 h (mean, 3.7 h), 14 h (mean, 4.3 h), and 24 h (mean, 7.3 h) after overdose on the IR, SR, and XL preparations, respectively.

Electroconvulsive Therapy

No report of spontaneous seizures was found in a study group of 619 patients. One patient who was excluded due to suspected neurosyphilis developed recurrent seizures 1 month after electroconvulsive therapy (ECT). Two patients in the control group had a single seizure with no relapse. ECT has not been found to cause epilepsy. Patients' underlying conditions may influence the development of seizures [38].

Antipsychotics

Both first-generation and second-generation antipsychotic medications can increase the chance of seizures. Hedges and colleagues [39] reviewed the published literature concerning the seizure-lowering effects of first- and second- generation antipsychotic medications, finding that rigorously controlled studies are relatively infrequent. Of the first-generation antipsychotic medications, chlorpromazine appears to be associated with the greatest risk of seizures, although other first-generation antipsychotics also lower seizure threshold. Conversely, molindone, haloperidol, fluphenazine, pimozide, and trifluoperazine are associated with a lower risk of seizure induction. Clozapine is the second-generation antipsychotic agent most frequently associated with seizures, with risperidone appearing to confer a relatively low risk, even in overdose [39].

First-Generation Antipsychotics

With the exception of chlorpromazine, the risk of seizures from first-generation antipsychotics ranges between 0.5 and 0.9 % [39]. In patients treated with chlorpromazine the risk increases to 1.2 %, especially in patients treated for an organic disease, whose risk is 2 %. The risk is dose-dependent (9 % for doses ≥1000 mg). The biochemical basis of the epileptogenic effect of antipsychotics can be attributed to the dopamine-blocking properties of these drugs [30].

Clozapine

Clozapine-induced seizures may occur at any dose; the risk increases with dose and goes up to 4 % at ≥600 mg/day. Some authors advocated that patients on that dose regimen have anticonvulsants added as a primary prophylactic measure [40]. The author discusses the pitfalls of this recommendation and highlights that seizures are better predicted by high serum concentration (1300 ng/ml) rather than dose alone, and that serum concentration is strongly influenced by gender, age, smoking habit, drug-drug interactions and variations in the 1A2, 2D6, and 3A4 genotypes [40].

Seizures, Alcohol, and Illicit Drugs

In recent times, psychiatric disorders as psychosis, ADHD, mood and personality disorders can be triggered by street drug/alcohol misuse [41], even if this correlation has not been found in all studies [42]. Alcohol/illicit drug abuse or dependence may worsen seizure control or even directly cause seizures. The potentially serious seizure outcomes from any of these compounds may cause seizures either acutely or on withdrawal [43]. Their use may also reduce effectiveness of antiepileptic drugs. In case of seizures onset in patients with a psychiatric disorder, a current/past alcohol/illicit drug (in particular cocaine or new compounds) misuse should be investigated.

Conclusion

In light of these findings, the correlation between epilepsy and psychiatric disorders is evident, indicating a bidirectional relationship and common underlying mechanisms. A specific attention should be given for alcohol drug misuse. The risk of seizures should be taken into consideration by the psychiatrist, because it could be the result of the disorder itself or of its treatment. In patients with a history of seizures, antipsychotics should be used carefully even if an increased risk for seizures is evident for clozapine, phenothiazines, olanzapine and, less, quetiapine. Antipsychotics with a low seizure potential should be however preferred. In therapeutic doses, antidepressants are safe and increase the seizure threshold. In light of these results, in patients with epilepsy and a comorbid depression, antidepressants should be used (even if with adequate monitoring): SSRI and SNRI should be preferred to TCA and bupropion.

References

1. Adelöw C, Andersson T, Ahlbom A, Tomson T. Hospitalization for psychiatric disorders before and after onset of unprovoked seizures/epilepsy. Neurology. 2012;78(6):396–401.
2. Hesdorffer DC, Ishihara L, Mynepalli L, Webb DJ, Weil J, Hauser WA. Epilepsy, suicidality, and psychiatric disorders: a bidirectional association. Ann Neurol. 2012;72(2):184–91.
3. American Psychiatric Association. Diagnostic and statistical manual of mental disorders. 5th ed. Washington, DC: American Psychiatric Press; 2013.
4. World Health Organization. The ICD-10. Classification of mental and behavioural disorders, clinical descriptions and diagnostic guidelines. Geneva: WHO press; 1992.
5. Cornaggia CM, Beghi M, Provenzi M, Beghi E. Correlation between cognition and behavior in epilepsy. Epilepsia. 2006;47(s2):34–9.
6. Oeseburg B, Dijkstra GJ, Groothoff JW, Reijneveld SA, Jansen DE. Prevalence of chronic health conditions in children with intellectual disability: a systematic literature review. Intellect Dev Disabil. 2011;49(2):59–85.
7. Lund J. Epilepsy and psychiatric disorder in the mentally retarded adult. Acta Psychiatr Scand. 1985;72(6):557–62.
8. Jenkins LK, Brown SW. Some issues in the assessment of epilepsy occurring in the context of learning disability in adults. Seizure. 1992;1(1):49–55.
9. Mariani E, Ferini-Strambi L, Sala M, Erminio C, Smirne S. Epilepsy in institutionalized patients with encephalopathy: clinical aspects and nosological considerations. Am J Ment Retard. 1993;98(Suppl):27–33.
10. Amiet C, Gourfinkel-An I, Bouzamondo A, Tordjman S, Baulac M, Lechat P, et al. Epilepsy in autism is associated with intellectual disability and gender: evidence from a meta-analysis. Biol Psychiatry. 2008;64(7):577–82.
11. Bolton PF, Carcani-Rathwell I, Hutton J, Goode S, Howlin P, Rutter M. Epilepsy in autism: features and correlates. Br J Psychiatry. 2011;198(4):289–94.
12. Danielsson S, Gillberg IC, Billstedt E, Gillberg C, Olsson I. Epilepsy in young adults with autism: a prospective population-based follow-up study of 120 individuals diagnosed in childhood. Epilepsia. 2005;46(6):918–23.
13. Austin JK, Harezlak J, Dunn DW, Huster GA, Rose DF, Ambrosius WT. Behavior problems in children before first recognized seizure. Pediatrics. 2001;107:115–22.
14. Hesdorffer DC, Ludvigsson P, Olafsson E, Gudmundsson G, Kjartansson O, Hauser WA. ADHD as a risk factor for incident unprovoked seizures and epilepsy in children. Arch Gen Psychiatry. 2004;61(7):731–6.

15. Kanner AM. Depression and epilepsy: a review of multiple facets of their close relation. Neurol Clin. 2009;27(4):865–80.
16. Forsgren L, Nyström L. An incident case-referent study of epileptic seizures in adults. Epilepsy Res. 1990;6(1):66–81.
17. Hesdorffer DC, Lúdvígsson P, Hauser WA, Olafsson E, Kjartansson O. Co-occurrence of major depression or suicide attempt with migraine with aura and risk for unprovoked seizure. Epilepsy Res. 2007;75(2-3):220–3.
18. Hesdorffer DC, Hauser WA, Olafsson E, Ludvigsson P, Kjartansson O. Depression and suicide attempt as risk factors for incident unprovoked seizures. Ann Neurol. 2006;59(1):35–41.
19. Hesdorffer DC, Hauser WA, Annegers JF, Cascino G. Major depression is a risk factor for seizures in older adults. Ann Neurol. 2000;47:246–9.
20. Kanner AM, Schachter SC, Barry JJ, Hesdorffer DC, Mula M, Trimble M, et al. Depression and epilepsy: epidemiologic and neurobiologic perspectives that may explain their high comorbid occurrence. Epilepsy Behav. 2012;24(2):156–68.
21. Danzer SC. Depression, stress, epilepsy and adult neurogenesis. Exp Neurol. 2012;233(1):22–32.
22. Epps SA, Kahn AB, Holmes PV, Boss-Williams KA, Weiss JM, Weinshenker D. Antidepressant and anticonvulsant effects of exercise in a rat model of epilepsy and depression comorbidity. Epilepsy Behav. 2013;29(1):47–52.
23. Mula M, Marotta AE, Monaco F. Epilepsy and bipolar disorders. Expert Rev Neurother. 2010;10(1):13–23.
24. Mazza M, Di Nicola M, Della Marca G, Janiri L, Bria P, Mazza S. Bipolar disorder and epilepsy: a bidirectional relation? Neurobiological underpinnings, current hypotheses, and future research directions. Neuroscientist. 2007;13(4):392–404.
25. Danielyan A, Nasrallah HA. Neurological disorders in schizophrenia. Psychiatr Clin North Am. 2009;32(4):719–57.
26. Makikyro T, Karvonen JT, Hakko H, et al. Comorbidity of hospital-treated psychiatric and physical disorders with special reference to schizophrenia: a 28 year follow-up of the 1966 northern Finland general population birth cohort. Public Health. 1998;112(4):221–8.
27. Engel J, Wilson C, Lopez-Rodriguez F. Limbic connectivity: anatomical substrates of behavioural disturbances in epilepsy. In: Trimble M, Schmitz B, editors. The neuropsychiatry of epilepsy. Cambridge: Cambridge University Press; 2002. p. 18–37.
28. Landolt H. Some clinical EEG correlations in epileptic psychoses (twilight states). EEG Clin Neurophysiol. 1953;5:121.
29. Krishnamoorthy ES, Trimble MR. Forced normalization: clinical and therapeutic relevance. Epilepsia. 1999;40 Suppl 10:57–64.
30. Ruffmann C, Bogliun G, Beghi E. Epileptogenic drugs: a systematic review. Expert Rev Neurother. 2006;6(4):575–89. Review.
31. Alper K, Schwartz KA, Kolts RL, Khan A. Seizure incidence in psychopharmacological clinical trials: an analysis of Food and Drug Administration (FDA) summary basis of approval reports. Biol Psychiatry. 2007;62(4):345–54.
32. Judge BS, Rentmeester LL. Antidepressant overdose-induced seizures. Psychiatr Clin North Am. 2013;36(2):245–60.
33. Reichert C, Reichert P, Monnet-Tschudi F, Kupferschmidt H, Ceschi A, Rauber-Lüthy C. Seizures after single-agent overdose with pharmaceutical drugs: analysis of cases reported to a poison center. Clin Toxicol (Phila). 2014;52(6):629–34.
34. Bailey B, Buckley NA, Amre DK. A meta-analysis of prognostic indicators to predict seizures, arrhythmias or death after tricyclic antidepressant overdose. J Toxicol Clin Toxicol. 2004;42(6):877–88.
35. Jabbari B, Bryan GE, March EE, et al. Incidence of seizures with tricyclic and tetracyclic antidepressants. Arch Neurol. 1985;42:480–1.
36. Gartlehner G, Thieda P, Hansen RA, Gaynes BN, Deveaugh-Geiss A, et al. Comparative risk for harms of second-generation antidepressants: a systematic review and meta-analysis. Drug Saf. 2008;31(10):851–65.

37. Isbister GK, Bowe SJ, Dawson A, Whyte IM. Relative toxicity of selective serotonin reuptake inhibitors (SSRIs) in overdose. J Toxicol Clin Toxicol. 2004;42(3):277–85.
38. Ray AK. Does electroconvulsive therapy cause epilepsy? J ECT. 2013;29(3):201–5.
39. Hedges D, Jeppson K, Whitehead P. Antipsychotic medication and seizures: a review. Drugs Today (Barc). 2003;39(7):551–7.
40. Caetano D. Use of anticonvulsants as prophylaxis for seizures in patients on clozapine. Australas Psychiatry. 2014;22(1):78–83.
41. Gururajan A, Manning EE, Klug M, van den Buuse M. Drugs of abuse and increased risk of psychosis development. Aust N Z J Psychiatry. 2012;46(12):1120–35.
42. Sordo L, Indave BI, Degenhardt L, Barrio G, Kaye S, et al. A systematic review of evidence on the association between cocaine use and seizures. Drug Alcohol Depend. 2013;133(3):795–804.
43. Leach JP, Mohanraj R, Borland W. Alcohol and drugs in epilepsy: pathophysiology, presentation, possibilities, and prevention. Epilepsia. 2012;53 Suppl 4:48–57.

Chapter 17
The Role of Epilepsy Surgery

Genevieve Rayner and Sarah J. Wilson

Abstract While seizure control is an obvious goal of epilepsy surgery, the postsurgical period can have the paradoxical effect of worsening an individual's psychiatric function. This chapter systematically reviews the literature relating to neuropsychiatric outcomes of epilepsy surgery, revealing that there is a heightened risk for psychopathology both before and after surgery. This commonly takes the form of depression, anxiety, and psychosocial adjustment difficulties, and can emerge in patients with no prior psychiatric history.

From this review a compelling case arises for the routine provision of presurgical psychiatric and psychosocial evaluation, in addition to postsurgical follow-up and rehabilitation. Pre-surgery, this evaluation can shape the team's understanding of surgical candidacy and the patient's capacity for informed consent. Moreover, it provides a prime opportunity for managing the sometimes-unrealistic expectations that patients and their families harbor for postsurgery life. While preexisting psychopathology is a risk factor for poor seizure and psychosocial outcomes, it is not a contraindication to surgery when the treating team has the capacity to treat it proactively. Post surgery, efficacious treatment of psychiatric comorbidity increases the likelihood of seizure freedom, as well as optimizing psychosocial functioning and quality of life. By contrast, failure to treat can allow psychiatric comorbidity to persist or escalate, and psychological difficulties to develop as the patient adjusts to life after surgery.

Electronic supplementary material The online version of this chapter (doi:10.1007/978-3-319-22159-5_17) contains supplementary material, which is available to authorized users.

G. Rayner, PhD (✉)
Melbourne School of Psychological Sciences, The University of Melbourne, Redmond Barry Building, Parkville, VIC, 3010, Australia

The Florey Institute of Neuroscience and Mental Health, Melbourne, VIC, Australia
e-mail: raynerg@unimelb.edu.au

S.J. Wilson, PhD
Melbourne School of Psychological Sciences, The University of Melbourne, Redmond Barry Building, Parkville, VIC, 3010, Australia

The Florey Institute of Neuroscience and Mental Health, Melbourne, VIC, Australia

Comprehensive Epilepsy Programme, Austin Health, Heidelberg, VIC, Australia
e-mail: sarahw@unimelb.edu.au

M. Mula (ed.), *Neuropsychiatric Symptoms of Epilepsy*, Neuropsychiatric Symptoms of Neurological Disease, DOI 10.1007/978-3-319-22159-5_17

Keywords Epilepsy • Surgery • Mood • Depression • Anxiety • Psychosis • Psychogenic nonepileptic seizures • Adjustment • Rehabilitation

Introduction

Epilepsy is one of the most common neurological disorders, with approximately 70 million sufferers worldwide [1]. Focal seizures occur within brain networks localized to one hemisphere of the brain [2] and are drug resistant in up to one third of individuals [3]. Poorly controlled seizures habitually interrupt day-to-day life and are associated with a substantial disease burden. In particular, drug-resistant epilepsy is commonly comorbid with cognitive impairment and psychiatric disturbance, and can be accompanied by a raft of psychosocial restrictions including an inability to drive, unemployment and underemployment, financial dependence, strained family dynamics, social isolation, and stigmatization [3–6]. Of the focal syndromes, temporal lobe epilepsy (TLE) is the most prevalent. It is also the most relevant to this chapter because it follows a chronic, drug-resistant course in >70 % of individuals [7–9].

Anticonvulsant drugs are not the only treatment option for focal epilepsy. Based on empirical research [3, 6, 10], international guidelines now recommend that after the failure of two antiepileptic drugs clinicians should consider a patient's suitability for surgery to remove epileptogenic brain tissue [11]. Anterior temporal lobectomy (ATL) is the prototypical intervention for TLE and is used in epilepsy centers worldwide. It typically comprises a 6.0–6.5 cm resection of the anterior lateral nondominant temporal lobe, or 4.0–4.5 cm of the dominant temporal lobe. The mesial resection includes the amygdala and, at a minimum, the anterior 1.0–3.0 cm of the hippocampus (most commonly, 4.0 cm) [7]. In support of its therapeutic efficacy, two randomized controlled trials have shown that ATL is superior to ongoing medical therapy in terms of seizure control and quality of life, with around two thirds of patients rendered seizure-free compared to <9 % of patients who continue on medical treatment [7, 8]. Importantly, rates of seizure freedom or improvement after surgery remain relatively stable over the long-term (i.e., >15 years), and the vast majority of patients (92 %) consider epilepsy surgery worthwhile throughout this period regardless of seizure outcome [12]. Current guidelines strongly recommend early surgical intervention to maximize a patient's chances of achieving seizure freedom [13].

The success of epilepsy surgery depends on more than just the alleviation of seizures [14]. Given the psychosocial limitations that accompany drug-resistant epilepsy, many patients see surgery as an opportunity to engage in life more fully, envisaging themselves enjoying liberties such as driving and independence; being employed; feeling happier, cleverer, and more in control; enjoying better family relationships; and having a better memory [14–16]. They may also harbor hopes that surgery will lead to the remission of a preexisting psychiatric condition [16]. Meanwhile, family members may assume that surgery will lessen the burden on them to support and care for the patient, and, in some cases, patients or partners alike may view seizure relief as an opportunity to leave an unhappy relationship. The reality, however, is that seizure freedom does not always engender such changes in the postoperative period [15].

Failure to meet preoperative expectations can leave patients feeling that surgery was unsuccessful [16], and the subsequent disappointment of postoperative realities may lead to unfavorable longer-term psychiatric outcomes [17]. The process of adjustment following ATL has been carefully documented, and primarily depends on managing preoperative expectations of surgery, postoperative mood and seizure outcome, as well as the patient's capacity to discard roles associated with chronic epilepsy and learn to become well [18, 19]. This process and its clinical manifestations are known as the burden of normality, and will be discussed in greater detail later in this chapter.

Neuropsychiatric Outcomes of Epilepsy Surgery

The surgical setting can play an influential role in the persistence, remission, or emergence of neuropsychiatric symptoms in certain individuals [20, 21]. Following surgery, between 32 and 68 % of adult patients will experience clinically significant psychopathology [22–27]. These overall rates, however, may conceal the onset of de novo psychopathology in the months shortly after surgery, conservatively estimated to occur in ~20 % of patients [26–28]. Alternatively, in patients with a preexisting psychiatric condition, symptoms have been noted to resolve in around 15–30 % [29] but up to 87 % [25] of patients after surgery. In an attempt to address the large variability in the rates of symptom occurrence, a recent systematic review of 13 studies by Macrodimitris and colleagues [30] concluded that patients typically experience an improvement in their psychiatric functioning post surgery or, at the very least, avoid a worsening of their neuropsychiatric symptoms.

The aim of this chapter is to systematically review the available literature examining neuropsychiatric outcomes for the four most common disorders following resective epilepsy surgery, namely, depression, anxiety, psychosis, and somatic symptom disorders. Databases Medline, PubMed, and EmBase were searched for peer-reviewed studies published in English between 1980 and 2015 using the following search terms: *psych*, outcome,* and *epilepsy surgery*. This identified a total of 1076 studies.

After 355 duplicates were removed, studies were excluded if (1) participants were aged ≤16 years at surgery, (2) they did not contain original empirical data, or (3) they did not report sufficient methodological detail (e.g., sample size, frequency or prevalence statistics, etc.). Inclusion criteria comprised use of (1) formal psychiatric assessment after surgery with contemporary nosology (i.e., DSM or ICD classification criteria) or (2) quantitative measures of psychiatric symptomatology (e.g., the Beck Depression Inventory, the State-Trait Anxiety Inventory) to assess depressive, anxious, psychotic, or somatic symptoms and/or disorder. This resulted in a

Table 17.1 Summary of the results of the systematic literature review [17, 31–40]

	Depression	Anxiety	Psychosis	Somatoform
No. of studies	26	12[a]	12[b]	3[c]
Design				
Prospective	18 (69 %)	9 (75 %)	2 (17 %)	0
Retrospective	8 (31 %)	3 (25 %)	10 (83 %)	3 (100 %)
Cross-sectional	0	0	0	0
Sample type				
Case series (i.e., $N \leq 10$)	1 (4 %)	0	5 (42 %)	1 (33 %)
Mode of classification				
Expert diagnosis	12 (46 %)	6 (50 %)	12 (100 %)	3 (100 %)
Self-report symptomatology only	14 (54 %)	6 (50 %)	0	0
Follow-up period (months)				
Range	1.5–60	1.5–96	12–264	24–56
Median	12	24	24	N/A

[a]Including ten studies overlapping with the depression outcome studies [17, 31, 32, 34–40]
[b]Including two studies overlapping with the depression/anxiety outcome studies [31, 33]
[c]Including one study overlapping with the depression/anxiety/psychosis outcome studies [31]

total of 41 outcome studies included in the review, published between 1989 and 2014. Of these, 56 % used psychiatric classification criteria to diagnose psychopathology; 45 % employed longitudinal, prospective follow-up experimental designs; and ~15 % were case studies or case series. Across the studies, the period of post-surgical follow-up spanned 1.5 months to 22 years, although the most common time frame occurred within the first 24 months after surgery. Table 17.1 summarizes the methodological properties of the studies captured by the systematic literature review, stratified by disorder. It reveals that depression remains the most commonly studied neuropsychiatric sequelae of epilepsy surgery.

Depressive Symptoms and Disorders

Presurgery Prevalence

Depressed mood is the most prominent psychiatric symptom of epilepsy [41]. Research suggests that between 17 and 55 % of people with drug-resistant epilepsy endorse clinically significant depressive symptoms [17, 42–46], with 43 % higher odds of developing depression than healthy controls after adjusting for demographic factors [47]. Of the 41 studies reviewed, 26 examined the occurrence of depressive symptoms surrounding epilepsy surgery (Table S17.1). Most of these were longitudinal studies prospectively following up patients for around a year after surgery, with a roughly even split of expert classification of depression versus self-reported symptomatology based on questionnaires. These studies indicate that prior to epilepsy surgery, between 16 and 40 % of surgical candidates show elevated rates of depressive symptoms and disorder [17, 29, 31–36, 48–51]. Following surgery, preoperative depressive symptoms remit for around half of these patients [29] within 3–6 months of surgery [36, 52].

Postsurgery Course

Most prospective studies indicate that after epilepsy surgery, around 20–30 % of patients experience unipolar major depression [17, 27, 29, 31, 37, 50, 51, 53–55], although Malmgren and colleagues [48] reported expert-diagnosed rates of postoperative mood disorder as high as 68 %. Most postsurgical depression is diagnosed within the first 3 months of surgery [26, 33, 38, 50]. The importance of continued monitoring for all patients throughout the early postoperative period is underscored by the statistic that between 10 and 50 % of individuals with postoperative depression have no preexisting psychiatric history [22, 23, 26, 27, 29, 33, 37, 38, 50, 53, 56, 57]. The emergence of de novo depression after epilepsy surgery may be especially common in patients with a mesial temporal lobe focus, and is typically heralded by significant postoperative irritability as well as marital tension and conflict [58]. Depressive disorder after epilepsy surgery is of critical clinical concern. Not only does postoperative depression limit the patient's ability to take full advantage of the benefits of seizure freedom or improvement [59], suicide rates after epilepsy surgery are around 13 times higher in postsurgical patients than in the broader US population, and commonly take place in the context of excellent seizure control [55, 60].

While depression after epilepsy surgery may conform to DSM-type criteria, Blumer et al. [22] have suggested that patients can also present with "dysphoric disorders with prominent depressive mood." Symptoms of this form of depression are intermittent and pleomorphic, comprising depressed mood, anergia, irritability, pain, insomnia, euphoria, fear, and anxiety. Depressive symptoms after epilepsy surgery typically persist for at least 3–6 months [26, 33, 38, 50], before steadily declining across a 24-month follow-up period [33, 50]. Regardless of the symptomatology, moderate to severe levels of depressive symptoms continue in about 15 % of patients who experience recurrent seizures and 8 % who are seizure free [32, 55]. Encouragingly, postoperative depression and dysphoric disorders show good remittance with pharmacological treatment [22].

Risk Factors for Depression After Epilepsy Surgery

Catalysts for deteriorating mood after epilepsy surgery encompass psychosocial, psychiatric, and neurobiological factors (Table 17.2). Psychosocially, risk factors for postoperative depression include maladaptive personality traits (primarily dependent and avoidant traits), financial dependence, adjustment difficulties in

Table 17.2 Risk factors for depressive symptoms after adult epilepsy surgery [24, 26, 27, 29, 37, 50, 53, 54, 58, 59, 62–68]

Neurobiological antecedents	
Bilateral EEG abnormalities	Anhoury et al. [62]; Carran et al. [53]; de Araújo Filho et al. [29]
Larger resection	Anhoury et al. [62]
Secondarily generalized seizures	Cleary et al. [63]; Carran et al. [53]
More frequent seizures presurgery	Desai et al. [27]
Abnormal contralateral hippocampal volume	Paparrigopoulos et al. [64]; Wrench et al. [58]
Younger age at surgery	Moss et al. [37]
Psychiatric and psychosocial antecedents	
High neuroticism and low extraversion	Wilson et al. [65]
Preoperative personality disorder [PD], chiefly Cluster C (Avoidant, Dependent, or Obsessive-Compulsive PD) or Cluster B (Borderline, Antisocial, Histrionic, or Narcissistic PD)	Koch-Stoeker [66]
Preoperative psychiatric history	Malmgren et al. [24]; Quigg et al. [67]; Pintor et al. [68]; Wrench et al. [50]; Cleary et al. [26, 63]; de Araújo Filho et al. [29]
Poor postoperative family dynamics	Wrench et al. [50]
Difficulties adjusting to changed roles post surgery	Meador [54]; Wilson et al. [59]

adapting to new societal and family roles, and poor postoperative family dynamics. Most consistently, however, a preexisting psychiatric history is reported, with studies from psychiatric populations supporting the notion that cumulative disruption to brain structure, function, and cognitive processing from previous depressive episodes heightens the risk of symptom recurrence in the future [61].

Neurobiological risk factors for postoperative depression include bilateral EEG abnormalities in presurgical investigations, younger age at surgery, a larger resection, preoperative generalized seizures, more frequent preoperative seizures, and abnormal hippocampal volume in the contralateral hemisphere (Table 17.2). While it appears that postsurgical depression is not related to the histopathology of the epileptogenic lesion [24, 56, 62, 69], there is considerable ambiguity as to whether the laterality of the lesion is an important antecedent, with no compelling evidence either way: some studies show no effect of laterality [24, 32, 56, 62], while others suggest that a right-sided resection is a vulnerability factor for worsening mood after surgery [23, 37, 53, 67]. Overall, the neurobiological risk factors for depression after epilepsy surgery comprise markers of more chronic, severe, and widespread epileptogenic abnormality occurring alongside focal unilateral dysfunction in mesial temporal structures.

Finally, specific risk factors for persistent depressive symptoms at 24-months include older age, preoperative generalized seizures, a family history of seizures, as well as a family history of psychiatric illness [32]. The relationship between a family history of psychiatric disturbance and persistent depression is particularly noteworthy, indicating that depression after epilepsy surgery, like depression in the general population, likely has a genetic underpinning in some cases.

Depression and Seizure Outcome

Good psychiatric outcome for depressive disorders after epilepsy surgery is robustly linked to good seizure outcome, and vice versa. In particular, seizure remission is related to lower levels of depressive symptomatology following surgery [49, 52, 55, 70], while recurrent postoperative seizures are associated with depressive symptoms and disorders presenting both pre- [29, 70] and postsurgically [32, 53]. Very few studies report no link between depression and seizure outcome [17, 36], and none reviewed here associate depression after epilepsy surgery with seizure freedom.

Summary: Depression

- ~30 % of surgical patients have a lifetime history of depression.
- After surgery, 20–30 % of patients present with depression.
  - A significant proportion (up to 25 %) has no psychiatric history i.e., de novo depression.
- The most compelling risk factor for postsurgery depression is presurgery depression (~75 % preexisting history across the lifespan).
- Neurobiological risk factors for postsurgery depression comprise markers of chronic, severe, and widespread epileptogenic abnormality, as well as younger age at surgery.
- Psychosocial risk factors for postsurgery depression comprise maladaptive personality traits, financial dependence, adjustment difficulties, and poor postoperative family dynamics.
- Seizure recurrence is linked to both pre- and postsurgery depression.

Anxiety Symptoms and Disorders

Presurgery Prevalence

Anxiety disorders are a somewhat heterogeneous group linked by abnormally elevated threat responses and a generalized dysregulation of negative affect. A population-based study estimated a lifetime prevalence of anxiety disorders in people with epilepsy at 22.8 % (versus 11 % in healthy controls) [41]. Moreover, patients may experience more than one form of anxiety disorder concurrently. This was illustrated in a study of 188 consecutive people with epilepsy that identified 49 patients (26 %) with a current anxiety disorder [71], of which 55 % had two or more anxiety disorders, while 57 % had a comorbid depressive episode, with the latter commonly occurring in anxious people with and without epilepsy. In a German study of 96 patients with drug-resistant epilepsy, the prevalence of anxiety was estimated at ~20 % [72].

Of the 41 studies identified in the current literature review, 12 examined the occurrence of anxiety symptoms surrounding epilepsy surgery, without delineating between subtypes of anxiety disorder (e.g., generalized anxiety disorder, agoraphobia, etc.) (Table S17.2). Most of the studies prospectively followed patients for 24 months after surgery, employing quantitative or linear measures of symptoms to an equal extent. These studies indicate that the prevalence of anxiety in presurgery epilepsy patients is commensurate with that of drug-resistant patients more broadly, meaning that 20–30 % of surgical candidates have a lifetime history of heightened or clinically significant anxiety [17, 27, 53, 73].

Postsurgery Course

The clinical trajectory of anxiety after adult epilepsy surgery typically shows a spike in anxious symptoms immediately following discharge from hospital [38]. In total, up to 28–42 % of patients may be diagnosed with an anxiety disorder in the early phase of surgical recovery [17, 27, 37], with around 27–46 % of these diagnoses comprising de novo symptomatology in people who were psychologically well before surgery [17, 34, 55, 73]. The studies also indicate that many patients with preexisting anxiety experience a dramatic remission in their symptoms [36, 73], while no studies reported a worsening of preexisting anxiety symptoms after surgery. Post surgery, anxiety symptoms tend to steadily decline until subbaseline levels of anxiousness are reached around the 24-month mark [32, 38, 39, 68, 74].

Risk Factors for Anxiety After Epilepsy Surgery

Psychosocially, patients at the highest risk of developing anxiety disorders after epilepsy surgery are those with a previous history of affective disorders and adjustment difficulties [17, 68, 75, 76]. These adjustment difficulties were most prominent in patients with extratemporal lobe resections and took the form of psychological, sociological, and behavioral features of the burden of normality (see Table 17.3) [17]. Moreover, preoperative anxiety is a significant predictor of postsurgery anxiety and depression [37]. Together, these risk factors for anxiety after epilepsy surgery implicate longstanding and possibly genetic vulnerabilities to mood dysregulation, as well as poor psychological coping skills in response to a situation often requiring significant psychosocial change (see also the section "The process of psychological recovery after epilepsy surgery").

Table 17.3 Features of the burden of normality to canvass in rehabilitation after epilepsy surgery [19, 59]

Life domain	Features	Common issues for rehabilitation
Psychological	Changes in self-concept ("well self")	Sense of "cure" or "difference" Need to "prove" normality Increased expectations (from self or others) Lack of "excuse" of chronic illness Grieving the loss of epilepsy Sense of missed opportunities ("lost years") Need to make up for lost time
Behavioral	Changes in activities	"Overdoing it" (physical, vocational, social) "Underdoing it" (physical, vocational, social) Other somatic complaints Change in sex drive (typically increased) Nonadherence to anticonvulsants
Affective	Changes in mood	Euphoria, joy of "cure" Anxiety, increased "pressure" Depression, shame, guilt Frustration, regret
Sociological	Changes in family dynamics and social function	Changed role of the primary carer Attitudes of family members and friends Increased family conflict New vocational horizons Educational and vocational programs Employment opportunities, promotion New social horizons Driving Intimate and other friendships New social activities and networks

Neurobiologically, neuroimaging research shows that postoperative anxiety is associated with resection of an amygdala with normal volume [73] or a smaller ipsilateral hippocampal remnant following a left temporal lobe resection [64]. Together, these two studies suggest that significant disease in mesial temporal structures, or the resection of relatively healthy tissue, plays some role in the development of post-surgical anxiety. This is broadly consistent with functional imaging data in TLE patients showing that greater preoperative ipsilateral amygdala activation, presumably from a healthy structure, is associated with significantly increased anxiety symptoms after surgery [77]. The amygdala plays a central role in the limbic circuit responsible for threat reactivity. This circuit is thought to be modulated by the Affective Appraisal Network, which has nodes in the ventromedial prefrontal cortex, the posterior cingulate cortex and the hippocampus, and is involved in emotion generation and regulation, self-related cognition, long-term memory retrieval, and context-based modulation of conditioned fear [78]. Although speculative, neuroimaging of postoperative anxiety suggests that surgical disruption to anxiety-related brain networks may exacerbate or give rise to anxiety symptoms after surgery.

Anxiety and Seizure Outcome

The relationship between anxiety and seizure recurrence after epilepsy surgery remains ambiguous. This literature review identified one study showing that seizure freedom after surgery was related to lower postsurgery anxiety [40], and another suggesting that heightened anxiety was more likely to persist long-term in patients with ongoing seizures [32]. Three studies, however, did not find a relationship between seizure outcome and pre- or postsurgery anxiety [17, 36, 74]. Since all five of these studies were methodologically robust, employing prospective designs with sample sizes of 57–360 patients, further investigation is needed to clarify the issue.

Summary: Anxiety

- 20–30 % of surgical patients have a lifetime history of significant anxiety.
  - This is a predictor of postsurgery anxiety and depression.
- Around ~30 % of patients meet criteria for an anxiety disorder early postsurgery.
  - A significant proportion represent de novo anxiety symptoms.
- Neurobiological risk factors for postsurgery anxiety implicate dysregulation of the mesial temporal node of the Affective Appraisal Network.
- Other risk factors for postsurgery anxiety include previous episodes of depression/anxiety and poor coping skills.
- Links between perisurgical anxiety and seizure recurrence remain equivocal.

Psychotic Symptoms and Disorder

Pre-surgery Prevalence

The psychoses of epilepsy are also a heterogeneous group of disorders that differ according to the temporal relationship they have with seizures. Postictal psychosis (PIP) is a well-established psychiatric complication of focal epilepsy, occurring in around 7 % of patients with drug-resistant TLE [79, 80]. Symptoms such as thought disorder, hallucinations, and delusions typically emerge 12–72 h after a cluster of seizures and last from a few days to a few weeks [79, 81, 82]. A diagnosis of PIP can be made on the basis of a single psychotic episode. Clinical risk factors include a history of encephalitis or head injury, a family history of psychiatric illness, secondarily generalized seizures, and bilateral, extratemporal, or nonlocalized EEG abnormalities (see [63]). The diffuse nature of these risk factors, together with widespread dysfunction reported in neuropsychological and neuroimaging studies, implicates seizure-related dysfunction to networks in the anterior quadrant of the brain. Interictal forms of psychosis also present in between 2 and 9 % of people with epilepsy, and more closely resemble primary psychotic disorders, such as schizophrenia and schizoaffective disorder [83]. In fact, overall evidence suggests that schizophrenia-like psychosis is 6–12 times more likely to present in people with epilepsy than in the general population [83]. Specific to surgical candidates, a prospective study of 84 patients showed a 6 % prevalence rate for psychotic disorder before surgery, including interictal psychosis, PIP, or a combination of both, with their occurrence linked to a history of febrile convulsions and a left mesial temporal lobe focus [33].

Postsurgery Course

Of the 41 studies reviewed, 12 examined the occurrence of psychotic symptoms before or after surgery (Table S17.3). Approximately 40 % of these studies presented data on small series of individuals with psychosis (i.e., $n<10$), and the majority used retrospective designs and expert diagnosis to identify individuals with psychotic symptoms. The findings indicate that comorbid psychosis and epilepsy is not necessarily a contraindication to epilepsy surgery. The case series consistently describe TLE patients with psychotic disorders who were able to provide informed consent and comply with both preoperative investigations and postsurgical management [84–86].

Post surgery, in one study 50 % of patients experienced an immediate worsening of their preexisting psychotic symptoms before stabilizing, while other small case series focusing on PIP reported complete symptom remission in the context of good seizure control [33, 87]. Others studies report no remission of psychotic symptoms despite good seizure outcome and patient report of improved quality of life. In the largest study to date, Cleary et al. [63] followed up 20 patients with PIP for up to 48 months after surgery, relative to 60 TLE patients without a psychiatric history. They found that preexisting PIP did not affect a patient's chance for seizure freedom after surgery. In sum, these studies suggest that epilepsy surgery can often prompt a remission or stabilization of psychotic symptoms in the context of seizure relief.

There is also some evidence to suggest that in patients with chronic psychosis, surgery may trigger nonpsychotic psychopathology. For instance, in the study by Cleary and colleagues [63], patients with recurrent PIP (defined as ≥ two psychotic episodes) were up to nine times more likely to develop de novo psychopathology in the 4 years following surgery compared to patients with no psychiatric history after controlling for preoperative psychiatric status. These de novo disorders emerged in the first year after surgery and persisted for at least 6 months, often requiring pharmacological treatment. Diagnoses commonly included depressive or anxiety disorders, although three patients with recurrent PIP went on to develop primary (interictal) psychotic disorders after surgery. This lends support to Kanner's [88] assertion that epilepsy surgery is strongly *indicated* in patients with PIP to prevent ongoing seizures and the transition from PIP to a primary psychotic disorder. Together, the studies indicate that patients should be counseled that surgery can offer seizure relief, but may not improve the psychotic disorder. Moreover, patients with recurrent PIP should be advised of the risk of de novo psychopathology developing postsurgery and the need for regular psychiatric follow-up to manage any emergent neuropsychiatric symptoms.

Finally, de novo psychoses can emerge in around 3–5 % of patients after ATL [89, 90], typically in individuals who are seizure-free [86, 91, 92]. These disorders are characterized by prominent delusions, anxiety, irritability, aggression, and dysphoria [90]. Most cases of de novo psychosis emerge within the first 12 months [91] and may be successfully treated with low-dose antipsychotic medication [92].

Risk Factors for Psychosis After Epilepsy Surgery

In two small studies investigating the psychopathological correlates of psychosis after epilepsy surgery, patients who developed de novo psychosis or aggravation of preexisting psychoses showed schizoid or schizotypal personality traits before surgery [91, 93], providing preliminary evidence they may have developed psychotic disorders irrespective of epilepsy surgery.

The neurobiological mechanisms underpinning vulnerability to postsurgical psychosis remain less clear. Risk factors for de novo psychosis after epilepsy surgery include a family history of psychosis, undergoing surgery after the age of 30, preoperative bilateral functional and structural abnormalities, and epileptogenic pathology suggestive of cortical dysplasia or hamartoma [23, 94]. Together, these rather disparate determinants implicate a genetic vulnerability to psychosis as well as abnormal anatomical development.

Others ascribe the development of de novo psychosis in seizure-free patients to the phenomenon of "forced normalization." This is said to occur when acute neuropsychiatric symptoms briefly emerge during periods of dramatic seizure reduction, usually accompanied by an improvement in EEG activity [95]. Central to potential pathogenic mechanisms for forced normalization is the belief that there are antagonistic neurobiological processes that alternately give rise to either epilepsy or psychosis. These include

- Residual inhibitory electrical or neurochemical activity in subcortical limbic regions that does not exceed the seizure threshold, but nonetheless stimulates regions important to psychotic phenomena
- Functional changes to neurotransmitter systems that have antagonistic epileptogenic/antipsychotic effects
- Impaired ion channel function dysregulating limbic system excitability [96]

The concept of forced normalization, however, remains controversial due to a paucity of both systemic research and direct empirical evidence for any of its putative mechanisms.

Summary: Psychosis

- ~6 % of surgical candidates have a lifetime history of psychotic disorder.
- Epilepsy patients with comorbid psychosis commonly experience meaningful seizure improvement after surgery, and no worsening of their psychotic symptoms.
- De novo psychosis emerges in ~3–5 % patients after anterior temporal lobectomy.
- Putative neurobiological mechanisms for psychosis after surgery include so-called "forced normalization," preoperative bilateral functional, and structural brain abnormalities.
- Other Risk factors for postsurgery psychosis include a family history of psychosis, undergoing surgery after the age of 30, and preexisting schizoid or schizotypal personality traits.
- De novo psychosis after epilepsy surgery is linked to seizure freedom.

Somatic Symptom and Related Disorders

Presurgery Prevalence

A psychogenic nonepileptic seizure (PNES) is typically defined as a paroxysmal event that resembles an epileptogenic seizure to the observer, but is not accompanied by changes in EEG activity. Instead, psychological and emotional factors are strongly suspected to have caused the event [97]. Of the 41 studies reviewed here, three examined the occurrence of PNES before or after surgery (Table S17.4). In one study of 58 surgical candidates, PNES was evident in 3 % of TLE patients and 19 % of extratemporal patients before surgery. These patients were predominantly female (~75 %) and had risk factors typical of PNES, including a history of sexual and physical abuse, family and relationship problems, aggression, low IQ, as well as poor visual memory [98].

Postsurgery Course

Initial evidence suggests that preexisting PNES should not be considered a contraindication to epilepsy surgery in patients who also experience epileptogenic seizures. Reuber et al. [99] followed up 13 adult epilepsy patients with comorbid PNES and found that epilepsy surgery led to meaningful improvements in 11 patients. Seven became free of both epileptogenic and psychogenic seizures, two became free of epileptic seizures but continued to have infrequent psychogenic seizures, one reported major improvement in epileptogenic seizures and cessation of psychogenic attacks, and in one patient nondisabling epileptogenic seizures persisted at lower frequency but psychogenic seizures ceased. This study provides preliminary evidence that epilepsy surgery may have a beneficial impact on comorbid PNES, although the psychological or neurobiological mechanisms underpinning remission remain unclear.

The successful surgical treatment of epilepsy occasionally has a paradoxical outcome, namely, the development of PNES after surgery, including in patients who achieve good seizure control [100]. A study by Davies et al. ([101]; N=228) estimates a 3.5 % incidence of de novo PNES after surgery, with symptoms emerging anywhere between 6 weeks to 6 years after the procedure (M=23 weeks). PNES is the most widely studied somatic symptom disorder in the epilepsy literature. Such disorders are heterogeneous; however, in a unique addition to the literature Naga et al. [102] identified 10 patients who developed somatic symptom disorders other than PNES from a cohort of 450 patients with surgically remediable epilepsy (i.e., a prevalence rate of 2.2 %). After surgery, seven patients developed an undifferentiated somatic symptom disorder, one developed a pain disorder, one developed body dysmorphia, and one developed a combined pain disorder and body dysmorphia. All of the patients had undergone an ATL and nine had a right-lateralized resection, providing preliminary neurobiological evidence for the role of the right temporal lobe in emotional regulation and the interpretation and attribution of somatic sensations and perceptions.

Risk Factors for Somatic Symptom Disorders After Epilepsy Surgery

Risk factors for the development of PNES after epilepsy surgery include a preexisting neuropsychiatric disorder, physical complications from surgery (such as a bone flap infection), and low IQ [100, 101]. Females are again overrepresented, with 8.5 % of female patients with a preoperative psychiatric diagnosis developing PNES after surgery [103]. These risk factors suggest that de novo PNES after epilepsy surgery might be more prevalent in female patients who have diminished psychological or cognitive resources to cope with a serious physical complication of surgery or to manage the often complex process of adjustment that underpins the patient's transition from chronically ill to suddenly well.

The neurobiological importance of the right hemisphere in the emergence of somatic symptom disorders after surgery is supported by a study comparing 79 consecutive patients with PNES to 122 patients with epileptogenic seizures. Seventy-six percent of the PNES patients in this cohort had unilateral cerebral abnormalities on neuroimaging, of which 71 % were in the right hemisphere [104]. Together, these studies support the longstanding hypothesis that the right hemisphere is preferentially involved in the perception and processing of emotions and, when dysfunctional, fails to facilitate the acceptance of traumatic emotions and memories and resolve unpleasant feelings. There remains limited understanding, however, of the mechanism by which psychological stress can "convert" into somatic symptoms, with no investigation of this mechanism in patients presenting with PNES after epilepsy surgery.

Another possible neurobiological account of PNES after epilepsy surgery implicates abnormalities in the Cognitive Control Network, the self-referential Autobiographic Memory Network, and circuits mediating emotional expression, regulation and awareness such as the anxiety-related Affective Appraisal Network (i.e., anterior cingulate and ventromedial prefrontal cortices, insula, amygdala, vermis), and motor planning/coordination (supplementary motor area, cerebellum) to produce a deficit of conscious sensory or motor processing [105]. The authors concluded that aberrant neuroplasticity between the mesial prefrontal cortex and amygdala, mediated by chronic stress, may facilitate the development of functional neurological symptoms in a subset of patients. This mechanism, however, requires direct testing in patients who have undergone epilepsy surgery.

Somatic Symptom Disorders and Seizure Outcome

There has been no robust investigation into the relationship between de novo somatic symptom disorder and seizure outcome after surgery, although data reviewed here suggest that (1) preexisting PNES can be ameliorated by epilepsy surgery, and (2) de novo somatoform disorder can emerge in the context of seizure freedom. More prospective studies investigating the relationships between seizure recurrence and somatic symptom disorders, such as PNES, are warranted.

Summary: Somatic Symptom and Related Disorders

- 3–19 % of epilepsy surgery candidates have comorbid PNES.
  - Patients often show abolition of epileptogenic and psychogenic seizures after surgery.
- After surgery, ~3.5 % of patients develop de novo PNES.
- Initial studies suggests that following epilepsy surgery, around 2.2 % of patients will develop a de novo somatic symptom disorder (other than PNES).
- Neurobiological accounts of somatic symptom disorders implicate the involvement of the right hemisphere, and, more recently, the Cognitive Control Network and Autobiographic Memory Network as well as emotion regulation and motor processing networks.
- Other risk factors for de novo PNES include a preoperative psychiatric history, physical complications from surgery, and female gender.
- There is no evidence linking seizure outcome and perisurgical somatic symptom disorder.

Rare Neuropsychiatric Symptoms Surrounding Adult Epilepsy Surgery
Occasionally in the epilepsy literature, small case series or case studies appear to report on the more unusual neuropsychiatric symptoms and disorders that may emerge or resolve after epilepsy surgery in adults. These include apparent improvements in pathological rage after surgery [106, 107], exacerbation or remission of obsessive-compulsive features [86, 108, 109], development of a profound tic disorder [110, 111], emergence of pathological or intrusive hypersexuality ([111, 112]; see also Case Vignette 2), as well the development of de novo postoperative mania ([53]; $n = 16$). These studies provide initial evidence that epilepsy surgery can impact on more uncommon neuropsychiatric conditions, however the small case numbers limit our understanding of the underlying mechanisms that might give rise to these patterns of behavior following surgery.

The Process of Psychological Recovery After Epilepsy Surgery

Regardless of the personal attributes and coping skills of the individual, epilepsy surgery typically invokes a process of significant psychological adjustment. This process may be most intense in the 3–6 months immediately following surgery, but longer-term follow-up studies suggest that psychological adaptation and re-orientation continues to evolve for at least the first 24 months. In particular, research groups from the United States and Australia have carefully mapped the psychiatric sequelae of epilepsy surgery and shown that the first 24 months can be broadly divided into three phases of recovery [50, 59, 113].

An initial, medically focused phase occurs while the patient is recuperating in hospital from the physical stressors of neurosurgery. For patients with premorbid psychiatric vulnerabilities, any surgical complications or an early recurrence of seizures may trigger a decline in mental state, as seen in the emergence of PNES in patients with preexisting psychiatric diagnoses. Most patients, however, do not experience surgical complications and are focused on becoming well enough to be discharged from hospital.

Once home, the recovery period spanning 1–6 months post surgery can take several forms. Patients who are seizure-free must adapt to the sudden ablation of a pervasive and disabling condition that has often been present since early childhood [114], and essentially learn to be "normal." At the core of this lies a change in the patient's self-concept that can require adjustment across multiple life domains (see Table 17.3). Adaptation also takes place in the context of any "agendas" or expectations that patients and their families bring to surgery [114]. The weight of the changes expected from patients can sometimes lead to maladaptive behaviors that can undermine the potential benefits of seizure freedom. This process of adjustment and its pitfalls have been previously well characterized as the burden of normality [19, 59].

For patients who have only minimally incorporated epilepsy into their self-identity, the transition from "illness" to "wellness" may be relatively smooth. In contrast, patients who feel that they cannot live up to the expectations placed on them as a "normal" person may shirk their new responsibilities, focus on novel medical symptoms, or describe missing their epilepsy. Other patients may view themselves as "cured" and feel pressured to make up for lost time, which can manifest inappropriately as patients "overdoing it," trying to wean anticonvulsant medication against medical advice, or throwing off parental or domestic responsibilities because its "their time to live." Neuropsychiatric symptoms may emerge in this context, particularly when the patient's new life is not automatically cured of all preexisting problems, or else proves to be unexpectedly dissatisfying or unrealistic to achieve [114].

In contrast, patients with seizure recurrence are required to adjust to the perceived "failure" of their surgery [17, 59, 115, 116], with postoperative seizures occurring in 20–60 % of patients. In these patients there may be significant disappointment [89], with resignation toward ongoing seizures as well as frustration over continued restrictions on independence and the perceived futility of anticonvulsant drugs [116]. A qualitative study investigating the experience of seizure recurrence showed a prominence of psychological issues over medical concerns [116]. The most frequent themes expressed by patients related to (1) the perceived success of surgery, (2) medication options, (3) acceptance of seizure recurrence, and (4) levels of personal independence. However, patient sentiments were heterogeneous, with some reporting ambivalence about their outcome of surgery, while others used cognitive reframing and benefit-finding to achieve a sense of satisfaction despite seizure recurrence. Case Vignette 1 illustrates the postsurgery trajectory of a young woman with preoperative psychopathology and poor coping resources who experienced persistent postsurgery depression. Paradoxically, this patient reported "relief" when her seizures recurred after surgery, demonstrating the centrality of epilepsy to her sense of self and her life.

Case Vignette 1: "N.M."

Persistent Depression in the Context of Seizure Recurrence and Poor Psychosocial Coping

Medical and Seizure History. This 24-year-old woman had a history of fortnightly focal seizures since the age of eight. MRI did not show any definitive abnormality. PET scan showed a fairly striking area of decreased metabolism in the posterior temporo-occipital region. Intracranial video-EEG monitoring revealed that seizures seemed to arise from the right posterior temporal area. An EEG-fMRI study showed an exquisite area of increased BOLD signal in the posterior temporal region on the right. Neuropsychologically, no focal deficits were detected. It was agreed that she would be offered a resection of the gyrus highlighted by EEG-fMRI.

Psychiatric History. Formal psychiatric evaluation disclosed significant issues relating back to the bitter divorce of her parents, as well as current difficulties relating to her highly involved but acrimonious relationships with her mother and sister, and significant vocational and social limitations she attributed to being unable to drive. She was deemed to have features of a moderately severe depression, and at high risk for a further worsening of her mood post surgery. She was commenced on citalopram.

Postsurgery Follow-up. Within a few weeks of surgery family members witnessed a return of focal dyscognitive events, albeit at a reduced rate. She was irregularly compliant with both her antiepileptic and antidepressant medication, and her mood remained low and variable. While disappointed at one level by the postoperative events, at the 3-month review N.M. described some sense of "comfort" in the familiarity that she ascribes to her seizures (e.g., a feeling akin to "finding a child who you have lost at the shops"). She continued to struggle with the increased expectations others had of her. Against a background of disrupted education, limited vocational opportunity, and a recent failed personal relationship, N.M. was struggling to make future plans. The situation was complicated by family relationships characterized by high levels of conflict. Despite this she continued to live with her sister, while her mother lived next door. To direct enquiry, she regarded the surgery as having been successful by virtue of improved seizure control. She was attempting to make some gains in her level of independence but was bitterly resentful of the perceived ongoing overmanagerial behavior of others and her failure to be eligible for a driver's license. She was counseled at length about the nature and course of postoperative adjustment both for herself and those close to her and encouraged to seriously reconsider the benefits of formal psychological support, which she declined.

At 29 months post surgery, the clinical picture remains largely unchanged: ongoing seizures against a background of multiple, ongoing psychosocial stressors, enmeshed relationships, chronic low mood, poor adjustment, limited coping skills, and variable adherence/disclosure. N.M. has made no real psychosocial gains.

In the third phase of rehabilitation spanning 12–24 months post surgery, patients often attempt to reconcile their changed psychological and seizure status. One study that followed 89 patients for 24 months following ATL revealed two distinct patient pathways [59]. The majority of patients (58 %) reported good outcomes, characterized by improved family dynamics, enhanced vocational and social functioning, and driving by 24 months post surgery. A range of trajectories led to these outcomes, including the experience of early postoperative adjustment difficulties. Case Vignette 2 illustrates the case of a young mother who eventually attained a good outcome from surgery, after overcoming adjustment difficulties and depression in the early postoperative phase. As in the study by Wilson et al. [59], resolution of early anxiety and vocational change at 12 months were indicators of a good outcome at 24 months for this patient. The case also highlights the critical value of close clinical follow-up and prompt psychological and pharmacological treatment of neuropsychiatric symptoms when they emerge after epilepsy surgery.

In the second distinct pathway, 31 % of patients perceived their outcomes as poor, reporting affective disturbance and difficulties discarding sick role behaviors at 24 months after surgery.[1] For instance, sickness behaviors such as protracting the recommended physical limitations imposed by surgery (e.g., declining to do any housework 6–12 months after uncomplicated surgery "to play it safe"), or focusing on novel somatic or cognitive complaints may contribute to the patient shirking familial and social obligations associated with becoming well and cause significant family or relationship discord. Early anxiety that remained unresolved served as a key marker of these poor outcomes, illustrating how stressful and overwhelming some patients find adjusting to a new "well" identity. This study highlights the importance of looking for more individualized markers of longer-term outcomes, with the complexities of postoperative adjustment underscoring the need for a detailed follow-up and rehabilitation program for a significant period after epilepsy surgery [59, 113]. The form that such a follow-up program may take is discussed further below.

Case Vignette 2: "S.P."

Early Depressive Symptoms and Adjustment Difficulties in the Setting of Seizure Freedom

Medical and Seizure History. S.P. was a 34-year-old working mother of two who experienced up to six focal seizures per day since the age of 22 after she fell off her bicycle. MRI confirmed extensive damage to the right lateral temporal neocortex. Video EEG monitoring captured an ictal-rhythm over the right frontotemporal region. Using SPECT, ECD (technetium-99m-ethyl cysteinate dimer)-injected seizures showed hyperperfusion in the right temporal region. PET showed right temporal hypometabolism. Neuropsychological assessment was entirely normal. She elected to undergo an extended lateral temporal resection with removal of anterior hippocampus and uncus.

Psychiatric History. Routine preoperative psychiatric evaluation identified significant depressive symptoms over the preceding 6 months, manifesting as low mood, insomnia, reduced appetite, loss of energy, irritability, intermittent anger, fleeting suicidal ideation, and generally reduced coping ability. S.P. had reduced her working hours, and was worried about caring for her young daughter. These symptoms occurred against the background of a depressive episode following the death of her sister 5 years prior, for which she briefly saw a psychologist. The need to consider antidepressant medication was raised together with the value of relinking in with a local mental health professional, but S.P. declined both.

[1] The remaining 11 % of patients in the study reported minimal adjustment issues after surgery.

Postsurgery Follow-up. In the context of seizure freedom, by 1 month post surgery S.P. had developed some insight into her persistently low mood and the impact that it was having on her recovery and the dynamics of the family unit. Following liaison between our multidisciplinary Seizure Surgery Follow-Up and Rehabilitation Program and her local GP, she was prescribed citalopram and commenced cognitive behavioral therapy with a clinical psychologist.

At 3 months post surgery, S.P. described a significant improvement in her mood. In particular, she described feeling "re-invigorated" with a very positive outlook and a sense that she was back to being the person she was prior to seizure onset. She described having a renewed sense of freedom, personal control, and autonomy with a related reduction in her dependence on others. She expressed resentment at well-intentioned comments from others that she required ongoing care and supervision. She stated that seizure freedom had "given me my life back" and was eager to maximize all future opportunities. Her libido also suddenly significantly increased beyond what she had ever previously experienced but her sexual satisfaction was diminished, leading to frustration and more frequent demands for sex from her partner.

One year after resective surgery, S.P. remained completely seizure-free and considered herself "cured" of epilepsy. Her mood was now stable; she successfully weaned antidepressant medication after 6 months and was no longer attending psychological therapy. Her hypersexuality had now settled considerably. She described herself as a happier, more confident, easy going, "in control" individual no longer plagued with the self-doubt that characterized her preoperative disposition. She denied ruminating about the possibility of seizures. Psychosocially, the dynamics of the marital relationship underwent some adjustment in the context of changed roles stemming from seizure freedom, but eventually settled. She enjoyed the support of a close network of friends. S.P. made a successful, graded return to her former work position, has regained her driver's license, and remained very happy with her decision to have surgery.

Summary: The Trajectory of Psychological Recovery After Epilepsy Surgery

- Seizure-free patients must adjust from being chronically sick to suddenly well, often invoking the burden of normality.
- Patients with seizure recurrence report a different adjustment process where significant disappointment and psychological concerns are paramount. Patients describe using benefit-finding and cognitive reframing as a way of adaptively coping with their suboptimal outcome.
- Regardless of seizure outcome, successful adjustment after epilepsy surgery depends on the intrinsic coping capabilities of patients and their families as well as the support of their treating team.
- Failure to adjust to seizure freedom or seizure recurrence may lead to ongoing neuropsychiatric symptoms and reduced quality of life.

Clinical Considerations Surrounding Adult Epilepsy Surgery

The success of a patient's psychological adjustment to either seizure freedom or seizure recurrence depends on how the treating teams manage and support the patient through the rehabilitation process. The International League Against Epilepsy (ILAE) Commission on the Neuropsychiatric Aspects of Epilepsy developed a set of International Consensus Clinical Statements to provide clear guidelines about post-operative follow-up [117]. These statements recommend that every person undergoing epilepsy surgery should receive psychologically informed management and care through a formal postoperative follow-up and rehabilitation program. In addition to medical investigations, this comprehensive model of care should include preoperative psychiatric, neuropsychological, and psychosocial evaluation, the results of which are used to contribute to decisions about surgery and the planning and provision of postoperative care, particularly in the first 12–24 months after surgery so that psychopathology can be readily detected and treated promptly.

Before Epilepsy Surgery

Before epilepsy surgery, a detailed, face-to-face psychosocial assessment helps the treating team to gain an understanding of the way epilepsy has affected the patient and family over the lifespan, including the extent to which epilepsy forms part of the patient's identity and influences the structure and functioning of the family. The presurgery evaluation should also canvass patient and family views about surgery and expectations of postoperative life [114]. Unrealistic expectations often require psychoeducation and guided cognitive reframing in order to best prepare patients and families for the adjustment process after surgery, and to aid the patient to make a truly informed decision about surgery [15, 16]. The central tenant of this counseling should be that while the surgery may be able to provide seizure relief, it cannot be expected to resolve longstanding relationship, personality, social, or vocational limitations; improvement in these domains will require a concerted effort on the part of the patient in the postoperative rehabilitation phase. Psychoeducation about optimizing physical recovery after surgery should also be addressed in preoperative counseling, including the need to remain compliant with anticonvulsant or psychotropic medications until otherwise directed after surgery [114].

The presurgery evaluation also provides an opportunity to treat any neuropsychiatric disorders, recognizing that patients with preexisting psychopathology are among the most likely to experience poor psychiatric and seizure outcomes after surgery. This assessment should canvass not only current psychopathology, but also previous episodes of psychiatric illness that are currently asymptomatic [71]. In patients who have severe neuropsychiatric conditions that may compromise decision-making ability, surgery is not necessarily contraindicated, but rather specialist neurobehavioral assessment is required to determine the patient's capacity to comply with treatment and to provide fully informed consent for an elective procedure by weighing the risks of surgery against its potential therapeutic benefits [84, 117]. Psychosocial and neuropsychiatric issues identified in the presurgical evaluation require discussion by the treating team to determine the patient's suitability for epilepsy surgery, and what, if any treatment or support needs to be put into place before surgery.

Does Treating Neurobehavioral Disorder Improve Seizure Outcome After Surgery?
The impact of epilepsy surgery on psychopathology is tied to the recurrence of seizures after surgery. Namely, patients who are most likely to enjoy good seizure control after surgery are those with lower levels of psychopathology before and after the operation. This appears to be a bidirectional relationship. Preexisting neuropsychiatric symptoms such as anxiety, depression, and mania may significantly lower a patients' chance of achieving seizure freedom or improvement after surgery ([26, 29, 53, 62, 70, 109]; but see [44] for a null finding). Conversely, recurrent seizures after surgery are linked to the emergence, persistence, and exacerbation of psychopathology in the postoperative period [62, 70, 118]. The remission of psychiatric symptoms and disorders after surgery is associated with the complete absence of seizures following the procedure ([22, 33, 47, 49]; although see [17] for a null finding). Together, these findings make a compelling case for the prompt identification and treatment of neuropsychiatric symptoms both before and after epilepsy surgery, to maximize an individual's chances of achieving good seizure control and improved quality of life.

After Surgery

After surgery, even psychologically resilient patients may find the rehabilitation process challenging, and thus ideally, professional support should be offered to all candidates during the postoperative period [113]. Where possible, follow-up monitoring should include regular (i.e., 3–6 monthly) multidisciplinary reviews with both patients and their family members. The focus throughout the rehabilitation period is to canvass patient adjustment to life after surgery in the context of seizure outcome, including identification of adjustment difficulties, such as features of the burden of normality. This provides patients and their families with tailored counseling and where indicated, formal treatment. Wilson et al. [59] noted that liaison with members of the patient's broader social community is also useful, particularly employers and vocational services to ensure that a carefully graded return to work is enabled. For geographically isolated patients, a dedicated epilepsy nurse clinician or other such specialist is essential for providing regular telephone monitoring and support, with the advent of telemedicine providing a novel opportunity to approximate face-to-face reviews with the treating team. Ideally, the postsurgery follow-up program should be of sufficient length (i.e., ≥24 months) to allow problems to appear, with work by Wilson and colleagues [59] illustrating how the adjustment process continually evolves over this period.

Patients with a history of psychiatric disorder are especially vulnerable to the challenges of postoperative life. Moreover, the strong link between seizure recurrence and the emergence or persistence of psychopathology after surgery indicates that regular management and review is particularly relevant in patients who experience seizure recurrence [119]. A patient displaying signs of comorbid psychopathology will often warrant pharmacological and/or psychological interventions, with symptom remission achievable in up 60 % of patients treated with either pharmacotherapy or cognitive behavior therapy (see [120] for a review). While some clinicians may be concerned that psychotropic drugs can lower the seizure threshold, Blumer et al. [22] and others [92] illustrate that postoperative neuropsychiatric symptoms can be successfully treated with medication without risking seizure relapse. On the contrary, the evidence described above suggests that failure to treat psychopathology after epilepsy surgery may heighten the chance of seizure recurrence and undermine the patient's psychosocial functioning and quality of life (see Text Box).

Summary: Clinical Considerations

- Ideally, all patients considered for epilepsy surgery should have access to formal pre- and postsurgery psychosocial counseling.
- Before surgery, patient and family expectations of surgery should be canvassed and psychoeducation provided to reframe unrealistic hopes for surgery; patients should also be prepared for the postsurgical adjustment process.
- Preexisting psychiatric conditions should be stabilized with medical or psychological treatment before proceeding to surgery.
- After surgery, patient rehabilitation should be provided by specialized clinicians, such as (neuro)psychologists, psychiatrists, and epilepsy nurse clinicians.
- Ideally, all patients should be regularly monitored for at least 2 years for the emergence of de novo or dormant psychopathology, and prompt treatment provided.

Implications for Future Research

Despite the impact of psychiatric comorbidity described by patients and caregivers surrounding epilepsy surgery, Cleary et al. [63] estimate that less than 3 % of outcome studies have investigated the psychiatric comorbidity of surgery. Urgently warranted are more prospective, experimentally controlled studies to better delineate the prevalence and severity of psychiatric conditions occurring in the context of epilepsy surgery, and to identify specific predictors of psychiatric outcome after epilepsy surgery. In particular, despite the prevalence and day-to-day impact of anxiety in people with epilepsy [121], the current literature review illustrates that anxiety attracts relatively scant research attention (Table 17.1) and further research into the course of anxiety both before and after epilepsy surgery is warranted.

The provision of personalized medicine in epilepsy would greatly benefit from predictive modeling of postsurgery outcomes, including psychiatric risk for different disorders and their clinical *subtypes*, rather than for heterogeneous cohorts of broadly similar patients [9, 59]. This could improve precision in how patients are grouped in behavioral, genetic, or neuroimaging studies and should help prevent the effects of smaller subgroups from being "washed out" in larger heterogeneous samples.

The neurobiological aspects of postsurgery rehabilitation also warrant more careful delineation. First, behavioral and neuroimaging studies could throw more light onto the neurocognitive and affective networks underscoring psychiatric disturbance after epilepsy surgery. Longitudinal studies could relate patterns of cortical activation before and after surgery to out-of-scanner measures of cognition and mood to assess the neurobiological basis of any changes in the patient's neuropsychiatric status, and how this might vary in differing subtypes of patients. Such approaches provide a mean of identifying biomarkers of neuropsychiatric outcome, which, in turn, would enhance prognostic counseling and the provision of optimal treatment for patients undergoing epilepsy surgery. Although challenging to achieve, improved treatment of neuropsychiatric symptoms would increase the likelihood of seizure freedom and maximize the considerable psychosocial benefits afforded by epilepsy surgery.

References

1. Brodie MJ, Schachter SC, Kwan P. Fast facts: epilepsy. 4th ed. Oxford: Health Press Limited; 2009.
2. Berg AT, Berkovic SF, Brodie MJ, Buchhalter J, Cross JH, van Emde Boas W, et al. Revised terminology and concepts for organization of seizures and epilepsies: report of the ILAE Commission on Classification and Terminology, 2005–2009. Epilepsia. 2010;51:676–85.
3. Kwan P, Brodie MJ. Early identification of refractory epilepsy. N Engl J Med. 2000;342:314–9.
4. Lehrner J, Kalchmayr R, Serles W, Olbrich A, Pataraia E, Aull S, Bacher J, Leutmezer F, Gröppel G, Deecke L, Baumgartner C. Health-related quality of life (HRQOL), activity of daily living (ADL) and depressive mood disorder in temporal lobe epilepsy patients. Seizure. 1999;8:88–92.
5. de Boer HM, Mula M, Sander JW. The global burden and stigma of epilepsy. Epilepsy Behav. 2008;12:540–6.
6. Kwan P, Schachter SC, Brodie MJ. Drug-resistant epilepsy. N Engl J Med. 2011;365:919–26.
7. Wiebe S, Blume WT, Girvin JP, Eliasziw M, Effectiveness and Efficiency of Surgery for Temporal Lobe Epilepsy Study Group. A randomized, controlled trial of surgery for temporal-lobe epilepsy. N Engl J Med. 2001;345:311–8.

8. Elger CE, Helmstaedter C, Kurthen M. Chronic epilepsy and cognition. Lancet Neurol. 2004;3:663–72.
9. Micallef S, Spooner CG, Harvey AS, Wrennall JA, Wilson SJ. Psychological outcome profiles in childhood-onset temporal lobe epilepsy. Epilepsia. 2010;51:2066–73.
10. Kilpatrick C, O'Brien T, Matkovic Z, Cook M, Kaye A. Preoperative evaluation for temporal lobe surgery. J Clin Neurosci. 2003;10:535–9.
11. Kwan P, Arzimanoglou A, Berg AT, Brodie MJ, Allen Hauser W, Mathern G, et al. Definition of drug resistant epilepsy: consensus proposal by the ad hoc Task Force of the ILAE Commission on Therapeutic Strategies. Epilepsia. 2010;51:1069–77.
12. Wasade VS, Elisevich K, Tahir R, Smith B, Schultz L, et al. Long-term seizure and psychosocial outcomes after resective surgery for intractable epilepsy. Epilepsy Behav. 2015;43:122–7.
13. Englot DJ, Chang EF. Rates and predictors of seizure freedom in resective epilepsy surgery: an update. Neurosurg Rev. 2014;37:389–404.
14. Baxendale S. The impact of epilepsy surgery on cognition and behaviour. Epilepsy Behav. 2008;12:592–9.
15. Baxendale SA, Thompson PJ. "If I didn't have epilepsy …": patient expectations of epilepsy surgery. J Epilepsy. 1996;9:274–81.
16. Wilson SJ, Saling MM, Kincade P, Bladin PF. Patient expectations of temporal lobe surgery. Epilepsia. 1998;39:167–74.
17. Wrench J, Wilson SJ, Bladin PF. Mood disturbance before and after seizure surgery: a comparison of temporal and extratemporal resections. Epilepsia. 2004;45:534–43.
18. Wilson SJ, Saling MM, Lawrence J, Bladin PF. Outcome of temporal lobectomy: expectations and the prediction of perceived success. Epilepsy Res. 1999;36:1–14.
19. Wilson S, Bladin P, Saling M. The "burden of normality": concepts of adjustment after surgery for seizures. J Neurol Neurosurg Psychiatry. 2001;70:649–56.
20. Wrench JM, Matsumoto R, Inoue Y, Wilson SJ. Current challenges in the practice of epilepsy surgery. Epilepsy Behav. 2011;22:23–31.
21. Bell B, Lin JJ, Seidenberg M, Hermann B. The neurobiology of cognitive disorders in temporal lobe epilepsy. Nat Rev Neurol. 2011;7:154–64.
22. Blumer D, Wakhlu S, Davies K, Hermann B. Psychiatric outcome of temporal lobectomy for epilepsy: incidence and treatment of psychiatric complications. Epilepsia. 1998;39:478–86.
23. Glosser G, Zwil AS, Glosser DS, O'Connor MJ, Sperling MR. Psychiatric aspects of temporal lobe epilepsy before and after anterior temporal lobectomy. J Neurol Neurosurg Psychiatry. 2000;68:53–8.
24. Taft C, Sager Magnusson E, Ekstedt G, Malmgren K. Health-related quality of life, mood, and patient satisfaction after epilepsy surgery in Sweden—A prospective controlled observational study. Epilepsia. 2014;55:878–85.
25. Cankurtaran ES, Ulug B, Saygi S, Tiryaki A, Akalan N. Psychiatric morbidity, quality of life, and disability in mesial temporal lobe epilepsy patients before and after anterior temporal lobectomy. Epilepsy Behav. 2005;7:116–22.
26. Cleary RA, Thompson PJ, Fox Z, Foong J. Predictors of psychiatric and seizure outcome following temporal lobe epilepsy surgery. Epilepsia. 2012;53:1705–12.
27. Desai S, Shukla G, Goyal V, Srivastava A, Srivastava MV, Tripathi M, et al. Changes in psychiatric comorbidity during early postsurgical period in patients operated for medically refractory epilepsy – a MINI-based follow-up study. Epilepsy Behav. 2014;32:29–33.
28. Sokic DV, Bascarevic V, Ristic A, Parojcic A, Vojvodic N, et al. Influence of psychiatric comorbidity on temporal lobe epilepsy surgery outcome. Epilepsia. 2013;54:111.
29. de Araújo Filho GM, Gomes FL, Mazetto L, Marinho MM, Tavares IM, Caboclo LO, et al. Major depressive disorder as a predictor of a worse seizure outcome one year after surgery in patients with temporal lobe epilepsy and mesial temporal sclerosis. Seizure. 2012;21:619–23.
30. Macrodimitris S, Sherman EM, Forde S, Tellez-Zenteno JF, Metcalfe A, Hernandez-Ronquillo L, et al. Psychiatric outcomes of epilepsy surgery: a systematic review. Epilepsia. 2011;52:880–90.

31. Baird AD, Wilson SJ, Bladin PF, Saling MM, Reutens DC. Sexual outcome after epilepsy surgery. Epilepsy Behav. 2003;4:268–78.
32. Devinsky O, Barr WB, Vickrey BG, Berg AT, Bazil CW, Pacia SV, et al. Changes in depression and anxiety after resective surgery for epilepsy. Neurology. 2005;65:1744–9.
33. Hellwig S, Mamalis P, Feige B, Schulze-Bonhage A, van Elst LT. Psychiatric comorbidity in patients with pharmacoresistant focal epilepsy and psychiatric outcome after epilepsy surgery. Epilepsy Behav. 2012;23:272–9.
34. Velez AM, Gherman E, Szabo CA. Does hippocampal sclerosis correlates with depression in patients with medically refractory epilepsy? Epilepsy Curr. 2013;13:256–7.
35. Hamid H, Blackmon K, Cong X, Dziura J, Atlas LY, Vickrey BG, et al. Mood, anxiety, and incomplete seizure control affect quality of life after epilepsy surgery. Neurology. 2014;82:887–94.
36. Spencer SS, Berg AT, Vickrey BG, Sperling MR, Bazil CW, Shinnar S, et al. Multicenter Study of Epilepsy Surgery. Initial outcomes in the Multicenter Study of Epilepsy Surgery. Neurology. 2003;61:1680–5.
37. Moss K, O'Driscoll K, Eldridge P, Varma T, Wieshmann UC. Risk factors for early postoperative psychiatric symptoms in patients undergoing epilepsy surgery for temporal lobe epilepsy. Acta Neurol Scand. 2009;120:176–81.
38. Ring HA, Moriarty J, Trimble MR. A prospective study of the early postsurgical psychiatric associations of epilepsy surgery. J Neurol Neurosurg Psychiatry. 1998;64:601–4.
39. Meldolesi GN, Di Gennaro G, Quarato PP, Esposito V, Grammaldo LG, Morosini P, et al. Changes in depression, anxiety, anger, and personality after resective surgery for drug-resistant temporal lobe epilepsy: a 2-year follow-up study. Epilepsy Res. 2007; 77:22–30.
40. Pauli E, Daeubler C, Schwarz M, Stefan H. Emotional-affective and personality aspects in temporal lobe epilepsy: postoperative changes. Epilepsia. 2009;50:6–7.
41. Tellez-Zenteno JF, Patten SB, Jetté N, Williams J, Wiebe S. Psychiatric comorbidity in epilepsy: a population-based analysis. Epilepsia. 2007;48:2336–44.
42. Boylan LS, Flint LA, Labovitz DL, Jackson SC, Starner K, Devinsky O. Depression but not seizure frequency predicts quality of life in treatment-resistant epilepsy. Neurology. 2004;62:258–61.
43. Jones JE, Watson R, Sheth R, Caplan R, Koehn M, et al. Psychiatric comorbidity in children with new onset epilepsy. Dev Med Child Neurol. 2007;49:493–7.
44. Adams SJ, O'Brien TJ, Lloyd J, Kilpatrick CJ, Salzberg MR, Velakoulis D. Neuropsychiatric morbidity in focal epilepsy. Br J Psychiatry. 2008;192:464–9.
45. Canuet L, Ishii R, Pascual-Marqui RD, Iwase M, Kurimoto R, Aoki Y, et al. Resting-state EEG source localization and functional connectivity in schizophrenia-like psychosis of epilepsy. PLoS One. 2011;6, e27863.
46. Ertekin BA, Kulaksizoğlu IB, Ertekin E, Gürses C, Bebek N, et al. A comparative study of obsessive-compulsive disorder and other psychiatric comorbidities in patients with temporal lobe epilepsy and idiopathic generalized epilepsy. Epilepsy Behav. 2009;14:634–9.
47. Fuller-Thomson E, Brennenstuhl S. The association between depression and epilepsy in a nationally representative sample. Epilepsia. 2009;50:1051–8.
48. Malmgren K, Starmark JE, Ekstedt G, Rosén H, Sjöberg-Larsson C. Nonorganic and organic psychiatric disorders in patients after epilepsy surgery. Epilepsy Behav. 2002;3:67–75.
49. Witt JA, Hollmann K, Helmstaedter C. The impact of lesions and epilepsy on personality and mood in patients with symptomatic epilepsy: a pre- to postoperative follow-up study. Epilepsy Res. 2008;82:139–46.
50. Wrench JM, Rayner G, Wilson SJ. Profiling the evolution of depression after epilepsy surgery. Epilepsia. 2011;52:900–8.
51. Lackmayer K, Lehner-Baumgartner E, Pirker S, Czech T, Baumgartner C. Preoperative depressive symptoms are not predictors of postoperative seizure control in patients with mesial temporal lobe epilepsy and hippocampal sclerosis. Epilepsy Behav. 2013; 26:81–6.

52. Hermann BP, Whitman S. Psychosocial predictors of interictal depression. J Epilepsy. 1989;2:231–7.
53. Carran MA, Kohler CG, O'Connor MJ, Bilker WB, Sperling MR. Mania following temporal lobectomy. Neurology. 2003;61:770–4.
54. Meador K. Psychiatry problems after epilepsy surgery. Epilepsy Curr. 2005;5:28–9.
55. Hamid H, Devinsky O, Vickrey BG, Berg AT, Bazil CW, Langfitt JT, et al. Suicide outcomes after resective epilepsy surgery. Epilepsy Behav. 2011;20:462–4.
56. Naylor AS, Rogvi-Hansen Bá, Kessing L, Kruse-Larsen C. Psychiatric morbidity after surgery for epilepsy: short-term follow up of patients undergoing amygdalohippocampectomy. J Neurol Neurosurg Psychiatry. 1994;57:1375–81.
57. Dulay MF, York MK, Soety EM, Hamilton WJ, Mizrahi EM, Goldsmith IL, et al. Memory, emotional and vocational impairments before and after anterior temporal lobectomy for complex partial seizures. Epilepsia. 2006;47:1922–30.
58. Wrench JM, Wilson SJ, O'Shea MF, Reutens DC. Characterising de novo depression after epilepsy surgery. Epilepsy Res. 2009;83:81–8.
59. Wilson SJ, Bladin PF, Saling MM, Pattison PE. Characterizing psychosocial outcome trajectories following seizure surgery. Epilepsy Behav. 2005;6:570–80.
60. Pompili M, Girardi P, Tatarelli R. Death from suicide versus mortality from epilepsy in the epilepsies: a meta-analysis. Epilepsy Behav. 2006;9:641–8.
61. Marchetti I, Koster EH, Sonuga-Barke EJ, De Raedt R. The default mode network and recurrent depression: a neurobiological model of cognitive risk factors. Neuropsychol Rev. 2012;22:229–51.
62. Anhoury S, Brown RJ, Krishnamoorthy ES, Trimble MR. Psychiatric outcome after temporal lobectomy: a predictive study. Epilepsia. 2000;41:1608–15.
63. Cleary RA, Thompson PJ, Thom M, Foong J. Postictal psychosis in temporal lobe epilepsy: risk factors and postsurgical outcome? Epilepsy Res. 2013;106:264–72.
64. Paparrigopoulos T, Ferentinos P, Brierley B, Shaw P, David AS. Relationship between postoperative depression/anxiety and hippocampal/amygdala volumes in temporal lobectomy for epilepsy. Epilepsy Res. 2008;81:30–5.
65. Wilson SJ, Wrench JM, McIntosh AM, Bladin PF, Berkovic SF. Personality development in the context of intractable epilepsy. Arch Neurol. 2009;66:68–72.
66. Koch-Stoecker S. Personality disorders as predictors of severe postsurgical psychiatric complications in epilepsy patients undergoing temporal lobe resections. Epilepsy Behav. 2002;3:526–31.
67. Quigg M, Broshek DK, Heidal-Schiltz S, Maedgen JW, Bertram 3rd EH. Depression in intractable partial epilepsy varies by laterality of focus and surgery. Epilepsia. 2003;44:419–24.
68. Pintor L, Bailles E, Fernández-Egea E, Sánchez-Gistau V, Torres X, Carreño M, et al. Psychiatric disorders in temporal lobe epilepsy patients over the first year after surgical treatment. Seizure. 2007;16:218–25.
69. Siegel AM, Cascino GD, Fessler AJ, So EL, Meyer FB. Psychiatric co-morbidity in 75 patients undergoing epilepsy surgery: lack of correlation with pathological findings. Epilepsy Res. 2008;80:158–62.
70. Metternich B, Wagner K, Brandt A, Kraemer R, Buschmann F, et al. Preoperative depressive symptoms predict postoperative seizure outcome in temporal and frontal lobe epilepsy. Epilepsy Behav. 2009;16:622–8.
71. Kanner AM, Barry JJ, Gilliam F, Hermann B, Meador KJ. Anxiety disorders, subsyndromic depressive episodes, and major depressive episodes: do they differ on their impact on the quality of life of patients with epilepsy? Epilepsia. 2010;51:1152–8.
72. Brandt C, Schoendienst M, Trentowska M, May TW, Pohlmann-Eden B, Tuschen-Caffier B, et al. Prevalence of anxiety disorders in patients with refractory focal epilepsy – a prospective clinic based survey. Epilepsy Behav. 2010;17:259–63.
73. Halley SA, Wrench JM, Reutens DC, Wilson SJ. The amygdala and anxiety after epilepsy surgery. Epilepsy Behav. 2010;18:431–6.

74. Mattsson P, Tibblin B, Kihlgren M, Kumlien E. A prospective study of anxiety with respect to seizure outcome after epilepsy surgery. Seizure. 2005;14:40–5.
75. Mintzer S, Lopez F. Comorbidity of ictal fear and panic disorder. Epilepsy Behav. 2002;3:330–7.
76. Foong J, Flugel D. Psychiatric outcome of surgery for temporal lobe epilepsy and presurgical considerations. Epilepsy Res. 2007;75:84–96.
77. Bonelli SB, Powell R, Yogarajah M, Thompson PJ, Symms MR, et al. Preoperative amygdala fMRI in temporal lobe epilepsy. Epilepsia. 2009;50:217–27.
78. Etkin A, Wager TD. Brain systems underlying anxiety disorders: a view from neuroimaging. In: Simpson HB, Schneier F, Neria Y, Lewis-Fernandez R, editors. Anxiety disorders: theory, research and clinical perspectives. Cambridge: Cambridge Medicine; 2010.
79. Kanner AM, Stagno S, Kotagal P, Morris HH. Postictal psychiatric events during prolonged video-electroencephalographic monitoring studies. Arch Neurol. 1996;53:258–63.
80. Alper K, Devinsky O, Westbrook L, Luciano D, Pacia S, et al. Premorbid psychiatric risk factors for postictal psychosis. J Neuropsychiatry Clin Neurosci. 2001;13:492–9.
81. Devinsky O, Abramson H, Alper K, FitzGerald LS, Perrine K, et al. Postictal psychosis: a case control series of 20 patients and 150 controls. Epilepsy Res. 1995;20:247–53.
82. Leutmezer F, Podreka I, Asenbaum S, Pietrzyk U, Lucht H, Back C, et al. Postictal psychosis in temporal lobe epilepsy. Epilepsia. 2003;44:582–90.
83. Sachdev P. Schizophrenia-like psychosis and epilepsy: the status of the association. Am J Psychiatry. 1998;155:325–36.
84. Reutens DC, Savard G, Andermann F, Dubeau F, Olivier A. Results of surgical treatment in temporal lobe epilepsy with chronic psychosis. Brain. 1997;120:1929–36.
85. Marchetti RL, Fiore LA, Valente KD, Gronich G, Nogueira AB, Tzu WH. Surgical treatment of temporal lobe epilepsy with interictal psychosis: results of six cases. Epilepsy Behav. 2003;4:146–52.
86. Barbieri V, Gozzo F, Schiariti MP, Lo Russo G, Sartori I, Castana L, et al. One-year postsurgical follow-up of 12 subjects with epilepsy and interictal psychosis. Epilepsy Behav. 2011;22:385–7.
87. da Conceição PO, de Araujo Filho GM, Mazetto L, Alonso NB, Yacubian EM. Safety of video-EEG monitoring and surgical outcome in patients with mesial temporal sclerosis and psychosis of epilepsy. Seizure. 2012;21:583–7.
88. Kanner AM. Does a history of postictal psychosis predict a poor postsurgical seizure outcome? Epilepsy Curr. 2009;9:96–7.
89. Bladin PF. Psychosocial difficulties and outcome after temporal lobectomy. Epilepsia. 1992;33:898–907.
90. Mayanagi Y, Watanabe E, Nagahori Y, Nankai M. Psychiatric and neuropsychological problems in epilepsy surgery: analysis of 100 cases that underwent surgery. Epilepsia. 2001;42:19–23.
91. Shaw P, Mellers J, Henderson M, Polkey C, David AS, Toone BK. Schizophrenia-like psychosis arising de novo following a temporal lobectomy: timing and risk factors. J Neurol Neurosurg Psychiatry. 2004;75:1003–8.
92. Calvet E, Caravotta PG, Scévola L, Teitelbaum J, Seoane E, et al. Psychosis after epilepsy surgery: report of three cases. Epilepsy Behav. 2011;22:804–7.
93. Inoue Y, Mihara T. Psychiatric disorders before and after surgery for epilepsy. Epilepsia. 2001;42:13–8.
94. Taylor DC. Factors influencing the occurrence of schizophrenia-like psychosis in patients with temporal lobe epilepsy. Psychol Med. 1975;5:249–54.
95. Krishnamoorthy ES, Trimble MR. Forced normalization: clinical and therapeutic relevance. Epilepsia. 1999;40:57–64.
96. Krishnamoorthy ES, Trimble MR, Sander JW, Kanner AM. Forced normalization at the interface between epilepsy and psychiatry. Epilepsy Behav. 2002;3:303–8.

97. Bodde NM, Brooks JL, Baker GA, Boon PA, Hendriksen JG, et al. Psychogenic non-epileptic seizures – definition, etiology, treatment and prognostic issues: a critical review. Seizure. 2009;18:543–53.
98. Reuber M, Qurishi A, Bauer J, Helmstaedter C, Fernandez G, et al. Are there physical risk factors for psychogenic non-epileptic seizures in patients with epilepsy? Seizure. 2003;12:561–7.
99. Reuber M, Kurthen M, Fernández G, Schramm J, Elger CE. Epilepsy surgery in patients with additional psychogenic seizures. Arch Neurol. 2002;59:82–6.
100. Ney GC, Barr WB, Napolitano C, Decker R, Schaul N. New-onset psychogenic seizures after surgery for epilepsy. Arch Neurol. 1998;55:726–30.
101. Davies KG, Blumer DP, Lobo S, Hermann BP, Phillips BL, Montouris GD. De novo nonepileptic seizures after cranial surgery for epilepsy: incidence and risk factors. Epilepsy Behav. 2000;1:436–43.
102. Naga AA, Devinsky O, Barr WB. Somatoform disorders after temporal lobectomy. Cogn Behav Neurol. 2004;17:57–61.
103. Markoula S, de Tisi J, Foong J, Duncan JS. De novo psychogenic nonepileptic attacks after adult epilepsy surgery: an underestimated entity. Epilepsia. 2013;54:e159–62.
104. Devinsky O, Mesad S, Alper K. Nondominant hemisphere lesions and conversion nonepileptic seizures. J Neuropsychiatry Clin Neurosci. 2001;13:367–73.
105. Perez DL, Dworetzky BA, Dickerson BC, Leung L, Cohn R, et al. An integrative neurocircuit perspective on psychogenic nonepileptic seizures and functional movement disorders: neural functional unawareness. Clin EEG Neurosci. 2015;46:4–15.
106. Sachdev P, Smith JS, Matheson J, Last P, Blumbergs P. Amygdalo-hippocampectomy for pathological aggression. Aust N Z J Psychiatry. 1992;26:671–6.
107. Ng YT, Hastriter EV, Wethe J, Chapman KE, Prenger EC, Prigatano GP, et al. Surgical resection of hypothalamic hamartomas for severe behavioral symptoms. Epilepsy Behav. 2011;20:75–8.
108. Kulaksizoglu IB, Bebek N, Baykan B, Imer M, Gürses C, Sencer S, et al. Obsessive-compulsive disorder after epilepsy surgery. Epilepsy Behav. 2004;5:113–8.
109. Guarnieri R, Walz R, Hallak JE, Coimbra E, de Almeida E, Cescato MP, et al. Do psychiatric comorbidities predict postoperative seizure outcome in temporal lobe epilepsy surgery? Epilepsy Behav. 2009;14:529–34.
110. Chemali Z, Bromfield E. Tourette's syndrome following temporal lobectomy for seizure control. Epilepsy Behav. 2003;4:564–6.
111. Baird AD, Wilson SJ, Bladin PF, Saling MM, Reutens DC. Hypersexuality after temporal lobe resection. Epilepsy Behav. 2002;3:173–81.
112. Devinsky J, Sacks O, Devinsky O. Kluver-Bucy syndrome, hypersexuality, and the law. Neurocase. 2010;16:140–5.
113. Koch-Stoecker S, Schmitz B, Kanner AM. Treatment of postsurgical psychiatric complications. Epilepsia. 2013;54:46–52.
114. Bladin PF, Wilson SJ, Saling MM, McIntosh PK, O'Shea MF. Outcome assessment in seizure surgery: the role of postoperative adjustment. J Clin Neurosci. 1999;6:313–8.
115. Fernando DK, McIntosh AM, Bladin PF, Wilson SJ. Common experiences of patients following suboptimal treatment outcomes: implications for epilepsy surgery. Epilepsy Behav. 2014;33:144–51.
116. Shirbin CA, McIntosh AM, Wilson SJ. The experience of seizures after epilepsy surgery. Epilepsy Behav. 2009;16:82–5.
117. Kerr MP, Mensah S, Besag F, de Toffol B, Ettinger A, Kanemoto K, et al. International consensus clinical practice statements for the treatment of neuropsychiatric conditions associated with epilepsy. Epilepsia. 2011;52:2133–8.
118. Reid K, Herbert A, Baker GA. Epilepsy surgery: patient-perceived long-term costs and benefits. Epilepsy Behav. 2004;5:81–7.

119. McIntosh AM, Wilson SJ, Berkovic SF. Seizure outcome after temporal lobectomy: current research practice and findings. Epilepsia. 2001;42:1288–307.
120. Kanner AM. The treatment of depressive disorders in epilepsy: what all neurologists should know. Epilepsia. 2013;54:3–12.
121. Johnson EK, Jones JE, Seidenberg M, Hermann BP. The relative impact of anxiety, depression, and clinical seizure features on health-related quality of life in epilepsy. Epilepsia. 2004;45:544–50.
122. Derry PA, Rose KJ, McLachlan RS. Moderators of the effect of preoperative emotional adjustment on postoperative depression after surgery for temporal lobe epilepsy. Epilepsia. 2000;41:177–85.
123. Maixner D, Sagher O, Bess J, Edwards J. Catatonia following surgery for temporal lobe epilepsy successfully treated with electroconvulsive therapy. Epilepsy Behav. 2010;19:528–32.
124. Quigg M, Broshek DK, Barbaro NM, et al. Neuropsychological outcomes after Gamma Knife radiosurgery for mesial temporal lobe epilepsy: a prospective multicenter study. Epilepsia. 2011;52:909–16.
125. Salzberg M, Taher T, Davie M, Carne R, Hicks RJ, Cook M, et al. Depression in temporal lobe epilepsy surgery patients: an FDG-PET study. Epilepsia. 2006;47:2125–30.
126. Suchy Y, Chelune G. Postsurgical changes in self-reported mood and Composite IQ in a matched sample of patients with frontal and temporal lobe epilepsy. J Clin Exp Neuropsychol. 2001;23:413–23.
127. da Conceição PO, Nascimento PP, Mazetto L, Alonso NB, Yacubian EM, de Araujo Filho GM. Are psychiatric disorders exclusion criteria for video-EEG monitoring and epilepsy surgery in patients with mesial temporal sclerosis? Epilepsy Behav. 2013;27:310–4.
128. D'Alessio L, Scévola L, Fernandez Lima M, Oddo S, Solís P, Seoane E, et al. Psychiatric outcome of epilepsy surgery in patients with psychosis and temporal lobe drug-resistant epilepsy: a prospective case series. Epilepsy Behav. 2014;37:165–70.
129. Louis S, Basha M, Mittal S, Lobe J, Shah A. Are patients with postictal psychiatric episodes at increased risk for developing psychiatric co-morbidities after epilepsy surgery? Epilepsy Curr. 2012;13:397.

Chapter 18
The Role of Antiepileptic Drugs

Mahinda Yogarajah and Marco Mula

Abstract Antiepileptic drugs (AEDs) suppress seizures by acting on a variety of mechanisms and molecular targets involved in the regulation of neuronal excitability. These include inhibitory (GABAergic) and excitatory (glutamatergic) neurotransmission, as well as ion (sodium and calcium) conductance through voltage-gated channels. However, these mechanisms and targets are also implicated in the regulation of mood and behavior, which may explain why each AED is associated with specific psychotropic effects. This chapter will discuss the role of mechanisms and molecular targets of AEDs in mood and behavior, and review the positive and negative psychotropic effects of AEDs.

Keywords Epilepsy • Antiepileptic drugs • Depression • Psychosis • Anxiety • Anticonvulsant • Mania • Behavior

Abbreviations

AED	Antiepileptic drug
CBZ	Carbamazepine
EMA	European Medicines Agency
ESL	Eslicarbazepine
ETX	Ethosuximide
FDA	Food and Drug Administration
FLB	Felbamate
GBP	Gabapentin

M. Yogarajah, BSc, MBBS, MRCP, PhD
Epilepsy Group, Atkinson Morley Regional Neuroscience Centre, St. George's University Hospitals NHS Foundation Trust, Blackshaw Road, London SW17 0QT, UK
e-mail: mahinda2@doctors.org.uk

M. Mula, MD, PhD (✉)
Epilepsy Group, Atkinson Morley Regional Neuroscience Centre, St. George's University Hospitals NHS Foundation Trust, Blackshaw Road, London SW17 0QT, UK

Institute of Medical and Biomedical Sciences, St George's University of London, London, UK
e-mail: mmula@sgul.ac.uk

M. Mula (ed.), *Neuropsychiatric Symptoms of Epilepsy*, Neuropsychiatric Symptoms of Neurological Disease, DOI 10.1007/978-3-319-22159-5_18

HRSA	Hamilton Rating Scale for Anxiety
LAC	Lacosamide
LEV	Levetiracetam
LTG	Lamotrigine
OXC	Oxcarbazepine
PGB	Pregabalin
PHT	Phenytoin
RTG	Retigabine
RUF	Rufinamide
STP	Stiripentol
TGB	Tiagabine
TPM	Topiramate
VGB	Vigabatrin
VPA	Valproate
ZNS	Zonisamide

Introduction

The introduction of nearly 15 new antiepileptic drugs (AEDs) in the past 20 years has significantly expanded the pharmacological armamentarium for epilepsy [1]. Although some of these agents offer appreciable advantages in terms of pharmacokinetics, tolerability, and lower drug interaction potential, improvements in clinical outcome have fallen short of expectations, with no more than 15–20 % of patients refractory to older AEDs attaining seizure freedom without unacceptable toxicity [2]. In addition, AEDs are still characterized by treatment-emergent psychiatric adverse effects that have a considerable impact on quality of life and compliance to treatment [3]. However, AEDs have also potential positive effects as demonstrated by the wide use in psychiatric practice for a broad spectrum of psychiatric disorders. The primary application is in mood stabilization [4] but interesting data are also emerging for anxiety disorders [5] and withdrawal syndromes [6].

Any discussion of the psychotropic effect of AEDs must acknowledge that psychopathology in epilepsy has a multifactorial, biopsychosocial etiology, and AEDs constitute only one of several factors. In fact, it is often difficult to determine which psychopathological manifestations are due specifically to the drug therapy, and which may be due to other factors that can affect the patient. In addition, the mechanisms of action of several AEDs are not fully understood, and several AEDs have a diverse array of actions on biological systems, only some of which may be related to the desired antiseizure effect. In summary, therefore, the psychotropic effects of AEDs in epilepsy derive from a number of variables related to the single compound (i.e., mechanism of action), to the underling neurological condition (i.e., neurobiology of

Direct
(Drug-related)
- Mechanism of action of the drug
- Drug toxicity
- Drug withdrawal

Indirect
(Epilepsy-related)
- "Forced normalization"
- "Release phenomenon"
- Postictal and periictal psychoses
- Severity of the epilepsy
- Limbic system abnormalities

(Patient-related)
- Past psychiatric history
- Family psychiatric history

Fig. 18.1 Variables implicated in treatment-emergent psychiatric adverse events of antiepileptic drugs.

seizure control), and to the individual (i.e., family history or personal history of psychiatric disorders) (Fig. 18.1) [7].

In this chapter, we discuss the role of mechanisms and molecular targets of AEDs in mood and behavior, and review the positive and negative psychotropic effects of AEDs.

Mechanisms of Action of AEDs in Mood and Behavior

Because AEDs have a wide variety of mechanisms at the neurotransmitter level, it is not surprising that the psychotropic effects vary greatly from one drug to another. AEDs can modulate neuronal membrane polarity, neurotransmitter activity, neuronal firing, and discharge propagation [8]. They act principally by reducing glutamatergic excitation, potentiating GABAergic inhibition, and by blockade of voltage-gated Na^+ or Ca^{2+} channels, although a number of other mechanisms have also been identified. At a basic level, the psychotropic potential of AEDs can be divided into those that are positive and those that are negative. Our knowledge about positive or negative psychotropic properties of AEDs is not based on standardized or defined diagnostic criteria. There are no systematic data with respect to the older generation of compounds, such as barbiturates, phenytoin (PHT), or carbamazepine (CBZ), and data for the new generation of drugs are derived from drug trials that are primarily designed to test antiseizure efficacy. Therefore, the psychopathological phenomenology of psychiatric adverse effects of AEDs as well as their severity, time course, and relationship to seizures still remains partly unknown.

More than 15 years ago, Ketter et al. [9] suggested that two categories of drugs could be identified on the basis of their predominant psychotropic profile. Sedating drugs are characterized by adverse effects like fatigue, cognitive slowing, and weight gain, and are usually related to potentiation of gamma amino butyric acid (GABA) inhibitory neurotransmission. On the other hand, there are activating drugs with anxiogenic and antidepressant properties that determine attenuation of glutamate excitatory neurotransmission. The first group includes drugs such as barbiturates, valproate (VPA), gabapentin (GBP), tiagabine (TGB), and vigabatrin (VGB), while the second group includes felbamate and lamotrigine (LTG). Topiramate (TPM) can be considered a molecule with a mixed profile. The paradigm proposed by Ketter is straightforward, but in patients with epilepsy the epilepsy itself complicates the situation. In fact, the final psychotropic effect of AEDs is related to both direct and indirect mechanisms (Fig. 18.1). The former represent the main properties of the drug, and can be predicted using Ketter's theoretical framework. However, treatment-emergent psychiatric adverse events may also result from the effect of the drug on the epilepsy itself. In this regard, some phenomena, such as forced normalization or postictal psychosis, may be the result of AED changes altering the control of the seizures, without being related to a specific drug. Factors such as the severity of the epilepsy or the presence of limbic system abnormalities may also be of relevance. Therefore, prediction of the final psychotropic effect of any AED needs to take into account not only the pharmacological variable related to the mechanism of action, but also the final activity of the compound on the pathophysiology of the individual CNS disorder.

γ-Aminobutyric Acid (GABA) Transmission

Over the past 30 years, converging evidence from animal and human studies has suggested that GABAergic mechanisms may be implicated in the pathophysiology of mood disorders as demonstrated by basic science studies in experimental models of depression and in patients with major depressive disorders [10]. In addition, mood stressors can affect GABAergic function [10] and GABAergic dysfunction has also been reported in aggressive behavior [11], agitation, and hyperactivity [12]. In this regard, it is important to note that the abrupt discontinuation of benzodiazepines can be accompanied by severe seizure exacerbation and changes in mental status, including anxiety, agitation, confusion, depression, psychosis, and even delirium [13, 14]. It seems, thus, evident that any disruption in GABAergic function has profound behavioral correlates.

Among AEDs, those that potentiate GABAergic neurotransmission, either by interacting with $GABA_A$ receptors or by modifying the activity of enzymes and transporters involved in the turnover of GABA, are barbiturates, vigabatrin (VGB), stiripentol (STP), and tiagabine (TGB). However, robust GABAergic effects are also displayed by other compounds such as topiramate (TPM) and valproate (VPA).

Glutamate Transmission

The role of glutamatergic dysfunction in the pathophysiology of mood and behavioral disorders has gained attention only in recent years. Glutamatergic neurotransmission is an important component in the stress-responsive cascade of events ultimately leading to hippocampal and cortical alterations associated with mood disorders [15–17]. Stress increases extracellular glutamate concentrations [18] and alters glutamate receptor binding profiles and subunit expression in several brain regions [19, 20]. A number of studies show elevated glutamate levels in the plasma of patients with mood disorders [21, 22]. In addition, drugs altering the binding profile of glutamate receptors [17] or modulating glutamatergic neurotransmission have positive effects on mood and behavior [11, 17]. Inhibition of glutamatergic neurotransmission is the primary or secondary mechanism of action for a number of AEDs, but it is of particular relevance for felbamate (FLB), lamotrigine (LTG), and TPM.

Voltage-Gated Sodium Channels

There has been a tendency to investigate the role of neurotransmitter systems in the pathophysiology of mood and behavioral disorders [23, 24], whereas other systems, such as disturbances in sodium and calcium transport, have been examined to a lesser extent [24]. Nevertheless, evidence exists that sodium homeostasis is altered in mood disorders [25, 26]. Furthermore, several effective mood-stabilizing treatments reduce intracellular sodium concentrations or inhibit, through blockade of voltage-gated sodium channels, sodium influx [27]. Of note, blockade of voltage-gated sodium channels also results in inhibition of glutamate release [28], which is itself associated with positive effects on mood and behavior as described above. How such effect differs from the primary modulation of glutamate receptors is unknown and further studies in this area are urgently needed.

Many AEDs act primarily as sodium channel-blockers, including carbamazepine (CBZ), phenytoin (PHT), oxcarbazepine (OXC), eslicarbazepine acetate (ESL), lacosamide (LCM), and rufinamide (RUF). Of note, blockade of voltage-gated sodium channels is also an important mechanism of action for LTG, FLB, TPM, and zonisamide (ZNS).

Voltage-Gated Calcium Channels

Voltage-gated calcium channels are multimeric proteins composed of five coassembled subunits (α_1, α_2, β, γ, δ), which can be broadly classified into high-voltage-activated channels (further subgrouped as L-, R-, P/Q- and N-types) and low-voltage-activated channels (T-type). Evidence exists that these channels, particularly high-voltage-activated channels, may be implicated in the pathophysiology of mood disorders. Genetic variation in *CACNA1C*, a gene encoding the alpha 1C subunit of the L-type voltage-gated calcium channel, has been associated with bipolar disorder, depression, and schizophrenia [29]. In some experimental models, voltage-gated calcium channel antagonists display antidepressant properties [30, 31], whereas agonists lead to depressant-like effects [32]. Inhibition of voltage-gated calcium channels probably translates into a reduction in excitatory neurotransmission [33, 34], which may be ultimately responsible for positive effects on mood and behavior.

Ethosuximide (ETX) is a low-voltage-activated T-type channel-blocker, whereas gabapentin (GBP) and pregabalin (PGB) are high-voltage-activated calcium channel-blockers through interaction with the α_2-δ modulatory site. Blockade of voltage-gated calcium channels is also an important mechanism for lamotrigine (LTG) and zonisamide (ZNS) (Fig. 18.1).

Other Direct Drug-Related Mechanisms

The serotoninergic system is widely recognized to modulate a wide range of physiological functions, including mood and behavior. Decreased serotoninergic neurotransmission has been proposed to play a key role in the pathophysiology of affective disorders, and enhancement of serotoninergic neurotransmission is the primary mechanism of action for many psychotropic agents [35, 36]. An increase in extracellular serotonin has been observed with VPA [37], CBZ [38], OXC [39], TPM [40], and ZNS in experimental models [41], and in vitro for LTG [42].

The dopaminergic system has long been linked with mood and behavioral disorders. Increased dopaminergic neurotransmission appears to play a role in schizophrenia, mania, and aggressive behavior, whereas decreased dopaminergic function may be implicated in the pathophysiology of depression [11, 43, 44]. Dopaminergic neurotransmission is a major target for psychotropic agents [45]. AEDs may also modulate dopaminergic function, although seen mainly in experimental models. VPA stimulates brain dopamine turnover [46], whereas CBZ, OXC, TPM, and ZNS increase extracellular dopamine levels [39, 40, 47].

Other potential mechanisms described in mood disorders comprise a disruption in neural plasticity [48] such as inositol biosynthesis, the cyclic adenine monophosphate (c-AMP) response element-binding protein, the brain-derived neurotrophic factor (BDNF), the glycogen synthase kinase-3 (GSK-3), the extracellular signal-regulated kinase pathway, the arachidonic acid pathway, the cytoprotective protein bcl-2, and mitogen-activated protein kinases [48, 49]. Some mood stabilizers and antidepressants may act on these factors, ultimately attenuating or reversing disease-related impairments in neuronal plasticity, neurogenesis, or cell survival. The mood stabilizers VPA and, to a lesser extent, CBZ display similar actions on these target [49].

Finally, it is important to mention the peculiar modulation of SV2A protein by levetiracetam (LEV) [1], although the role of SV2A in psychiatric disorders is still unknown.

Indirect Mechanisms: Forced Normalization

In some patients with epilepsy, sudden suppression of seizures may act as a trigger for the precipitation of psychiatric symptoms, a phenomenon called "forced normalization." This concept was originally described by Heinrich Landolt, head of the

Swiss Epilepsy Centre in Zurich between 1955 and 1971 [50]. He reported EEG investigations of patients with epilepsy who had paroxysmal psychiatric disorders, using the newly introduced EEG and described a group of patients who had productive psychotic episodes with "paradoxical normalization" of the EEG. In other words, the abnormal EEGs of these patients improved or normalized during the time that they were psychotic. Landolt noted that the introduction of a particular class of drugs, the suximides, led to an increase in the number of cases [51]. During the same period, Gibbs [52] reported the occurrence of psychiatric problems in patients with temporal lobe epilepsy when seizures were suppressed with phenacemide and commented that this could sometimes happen with barbiturates and hydantoins [51]. Subsequently, Tellenbach [53] introduced the term "alternative psychosis" for the clinical phenomenon of the reciprocal relationship between abnormal mental states and seizures, which did not, as Landolt's term did, rely on EEG findings.

Since the early observations of Landolt, a number of patients with alternative psychosis have been documented [51, 54, 55]. In many of the series described, the precipitation of the abnormal behavioral state or the psychosis has been linked with the prescription of AEDs, but it is important to note that this phenomenon should not be restricted to drug-induced seizure control. In fact, it is likely that in patients who develop de novo psychosis following epilepsy surgery, forced normalization may play such a role. Indeed, a case of an alternative psychosis secondary to vagus nerve stimulation has also been reported [56].

Several psychopathological pictures including hypomania/mania, depression, and anxiety [51] have been linked to the forced normalization phenomenon, but psychosis is the most common [57]. Peter Wolf [58] noted that several clinical pictures including psychosis may evolve, and that the development of psychotic symptoms was preceded by premonitory symptoms, especially insomnia, anxiety, and social withdrawal. Wolf reported an association with generalized idiopathic epilepsies, and the prescription of ETX, highlighting again the importance of both generalized seizures, and the suximide drugs in the development of these behavioral problems [59]. Different authors speculated on the potential underlying mechanisms including on-going epileptic activity in limbic structures, inhibition surrounding the epileptic focus, an altered balance between excitatory and inhibitory neurotransmission [51]. At any rate, forced normalization has been reported with most AEDs, and may at least in part explain why certain AEDs have paradoxical effects in epilepsy compared to primary psychiatric disorders (e.g., exacerbating mood dysfunction in patients with epilepsy vs. improving affective disorders in psychiatric populations).

Negative Effects of AEDs

The most common negative effects of AEDs are depression, psychosis and irritability, aggression and behavioral change. Given the multiple mechanisms of action of most AEDs, it is unsurprising that each AED can have multiple psychotropic effects. The AEDs described below are categorized according to their most commonly reported effect.

Depression

Depression in epilepsy is a multifactorial problem with a number of variables being implicated [60–64]. For AED-related depressive symptoms, there is evidence for the following variables being relevant to the association: enhanced GABA neurotransmission, folate deficiency, polytherapy, the presence of hippocampal sclerosis, forced normalization and a past history of affective disorders [7].

AEDs that are particularly relevant in the occurrence of depression as a treatment-emergent adverse event include barbiturates [7], VGB [65], TGB [66], TPM [67], and ZON [68] (Fig. 18.2). All of these AEDs have varying degrees of GABAergic function, and it is of interest that some AEDs are more closely associated with depression than others, especially those with activity at the benzodiazepine-GABA receptor. In patients with psychiatric disorders without epilepsy, long-term treatment with benzodiazepines has also been reported as provoking depressive symptoms [69], and withdrawal can provoke a depressive illness [14]. Interestingly, an increasing number of clinical observations and experimental studies have shown that GABAergic mechanisms are involved in the pathogenesis of depression [70].

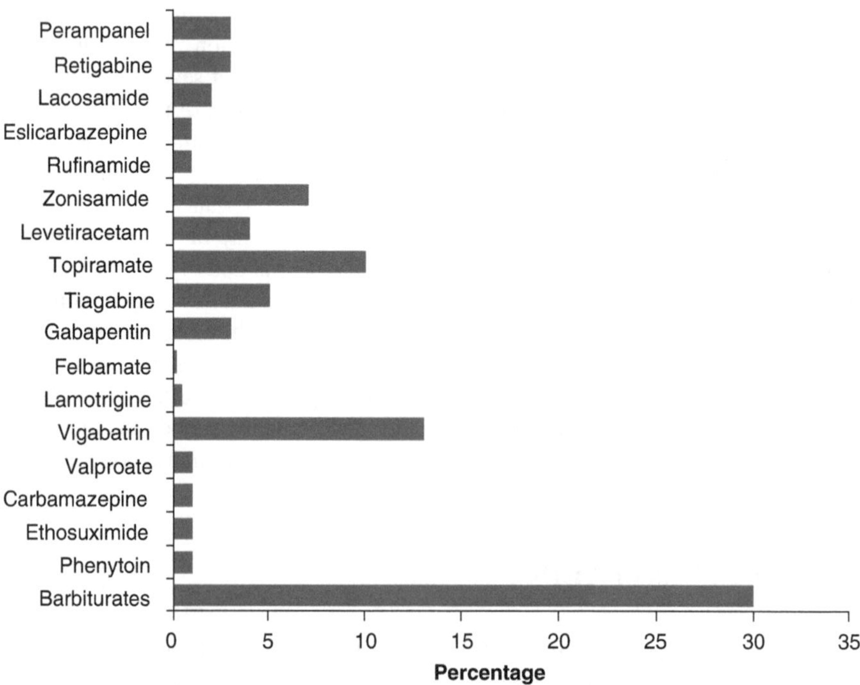

Fig. 18.2 Prevalence of depressive symptoms in controlled clinical trials of individual antiepileptic drugs

Barbiturates

One of the first studies on this subject was the one by Rodin et al. [71]. They stabilized 45 patients on a combination of PHT and either primidone or CBZ. After a 3-month period, those receiving CBZ were switched to primidone and vice versa. Over time, patients became clinically more depressed on a regime of primidone, and less so on CBZ. Subsequent studies corroborated these findings [72, 73]. In general terms, it is recognized that a long history of exposure to barbiturates may carry the greatest risk of depression, particularly in the setting of polytherapy, and a personal or family history of affective disorders [7]. Interestingly enough, in children and individuals with learning disabilities, the use of barbiturates can also induce a syndrome characterized by insomnia, hyperactivity, impulsiveness, and aggressive behavior [12, 74], similar to that described with benzodiazepines [14].

Vigabatrin

Treatment-emergent psychiatric problems with VGB have been extensively studied [75, 76]. In some patients, the onset of depression was linked with a dramatic control of seizure frequency (a form of forced normalization) [51, 58], while in others it was unrelated to this, but in the majority of cases, it appeared to be more common in patients with a past history of depression [76]. A meta-analysis of double-blind, placebo-controlled adjunctive-treatment trials in a total of 717 adult patients with drug-resistant partial epilepsy showed that VGB, compared to placebo, is associated with a higher incidence of depression (12.1 % vs. 3.5 %, $p<0.001$) and psychosis (2.5 % vs. 0.3 %, $p=0.028$) [65]. Depressive symptoms are often mild in severity and psychosis generally improves following dose adjustment or discontinuation of VGB. In addition, monotherapy trials showed an incidence of depression much lower (~5 %) [77]. However, it is also for this reason that the use of VGB became progressively limited to specific epileptic syndromes. As described for other GABAergic drugs, in pediatric populations, up to 14.2 % of patients develop paradoxical hyperactivity, agitation, insomnia, or aggressive behavior. As described for almost all AEDs, risk factors for treatment-emergent psychiatric adverse events include high starting and maintenance doses, a past psychiatric history, and a severe form of epilepsy [76, 78].

Topiramate

TPM has a broad-spectrum efficacy due to the multiple mechanisms of action. In fact, TPM potentiates GABAergic neurotransmission, inhibits voltage-gated sodium and calcium channels, kainate/α-amino-3-hydroxy-5-methylisoxazole-4-proprionic acid (AMPA)-type glutamate receptors and carbonic anhydrase. The variety of mechanisms may explain why TPM has "mixed" effects on mood and behavior [9].

Two healthy volunteer studies demonstrated that treatment with TPM was associated with the onset of depression and a significant augmentation in GABAergic neurotransmission [79, 80]. In patients with epilepsy, TPM has been associated with depression and behavior problems [67, 81]. In contrast to this, studies in patients with major depression suggest a potential positive effect of TPM. In a 10-week, randomized, double-blind, placebo-controlled trial of 64 patients with a major depressive disorder, TPM 200 mg/day monotherapy was associated with a 17 % improvement in the Hamilton Depression Rating Scale scores (from 23.1 to 19.2) compared to a 4 % improvement with placebo (from 22.9 to 22.0; $p=0.02$) [82]. Similar results were found for add-on TPM in treatment-resistant major depressive disorder [83]. TPM was also found to be effective for anger and aggression associated with depression [82] or borderline personality disorder [84, 85], whereas data in schizophrenia are conflicting [86–88]. Preliminary data also suggests that it may be useful in eating disorders [89]. Overall studies demonstrate that the psychotropic potential of TPM is likely to be large and polymorphous [90]. Further studies are definitely needed.

Tiagabine

TGB potentiates GABAergic neurotransmission by selectively inhibiting the GAT-1 GABA transporter, which is responsible for the uptake of GABA into neurons and surrounding glial cells after synaptic release. Data on the psychotropic profile of TGB are controversial. Although case-series and a few open-label studies suggest that this AED may have beneficial or no effects on mood and anxiety [91–93], the incidence of mood disorders across five randomized, double-blind, placebo-controlled, add-on trials was higher in patients taking TGB compared to those on placebo (5 % vs. 1 %) [94]. Nervousness was also more common with TGB than placebo (12 % vs. 3 %). Nevertheless, psychiatric problems appear to be mild to moderate, occur during titration, and abate spontaneously. The risk of TGB-induced psychiatric problems may be increased in patients with a personal history of mood disorders [7].

Zonisamide

ZNS is a second-generation AED that acts predominantly through blockade of voltage-gated sodium channels and inactivation of voltage-gated T-type calcium channels [95]. Other mechanisms, however, appear to be involved. ZNS binds to the GABA-benzodiazepine receptor complex [96], elevates brain levels of GABA [97], reduces extracellular release of glutamate [98], and inhibits carbonic anhydrase [95]. This broad mechanistic profile may underlie the variety of effects of this AED on mood and behavior. In patients with epilepsy receiving ZNS, the occurrence of treatment-emergent psychiatric adverse events may not be uncommon. In a single-center study of 544 patients, the incidence of adverse psychiatric effects severe enough to be associated with discontinuation of ZNS was 6.9 % [68]. The most common reason for discontinuation was depression ($n=11$), followed by aggressive behavior ($n=8$), psychosis ($n=6$), and irritability ($n=5$). Risk factors for discontinuation due to adverse psychiatric effects were past psychiatric history ($p=0.005$), symptomatic generalized epilepsy ($p=0.027$), and lower maximum ZNS serum concentration (mean = 17.9 mg/L vs. 34.7 mg/L, $p<0.001$).

AEDs, Indirect Factors, and Depression

In the pathogenesis of AED-induced depressive symptoms, a relevant role is played by the limbic structures [99]. There is growing evidence in literature that depression might be linked to small hippocampal volumes, and this association has been described in patients with epilepsy [100] but also in patients without epilepsy with a major depressive disorder [101, 102]. A case-control study of patients taking TPM showed that subjects with temporal lobe epilepsy and hippocampal sclerosis were more likely to develop depression than those with temporal lobe epilepsy and normal MRI, matched for starting dose and titration schedule of TPM [99]. Although patients with hippocampal sclerosis tend to be affected by more severe epilepsy, implying that treatment resistance is likely and that polytherapy may be prescribed, the hippocampal sclerosis itself appeared to be the main factor associated with the occurrence of depression [99].

Folate deficiency is another issue that may be of relevance regarding AEDs and depression. Patients in polytherapy are reported to have low serum, red cell, or cerebro-spinal fluid folate levels [103] and this deficit seems to be even greater in patients with epilepsy and psychopathology. It is known that folic acid plays a crucial role in several important central nervous system transmethylation reactions and is linked to monoamine metabolism [69]. In this regard, it is worth noting that AEDs with a positive impact on mood and behavior, such as CBZ or LTG, have minimal effects on folate levels [104]. On the contrary, it is established that barbiturates or PHT treatment can depress serum, red blood cell, or CSF folate levels in a high proportion of patients [105].

Psychosis

There is a considerable literature suggesting that the development of psychosis with AED therapy is associated with the forced normalization phenomenon in many cases [57]. Fischer et al. [106] and Roger et al. [107] described episodes of psychoses during treatment with ETX characterized by anxiety, depression, visual and auditory hallucinations, and intermittent impairment of consciousness, the EEG often reverting to normal. These episodes resolved with the discontinuation of the AED and seizure recurrence. Another study [108] described seven patients who had no previous psychiatric histories and whose behavioral problems emerged shortly after starting or altering AED therapy. Their EEGs, abnormal before treatment, normalized during the psychotic episodes. All patients had temporal lobe abnormalities on the EEG, but only two were on suxinimides.

Psychosis can, however, also be a direct effect of AEDs. Of the newer AEDs, psychoses have been noted, as a potential adverse event, in several cases, suggesting that this phenomenon is not drug-specific. Psychotic episodes have been described with felbamate (FBM) [109], TGB [66], TPM [110], VGB [111], ZON [112, 113], and levetiracetam (LVT) [54]. Although there is no clear evidence for LTG precipitating psychosis, there are at least some case reports that suggest that this might be a possibility [114]. In general terms, the frequency of psychoses during AED treatment seems to be in the region of 1–2 % and all described cases were difficult-to-treat patients undergoing add-on therapy.

With respect to specific AEDs, psychoses associated with VGB have been the most extensively studied. In a study by Thomas et al. [76], 30 % of patients who developed a psychosis during therapy with VGB had a previous history of psychosis and 60 % of them were seizure free. Since these early reports, the clinical significance of VGB-associated behavioral problems has been a matter of controversy and two meta-analyses have been published [65, 78]. Analyzing seven placebo-controlled European studies, Ferrie et al. [78] showed an overall occurrence of these complications of 3.4 % in the VGB group and 0.6 % in the placebo group. Another meta-analysis of American and non-American double-blind studies demonstrated that there is a significantly increased risk for psychosis, occurring in 2.5 % of patients treated with VGB compared to 0.3 % in the placebo group [65]. TGB has also been investigated, and placebo-controlled studies showed that the risk of psychoses was not significantly increased [115]. However, the paradoxical provocation of de novo nonconvulsive status epilepticus is a specific issue reported by different authors [116] and, in some selected cases, there may be a differential diagnosis with brief ictal psychotic episodes. In such an event, EEG investigations are essential.

In general terms, it seems that psychoses with newer AEDs occurred in early clinical trials, and were a reflection of two factors. Firstly, many of these trials included a dosing schedule that subsequently appeared to be too rapid, or with too high dosages. Secondly, in many cases the populations studied were composed largely of patients with very difficult-to-treat epilepsy and those who had temporal lobe epilepsy, a population of patients that are most susceptible to develop psychoses. In other words, certain AEDs appear more likely to be associated with a psychosis as treatment-emergent adverse event, although the latter tend to be seen in those patients who, in any case, are susceptible to develop psychopathology. With the introduction of other powerful drugs in the future, these complications need to be both evaluated and treated.

Aggressiveness, Irritability, and Personality Changes

One of the first studies investigating this issue was that by Reynolds and Travers [103] who studied 57 adult outpatients with chronic epilepsy for the presence or absence of behavioral changes or psychiatric disorders, looking at serum AEDs levels. Patients with behavioral problems had significantly higher levels of both phenobarbitone and PHT than those without, irrespective of seizure frequency. Since that time, there have been many studies about the effects of AEDs on cognitive function or mood, but few of them have specifically investigated the issue of changes in behavior. In general terms, drug-induced behavioral problems, including irritability and aggressive behavior, appear to be more frequent with polytherapy and in patients with severe epilepsy syndromes, where mental retardation or abnormalities in the limbic system might be present [117]. For this reason, the trend toward treating patients on monotherapy, particularly in this subgroup of more vulnerable patients, would seem important for the patient's overall well-being.

A wide spectrum of behavioral changes has been described with different molecules. For example, we have already mentioned the paradoxical effects of GABAergic AEDs in children ADHD-like symptoms [74, 118]. However, whether this is a class effect or not is still matter of debate as other studies have not demonstrated behavioral problems with phenobarbitone among children [119, 120]. As already mentioned, VGB showed the same paradoxical effect in children with learning disabilities [121]. However, LEV is the AED with the most consistent and widespread reports of behavioral changes and aggressivity.

Levetiracetam

Aggressive behavior and irritability have shown to be one of the main treatment-emergent psychiatric adverse events during therapy with LEV, occurring in about 5 % of patients [122]. The mechanism of action of LEV differs from that of currently available AEDs and appears to be mediated by binding to the synaptic vesicle protein SV2A [123]. LEV was initially postulated to have mood-stabilizing and anxiolytic properties [124, 125]. However, two randomized, double-blind, placebo-controlled trials failed to demonstrate the superiority of LEV over placebo in the treatment of bipolar depression [126] and generalized social anxiety disorder [127]. A negative trial has also been reported in impulsive aggression [128]. In a postmarketing, single, tertiary center study of 517 consecutive patients treated with LEV, 53 (10.1 %) experienced adverse psychiatric effects [129]. Thirteen (2.5 %) developed depression, 6 (1.2 %) psychotic symptoms, 19 (3.5 %) aggressive behavior, 12 (2.3 %) emotional lability, and 3 (0.6 %) other behavioral problems, such as agitation, anger/hostile behavior, and personality changes. Risk factors for developing adverse psychiatric effects included a history of febrile convulsions, a history of status epilepticus, and a previous psychiatric history [129]. Notably, there are several reports suggesting that status epilepticus and febrile convulsions may play a role in the epileptogenic process. The main hypothesis has involved neuronal loss and synaptic reorganization, mainly in the limbic system. These phenomena might explain the biological vulnerability of a subgroup of patients to psychiatric adverse events. Whether a faster titration schedule is also a risk factor is controversial [122, 129]. Of note, a recent study found an association between genetic variations in dopaminergic activity and the risk for adverse psychiatric effects during LEV therapy [130].

	Other indications	Potential benefits	Alert
PB		Anxiolytic, hypnotic	Major depression, ADHD
CBZ OXC ESL	Bipolar disorder, pain	Addiction, withdrawal syndrome, dyscontrol	ADHD
ETX	None	NK	None (?Psychosis)
FLB	None	NK	Major depression, anxiety disorders
GBP	Pain	Anxiety disorders	ADHD
LCM	None	NK	None
LTG	Bipolar disorder		?Anxiety disorders, ?ADHD
LEV	None	NK	Anxiety disorders, dyscontrol
PRP	None	NK	NK
PHT	None	Mania	Major depression
PGB	GAD, Pain		NK
TGB	None	NK	Major depression
TPM	Migraine	Binge eating disorder	Major depression
VPA	Bipolar disorder	?Anxiety disorders	None
VGB	None	NK	Major depression, psychosis
ZNM	None		Major depression, psychosis

Fig. 18.3 Indications of antiepileptic drugs outside epilepsy, potential beneficial and detrimental effects in epilepsy (*NK* not known, *GAD* generalized anxiety disorder)

Learning disabilities plays a special role in treatment-emergent psychiatric adverse events of AEDs mainly because can be frequently encountered in all types of epilepsy [131]. A single-center study pointed out that aggressive behavior is the main treatment-emergent psychiatric problem with LEV [129]. However, it was not more common in learning disabled patients as compared to the general population, suggesting that patients with learning disabilities are not generally more prone to develop psychiatric reactions of AEDs. However, in this special population of patients, specific phenomena such as the "release phenomenon" have to be considered [132]. This condition occurs when a patient who has been disabled by frequent seizures suddenly become seizure free without being sedated. As a consequence, these patients may have an increased propensity to misbehave (Fig. 18.3).

Positive Effects

An emerging theme that unifies epilepsy and primary psychiatric disorders is altered neuronal excitability, caused by abnormal expression and function of membrane ion channels [133]. For this reason, AEDs may be effective in the treatment of such conditions. Indeed, the European Medicines Agency (EMA) has approved the use of PGB in generalized anxiety disorder, while both the EMA and the Food and Drug Administration (FDA) have approved the use of CBZ, LTG, and VPA in bipolar disorders, although in different phases. Interestingly enough, all these AEDs are channel modulators. However, TPM and OXC, which are also sodium channel modulators, have failed to demonstrate efficacy in bipolar disorders. In fact, despite initial reports suggesting that TPM can be effective in bipolar and post-traumatic stress disorders, randomized controlled trials failed to demonstrate its superiority compared to placebo [134–137]. Promising data, although still preliminary, suggest some efficacy in obsessive-compulsive disorder [5] and eating disorders [89]. For OXC, initially, small, underpowered, and uncontrolled studies suggested that OXC may be useful in the acute treatment of mania, but conclusive evidence is lacking [49]. A randomized, double-blind, placebo-controlled trial in young patients with mania failed to detect significant differences between OXC and placebo [138]. Whether OXC is effective in the acute treatment of bipolar depression or the maintenance treatment of bipolar disorder is still undetermined [49, 139, 140]. The fact that OXC lacks positive psychotropic effects in comparison to its first-generation predecessor CBZ casts some doubts on the hypothesis that sodium channel blockade is a decisive factor for mood stabilization. On the other hand, preliminary evidence suggests that OXC may exert beneficial effects on behavioral disorders, particularly impulsive aggression [128].

Mood Stabilization Effects: Aggressiveness and Impulse Control

Sodium Valproate

Although its primary mechanism of action is yet to be identified, evidence exists that VPA raises brain levels of GABA. This may occur by acting at different stages of the metabolism of GABA: (1) inhibition of GABA transaminase, (2) inhibition of succinic semialdehyde dehydrogenase, and (3) activation of glutamic acid decarboxylase [141]. It should be noted, however, that other mechanisms have been linked to VPA, such as inhibition of glutamatergic neurotransmission, inhibition of T-type calcium currents, and, possibly, blockade of voltage-gated sodium channels [142]. VPA has also been shown to exert epigenetic effects by inhibiting histone deacetylase activity [143]. Overall, each of these mechanisms could contribute to its psychotropic properties.

VPA is an effective mood stabilizer and is approved by the FDA and EMA for the treatment of acute mania and mixed episodes [49]. Meta-analyses show that VPA is as effective as lithium in the treatment of acute mania [144] or acute depression [145] in bipolar disorders. In addition, VPA is effective in patients who do not respond to lithium, with a more rapid antimanic effect than lithium and therapeutic benefit within 3–5 days [146]. Although it has no maintenance indication in bipolar disorder, there is support for its use as a first-line agent for maintenance treatment as well [147, 148]. A recent Cochrane review of the role of VPA as maintenance treatment analyzed data from six randomized controlled trials ($n = 876$) and concluded that VPA was more effective than placebo in preventing study withdrawal due to any mood episode (RR 0.68, 95 % CI 0.49–0.93; number needed to treat for additional beneficial outcome = 8), but no difference in efficacy was found between VPA and lithium (RR 1.02, 95 % CI 0.87–1.20). However, VPA was well tolerated and associated with fewer participants dropping out of treatment for any cause when compared with placebo or lithium (RR 0.82, 95 % CI 0.71–0.95 and RR 0.87, 95 % CI 0.77–0.98, respectively). VPA also has beneficial effects on several behavioral problems, such as hostility, impulsivity, and aggression, which may arise in different clinical contexts [149].

Carbamazepine

CBZ is the prototypical sodium-channel blocking AED, and is approved by both the FDA and EMA for the treatment of acute manic and mixed episodes of bipolar I disorder [150]. In two multicenter, randomized, double-blind, placebo-controlled trials, 443 bipolar disorder patients with manic or mixed episodes were randomized to a flexible-dose (200–1600 mg/day) extended-release CBZ ($n = 225$) or placebo ($n = 220$) for a 3-week period [151, 152]. In both studies, the improvement in the Young Mania Rating Scale score (the primary efficacy end point) was greater with CBZ treatment than with placebo (first study, $p = 0.032$; second study, $p < 0.001$), and the CBZ arm had a higher responder rate compared to the placebo arm (52 % v 26 %, $p < 0.05$). CBZ also appears to be effective for maintenance treatment of bipolar disorder [49], although to a lesser extent when compared to lithium [153, 154]. CBZ seems to be a better alternative for atypical manifestations of bipolar disorder, such as rapid cycling course, mood-incongruent delusions, or other comorbid psychiatric/neurologic conditions [155]. CBZ may also be effective in unipolar depression [156], whereas its utility in schizophrenia is still uncertain [157].

Lamotrigine

LTG has indirect antiglutamatergic effects by acting at voltage-gated sodium channels to stabilize neuronal membranes and glutamate release [158, 159]. LTG has also been shown to modulate calcium conductance involved in the release of excitatory amino acids in the cortico-striatal pathway [160], and to affect potassium conductance [161]. It may also increase the production of kynurenic acid, an endogenous antagonist at the glycine binding site on the NMDA receptor [162]. Support for the use of LTG is most robust in the maintenance treatment of bipolar disorder in order to prevent the occurrence of mood episodes [163], and indeed it is licensed for this by both the FDA and EMA. However, LTG appears to be more effective in preventing the relapse of depression than mania or hypomania [164]. A pooled analysis ($n = 638$) of two randomized controlled trials demonstrated significantly increased time to intervention for a mood episode in LTG versus placebo ($p<0.001$) as well as lithium versus placebo ($p<0.001$), with no statistical difference between LTG and lithium monotherapy. However, the trial also demonstrated that LTG, but not lithium, was superior to placebo at prolonging time to intervention for a depressive episode (LTG, $p=0.009$; lithium, $p=0.120$). Notably, both LTG and lithium were statistically superior to placebo at prolonging the time to intervention for a manic, hypomanic, or mixed episode: median survival placebo, 86 days (95 % CI, 58–121); lithium, 184 days (95 % CI, 119–not calculable); and LTG, 197 days (95 % CI, 144–388), though lithium was superior to LTG ($p=0.030$). Although LTG is not FDA approved for the treatment of acute bipolar depression, there is some evidence to support a role in this context. A meta-analysis of individual patient data [165] ($n=1072$) from 5 randomized controlled trials demonstrated that LTG was better than placebo on several depression indices. On exploratory subgroup analysis, with groups divided by severity based on baseline depression scores, LTG was better than placebo only in individuals with more severe depressive symptoms at randomization. LTG seems to be effective in unipolar depression [166], at least in patients with epilepsy [167], whereas its usefulness in schizophrenia is still uncertain [168, 169]. LTG has also been shown to have beneficial effects on impulsivity and aggression [170, 171]. Interestingly, a paradoxical effect on such a direction has been described in patients with epilepsy and learning disabilities [172].

Phenytoin

PHT is an established AED with a robust capacity to bind to, and prolong the inactivation of, mammalian, voltage-gated sodium channels. Small randomized studies suggest that PHT may be useful in the treatment of bipolar disorder (acute therapy for manic episodes [173] and maintenance treatment [174]), major depressive disorder [175], and impulsive aggression [176]. However, larger studies are needed to confirm the effectiveness of PHT in these conditions.

Anxiety

Different drug groups have been successfully used in anxiety disorders but selective serotonin reuptake inhibitors (SSRIs) and serotonin noradrenalin reuptake inhibitors (SNRIs) still represent the gold standard for long-term treatment [177]. The role of GABAergic drugs in this scenario is of interest. Benzodiazepines represent the gold standard for the acute treatment because they have the advantage of a rapid onset of action. However, the long-term use can be complicated by the abuse liability, dependence, and withdrawal risk if they are not tapered properly. Interestingly enough, classic GABAergic AEDs showed not also to be ineffective in the long-term treatment of anxiety disorders, but, in some selected cases, showed even deleterious effects [178]. Although this may appear contradictory, it is probably due to the still limited insight in GABAergic neurotransmission.

At the moment, calcium channel blockers represent an emerging class of compounds that showed potential benefits in anxiety disorders. In reality, the use of this class of drugs is not completely original considering that older agents globally reduce widespread activating pathways.

Gabapentin

GBP modulates calcium currents by binding to the α_2-δ subunit of voltage-gated calcium channels [1]. In a double-blind, placebo-controlled, parallel-group trial, 69 patients with social phobia were randomized to flexible-dose (900–3600 mg/day) GBP ($n=34$) or placebo ($n=35$) for 14 weeks [179]. Compared to placebo, GBP was associated with a significant improvement in a number of measures such as the Liebowitz Social Anxiety Scale, the Brief Social Phobia Scale, and the Social Phobia Inventory. Initial open-label studies suggested that GBP could be effective in the treatment of bipolar disorder [49]. However, a randomized, double-blind, placebo-controlled, add-on trial failed to demonstrate the superiority of GBP over placebo in the acute therapy of mania [180]. Similar results were obtained in patients with refractory bipolar or unipolar mood disorders [181]. A small, randomized, double-blind, placebo-controlled trial suggested that adjunctive GBP may be useful in maintenance treatment of bipolar disorder [182], but larger studies are needed. As previously described for other AEDs, GBP showed a paradoxical effect in children and patients with severe intellectual disabilities with the occurrence of hyperactivity and aggression [183, 184].

Pregabalin

Similarly to GBP, PGB is a ligand for α_2-δ subunit of voltage-gated calcium channels. Several randomized, double-blind, placebo-controlled trials have found that PGB is effective in generalized anxiety disorder and social anxiety disorder, and it has been licensed by the EMA for use in the former condition [185–188]. Furthermore, studies comparing PGB to benzodiazepines [189], and to venlafaxine [190], in the acute and long-term treatment of anxiety, respectively, have demonstrated its efficacy. Other controlled studies suggest that PGB may be effective in the amelioration of comorbid depressive symptoms [191], especially in elderly subjects with generalized anxiety disorder [192]. In one study, 273 elderly patients with generalized anxiety disorder were randomized in a 2:1 ratio to flexible-dose (150–600 mg/day) PGB ($n=177$) or placebo ($n=96$) for 8 weeks [185]. PGB was associated with a greater improvement, starting in the 2nd week of treatment, in the Hamilton Rating Scale for Anxiety (HRSA) total scores as compared to placebo ($p<0.05$). Greater improvements were also found in the HRSA psychic and somatic anxiety factors and in the Hamilton Rating Scale for Depression total scores. Finally, the long-term efficacy of PGB in the treatment of generalized anxiety disorder has also been demonstrated [193]. Although a few reports suggest that PGB may be effective in other mood disorders [194, 195], evidence from randomized controlled trials is lacking. In patients with epilepsy, PGB does not appear to have significant negative effects on mood or behavior [196], although, again, depression has been reported in some patients [197].

Limitations of Current Literature

At this point it is important to emphasize that available data on psychotropic effects of AEDs in patients with epilepsy suffer from a number of methodological limitations. Many observations come from case reports or uncontrolled studies, and this limitation may be compounded by a lack of rigor in the definition and measurement of psychiatric events. Because psychiatric symptoms can be related to the epilepsy itself rather than to its treatment, establishing cause-effect relationships can be problematic. Data from controlled trials also suffer a number of limitations such as (1) the frequent use of an add-on design, so that any psychotropic effect could be attributable to pharmacodynamic or pharmacokinetic drug interactions; (2) the use of fixed doses and titration schedules, which often differ from those most commonly applied in clinical practice; (3) the exclusion of patients with comorbid psychiatric disorders and other high risk groups; (4) the follow-up period is often not sufficient to detect effects with a late onset; and (5) the lack of a standardized assessment. Indeed, the fact that data on the psychotropic effects of AEDs in epilepsy come from very heterogeneous sources (i.e., case reports, retrospective surveys, observational studies, controlled clinical trials with different designs and outcome measures) limits the ability to draw conclusions about the comparative effects of individual compounds. However, it seems evident that treatment-emergent psychiatric adverse events are more frequent in patients with epilepsy as compared to psychiatric disorders.

References

1. Mula M. New antiepileptic drugs: molecular targets. Cent Nerv Syst Agents Med Chem. 2009;9(2):79–86.
2. Johannessen Landmark C, Johannessen SI. Pharmacological management of epilepsy: recent advances and future prospects. Drugs. 2008;68(14):1925–39.
3. Perucca P, Carter J, Vahle V, Gilliam FG. Adverse antiepileptic drug effects: toward a clinically and neurobiologically relevant taxonomy. Neurology. 2009;72(14):1223–9.
4. Ettinger AB. Psychotropic effects of antiepileptic drugs. Neurology. 2006;67(11):1916–25.
5. Mula M, Pini S, Cassano GB. The role of anticonvulsant drugs in anxiety disorders: a critical review of the evidence. J Clin Psychopharmacol. 2007;27(3):263–72.
6. Spina E, Perugi G. Antiepileptic drugs: indications other than epilepsy. Epileptic Disord Int Epilepsy J Videotape. 2004;6(2):57–75.
7. Mula M, Sander JW. Negative effects of antiepileptic drugs on mood in patients with epilepsy. Drug Saf. 2007;30(7):555–67.

8. White HS, Smith MD, Wilcox KS. Mechanisms of action of antiepileptic drugs. Int Rev Neurobiol. 2007;81:85–110.
9. Ketter TA, Post RM, Theodore WH. Positive and negative psychiatric effects of antiepileptic drugs in patients with seizure disorders. Neurology. 1999;53(5 Suppl 2):S53–67.
10. Sanacora G, Saricicek A. GABAergic contributions to the pathophysiology of depression and the mechanism of antidepressant action. CNS Neurol Disord Drug Targets. 2007;6(2):127–40.
11. Comai S, Tau M, Gobbi G. The psychopharmacology of aggressive behavior: a translational approach: part 1: neurobiology. J Clin Psychopharmacol. 2012;32(1):83–94.
12. Loring DW, Marino S, Meador KJ. Neuropsychological and behavioral effects of antiepilepsy drugs. Neuropsychol Rev. 2007;17(4):413–25.
13. Hauser P, Devinsky O, De Bellis M, Theodore WH, Post RM. Benzodiazepine withdrawal delirium with catatonic features. Occurrence in patients with partial seizure disorders. Arch Neurol. 1989;46(6):696–9.
14. Olajide D, Lader M. Depression following withdrawal from long-term benzodiazepine use: a report of four cases. Psychol Med. 1984;14(4):937–40.
15. Sheline YI. Hippocampal atrophy in major depression: a result of depression-induced neurotoxicity? Mol Psychiatry. 1996;1(4):298–9.
16. Sapolsky RM. Glucocorticoids and hippocampal atrophy in neuropsychiatric disorders. Arch Gen Psychiatry. 2000;57(10):925–35.
17. Kendell SF, Krystal JH, Sanacora G. GABA and glutamate systems as therapeutic targets in depression and mood disorders. Expert Opin Ther Targets. 2005;9(1):153–68.
18. Bagley J, Moghaddam B. Temporal dynamics of glutamate efflux in the prefrontal cortex and in the hippocampus following repeated stress: effects of pretreatment with saline or diazepam. Neuroscience. 1997;77(1):65–73.
19. Nowak G, Ordway GA, Paul IA. Alterations in the N-methyl-D-aspartate (NMDA) receptor complex in the frontal cortex of suicide victims. Brain Res. 1995;675(1–2):157–64.
20. Bartanusz V, Aubry JM, Pagliusi S, Jezova D, Baffi J, Kiss JZ. Stress-induced changes in messenger RNA levels of N-methyl-D-aspartate and AMPA receptor subunits in selected regions of the rat hippocampus and hypothalamus. Neuroscience. 1995;66(2):247–52.
21. Altamura CA, Mauri MC, Ferrara A, Moro AR, D'Andrea G, Zamberlan F. Plasma and platelet excitatory amino acids in psychiatric disorders. Am J Psychiatry. 1993;150(11):1731–3.
22. Mauri MC, Ferrara A, Boscati L, Bravin S, Zamberlan F, Alecci M, et al. Plasma and platelet amino acid concentrations in patients affected by major depression and under fluvoxamine treatment. Neuropsychobiology. 1998;37(3):124–9.
23. Lerer B, Macciardi F. Pharmacogenetics of antidepressant and mood-stabilizing drugs: a review of candidate-gene studies and future research directions. Int J Neuropsychopharmacol Off Sci J Coll Int Neuropsychopharmacol CINP. 2002;5(3):255–75.
24. Vawter MP, Freed WJ, Kleinman JE. Neuropathology of bipolar disorder. Biol Psychiatry. 2000;48(6):486–504.
25. Naylor GJ, McNamee HB, Moody JP. Changes in erythrocyte sodium and potassium on recovery from a depressive illness. Br J Psychiatry. 1971;118(543):219–23.
26. Mendels J, Frazer A. Alterations in cell membrane activity in depression. Am J Psychiatry. 1974;131(11):1240–6.
27. El-Mallakh RS, Huff MO. Mood stabilizers and ion regulation. Harv Rev Psychiatry. 2001;9(1):23–32.
28. Farber NB, Jiang X-P, Heinkel C, Nemmers B. Antiepileptic drugs and agents that inhibit voltage-gated sodium channels prevent NMDA antagonist neurotoxicity. Mol Psychiatry. 2002;7(7):726–33.
29. Bhat S, Dao DT, Terrillion CE, Arad M, Smith RJ, Soldatov NM, et al. CACNA1C (Cav1.2) in the pathophysiology of psychiatric disease. Prog Neurobiol. 2012;99(1):1–14.
30. Mogilnicka E, Czyrak A, Maj J. Dihydropyridine calcium channel antagonists reduce immobility in the mouse behavioral despair test; antidepressants facilitate nifedipine action. Eur J Pharmacol. 1987;138(3):413–6.

31. Galeotti N, Bartolini A, Ghelardini C. Blockade of intracellular calcium release induces an antidepressant-like effect in the mouse forced swimming test. Neuropharmacology. 2006;50(3):309–16.
32. Sinnegger-Brauns MJ, Hetzenauer A, Huber IG, Renström E, Wietzorrek G, Berjukov S, et al. Isoform-specific regulation of mood behavior and pancreatic beta cell and cardiovascular function by L-type Ca^{2+} channels. J Clin Invest. 2004;113(10):1430–9.
33. Dooley DJ, Mieske CA, Borosky SA. Inhibition of K(+)-evoked glutamate release from rat neocortical and hippocampal slices by gabapentin. Neurosci Lett. 2000;280(2):107–10.
34. Quintero JE, Dooley DJ, Pomerleau F, Huettl P, Gerhardt GA. Amperometric measurement of glutamate release modulation by gabapentin and pregabalin in rat neocortical slices: role of voltage-sensitive Ca^{2+} $\alpha 2\delta$-1 subunit. J Pharmacol Exp Ther. 2011;338(1):240–5.
35. Kupfer DJ, Frank E, Phillips ML. Major depressive disorder: new clinical, neurobiological, and treatment perspectives. Lancet. 2012;379(9820):1045–55.
36. Schloss P, Williams DC. The serotonin transporter: a primary target for antidepressant drugs. J Psychopharmacol Oxf Engl. 1998;12(2):115–21.
37. Whitton PS, Oresković D, Jernej B, Bulat M. Effect of valproic acid on 5-hydroxytryptamine turnover in mouse brain. J Pharm Pharmacol. 1985;37(3):199–200.
38. Dailey JW, Reith ME, Yan QS, Li MY, Jobe PC. Carbamazepine increases extracellular serotonin concentration: lack of antagonism by tetrodotoxin or zero Ca^{2+}. Eur J Pharmacol. 1997;328(2–3):153–62.
39. Clinckers R, Smolders I, Meurs A, Ebinger G, Michotte Y. Hippocampal dopamine and serotonin elevations as pharmacodynamic markers for the anticonvulsant efficacy of oxcarbazepine and 10,11-dihydro-10-hydroxycarbamazepine. Neurosci Lett. 2005;390(1):48–53.
40. Yamamura S, Hamaguchi T, Ohoyama K, Sugiura Y, Suzuki D, Kanehara S, et al. Topiramate and zonisamide prevent paradoxical intoxication induced by carbamazepine and phenytoin. Epilepsy Res. 2009;84(2–3):172–86.
41. Okada M, Hirano T, Kawata Y, Murakami T, Wada K, Mizuno K, et al. Biphasic effects of zonisamide on serotonergic system in rat hippocampus. Epilepsy Res. 1999;34(2–3): 187–97.
42. Southam E, Kirkby D, Higgins GA, Hagan RM. Lamotrigine inhibits monoamine uptake in vitro and modulates 5-hydroxytryptamine uptake in rats. Eur J Pharmacol. 1998;358(1):19–24.
43. Diehl DJ, Gershon S. The role of dopamine in mood disorders. Compr Psychiatry. 1992;33(2):115–20.
44. Brown AS, Gershon S. Dopamine and depression. J Neural Transm Gen Sect. 1993;91(2–3):75–109.
45. Nutt DJ. The role of dopamine and norepinephrine in depression and antidepressant treatment. J Clin Psychiatry. 2006;67 Suppl 6:3–8.
46. Löscher W, Hönack D. Valproate and its major metabolite E-2-en-valproate induce different effects on behaviour and brain monoamine metabolism in rats. Eur J Pharmacol. 1996;299(1–3):61–7.
47. Okada M, Kaneko S, Hirano T, Mizuno K, Kondo T, Otani K, et al. Effects of zonisamide on dopaminergic system. Epilepsy Res. 1995;22(3):193–205.
48. Rogawski MA, Löscher W. The neurobiology of antiepileptic drugs for the treatment of non-epileptic conditions. Nat Med. 2004;10(7):685–92.
49. Grunze HCR. Anticonvulsants in bipolar disorder. J Ment Health Abingdon Engl. 2010;19(2):127–41.
50. Landolt H. Serial EEG investigations during psychotic episodes in epileptic patients and during schizophrenic attacks. In: Lorenz de Haas AM, editor. Lectures on Epilepsia. Amsterdam: Elsevier; 1958. p. 91–133.
51. Trimble MR, Schimtz B. Forced normalization and alternative psychoses of epilepsy. Petersfield: Wrightson Biomedical Publishing Ltd.; 1998.
52. Gibbs FA. Ictal and non-ictal psychiatric disorders in temporal lobe epilepsy. J Nerv Ment Dis. 1951;113(6):522–8.

53. Tellenbach H. Epilepsy as a convulsive disorder and as a psychosis. on alternative psychoses of paranoid nature in 'forced normlization' (Landolt) of the electroencephalogram of epileptics. Nervenarzt. 1965;36:190–202.
54. Krishnamoorthy ES, Trimble MR, Sander JWAS, Kanner AM. Forced normalization at the interface between epilepsy and psychiatry. Epilepsy Behav. 2002;3(4):303–8.
55. Seethalakshmi R, Krishnamoorthy ES. The complex relationship between seizures and behavior: an illustrative case report. Epilepsy Behav. 2007;10(1):203–5.
56. Gatzonis SD, Stamboulis E, Siafakas A, Angelopoulos E, Georgaculias N, Sigounas E, et al. Acute psychosis and EEG normalisation after vagus nerve stimulation. J Neurol Neurosurg Psychiatry. 2000;69(2):278–9.
57. Krishnamoorthy ES, Trimble MR. Forced normalization: clinical and therapeutic relevance. Epilepsia. 1999;40 Suppl 10:S57–64.
58. Wolf P. Acute behavioural symptomatology at disappearance of epileptiform EEG abnormality: paradoxical or forced normalization. In: Smith D, Treiman D, Trimble MR, editors. Neurobehavioural problems in epilepsy. New York: Raven Press; 1991.
59. Wolf P, Trimble MR. Biological antagonism and epileptic psychosis. Br J Psychiatry J Ment Sci. 1985;146:272–6.
60. Seethalakshmi R, Krishnamoorthy ES. Depression in epilepsy: phenomenology, diagnosis and management. Epileptic Disord Int Epilepsy J Videotape. 2007;9(1):1–10.
61. Gilliam F. The impact of epilepsy on subjective health status. Curr Neurol Neurosci Rep. 2003;3(4):357–62.
62. Harden CL, Maroof DA, Nikolov B, Fowler K, Sperling M, Liporace J, et al. The effect of seizure severity on quality of life in epilepsy. Epilepsy Behav. 2007;11(2):208–11.
63. Turky A, Beavis JM, Thapar AK, Kerr MP. Psychopathology in children and adolescents with epilepsy: an investigation of predictive variables. Epilepsy Behav. 2008;12(1):136–44.
64. Lambert MV, Robertson MM. Depression in epilepsy: etiology, phenomenology, and treatment. Epilepsia. 1999;40 Suppl 10:S21–47.
65. Levinson DF, Devinsky O. Psychiatric adverse events during vigabatrin therapy. Neurology. 1999;53(7):1503–11.
66. Trimble MR, Rüsch N, Betts T, Crawford PM. Psychiatric symptoms after therapy with new antiepileptic drugs: psychopathological and seizure related variables. Seizure. 2000;9(4):249–54.
67. Mula M, Trimble MR, Lhatoo SD, Sander JWAS. Topiramate and psychiatric adverse events in patients with epilepsy. Epilepsia. 2003;44(5):659–63.
68. White JR, Walczak TS, Marino SE, Beniak TE, Leppik IE, Birnbaum AK. Zonisamide discontinuation due to psychiatric and cognitive adverse events: a case-control study. Neurology. 2010;75(6):513–8.
69. Trimble MR. Biological psychiatry. 2nd ed. Chichester: Wiley; 1996.
70. Petty F. GABA and mood disorders: a brief review and hypothesis. J Affect Disord. 1995;34(4):275–81.
71. Rodin EA, Katz M, Lennox K. Differences between patients with temporal lobe seizures and those with other forms of epileptic attacks. Epilepsia. 1976;17(3):313–20.
72. Brent DA, Crumrine PK, Varma RR, Allan M, Allman C. Phenobarbital treatment and major depressive disorder in children with epilepsy. Pediatrics. 1987;80(6):909–17.
73. Lopez-Gomez M, Ramirez-Bermudez J, Campillo C, Sosa AL, Espinola M, Ruiz I. Primidone is associated with interictal depression in patients with epilepsy. Epilepsy Behav. 2005;6(3):413–6.
74. Vining EP, Mellitis ED, Dorsen MM, Cataldo MF, Quaskey SA, Spielberg SP, et al. Psychologic and behavioral effects of antiepileptic drugs in children: a double-blind comparison between phenobarbital and valproic acid. Pediatrics. 1987;80(2):165–74.
75. Ring HA, Crellin R, Kirker S, Reynolds EH. Vigabatrin and depression. J Neurol Neurosurg Psychiatry. 1993;56(8):925–8.
76. Thomas L, Trimble M, Schmitz B, Ring H. Vigabatrin and behaviour disorders: a retrospective survey. Epilepsy Res. 1996;25(1):21–7.

77. Chadwick D. Safety and efficacy of vigabatrin and carbamazepine in newly diagnosed epilepsy: a multicentre randomised double-blind study. Vigabatrin European Monotherapy Study Group. Lancet. 1999;354(9172):13–9.
78. Ferrie CD, Robinson RO, Panayiotopoulos CP. Psychotic and severe behavioural reactions with vigabatrin: a review. Acta Neurol Scand. 1996;93(1):1–8.
79. Martin R, Kuzniecky R, Ho S, Hetherington H, Pan J, Sinclair K, et al. Cognitive effects of topiramate, gabapentin, and lamotrigine in healthy young adults. Neurology. 1999;52(2):321–7.
80. Kuzniecky R, Ho S, Pan J, Martin R, Gilliam F, Faught E, et al. Modulation of cerebral GABA by topiramate, lamotrigine, and gabapentin in healthy adults. Neurology. 2002;58(3):368–72.
81. Mula M, Hesdorffer DC, Trimble M, Sander JW. The role of titration schedule of topiramate for the development of depression in patients with epilepsy. Epilepsia. 2009;50(5):1072–6.
82. Nickel C, Lahmann C, Tritt K, Muehlbacher M, Kaplan P, Kettler C, et al. Topiramate in treatment of depressive and anger symptoms in female depressive patients: a randomized, double-blind, placebo-controlled study. J Affect Disord. 2005;87(2–3):243–52.
83. Mowla A, Kardeh E. Topiramate augmentation in patients with resistant major depressive disorder: a double-blind placebo-controlled clinical trial. Prog Neuropsychopharmacol Biol Psychiatry. 2011;35(4):970–3.
84. Nickel MK, Nickel C, Kaplan P, Lahmann C, Mühlbacher M, Tritt K, et al. Treatment of aggression with topiramate in male borderline patients: a double-blind, placebo-controlled study. Biol Psychiatry. 2005;57(5):495–9.
85. Nickel MK, Nickel C, Mitterlehner FO, Tritt K, Lahmann C, Leiberich PK, et al. Topiramate treatment of aggression in female borderline personality disorder patients: a double-blind, placebo-controlled study. J Clin Psychiatry. 2004;65(11):1515–9.
86. Tiihonen J, Halonen P, Wahlbeck K, Repo-Tiihonen E, Hyvärinen S, Eronen M, et al. Topiramate add-on in treatment-resistant schizophrenia: a randomized, double-blind, placebo-controlled, crossover trial. J Clin Psychiatry. 2005;66(8):1012–5.
87. Afshar H, Roohafza H, Mousavi G, Golchin S, Toghianifar N, Sadeghi M, et al. Topiramate add-on treatment in schizophrenia: a randomised, double-blind, placebo-controlled clinical trial. J Psychopharmacol Oxf Engl. 2009;23(2):157–62.
88. Muscatello MRA, Bruno A, Pandolfo G, Micò U, Bellinghieri PM, Scimeca G, et al. Topiramate augmentation of clozapine in schizophrenia: a double-blind, placebo-controlled study. J Psychopharmacol Oxf Engl. 2011;25(5):667–74.
89. Leombruni P, Lavagnino L, Fassino S. Treatment of obese patients with binge eating disorder using topiramate: a review. Neuropsychiatr Dis Treat. 2009;5:385–92.
90. Mula M, Cavanna AE, Monaco F. Psychopharmacology of topiramate: from epilepsy to bipolar disorder. Neuropsychiatr Dis Treat. 2006;2(4):475–88.
91. Dodrill CB, Arnett JL, Shu V, Pixton GC, Lenz GT, Sommerville KW. Effects of tiagabine monotherapy on abilities, adjustment, and mood. Epilepsia. 1998;39(1):33–42.
92. Suppes T, Chisholm KA, Dhavale D, Frye MA, Altshuler LL, McElroy SL, et al. Tiagabine in treatment refractory bipolar disorder: a clinical case series. Bipolar Disord. 2002;4(5):283–9.
93. Rosenthal M. Tiagabine for the treatment of generalized anxiety disorder: a randomized, open-label, clinical trial with paroxetine as a positive control. J Clin Psychiatry. 2003;64(10):1245–9.
94. Leppik IE. Tiagabine: the safety landscape. Epilepsia. 1995;36 Suppl 6:S10–3.
95. Wroe SJ. Zonisamide. In: Shorvon S, Perucca E, Engel Jr J, editors. The treatment of epilepsy. 3rd ed. Oxford: Wiley-Blackwell; 2009. p. 713–20.
96. Mimaki T, Suzuki Y, Tagawa T, Karasawa T, Yabuuchi H. [3H]zonisamide binding in rat brain. Med J Osaka Univ. 1990;39(1–4):19–22.
97. Ueda Y, Doi T, Tokumaru J, Willmore LJ. Effect of zonisamide on molecular regulation of glutamate and GABA transporter proteins during epileptogenesis in rats with hippocampal seizures. Brain Res Mol Brain Res. 2003;116(1–2):1–6.

98. Okada M, Kawata Y, Mizuno K, Wada K, Kondo T, Kaneko S. Interaction between Ca^{2+}, K^{+}, carbamazepine and zonisamide on hippocampal extracellular glutamate monitored with a microdialysis electrode. Br J Pharmacol. 1998;124(6):1277–85.
99. Mula M, Trimble MR, Sander JWAS. The role of hippocampal sclerosis in topiramate-related depression and cognitive deficits in people with epilepsy. Epilepsia. 2003;44(12):1573–7.
100. Quiske A, Helmstaedter C, Lux S, Elger CE. Depression in patients with temporal lobe epilepsy is related to mesial temporal sclerosis. Epilepsy Res. 2000;39(2):121–5.
101. Bremner JD, Narayan M, Anderson ER, Staib LH, Miller HL, Charney DS. Hippocampal volume reduction in major depression. Am J Psychiatry. 2000;157(1):115–8.
102. Frodl T, Meisenzahl EM, Zetzsche T, Born C, Groll C, Jäger M, et al. Hippocampal changes in patients with a first episode of major depression. Am J Psychiatry. 2002;159(7):1112–8.
103. Reynolds EH, Travers RD. Serum anticonvulsant concentrations in epileptic patients with mental symptoms. A preliminary report. Br J Psychiatry J Ment Sci. 1974;124:440–5.
104. Sander JW, Patsalos PN. An assessment of serum and red blood cell folate concentrations in patients with epilepsy on lamotrigine therapy. Epilepsy Res. 1992;13(1):89–92.
105. Reynolds EH. Mental effects of antiepileptic medication: a review. Epilepsia. 1983;24 Suppl 2:S85–95.
106. Fischer M, Korskjaer G, Pedersen E. Psychotic episodes in Zarondan treatment. Effects and side-effects in 105 patients. Epilepsia. 1965;6(4):325–34.
107. Roger J, Grangeon H, Gueyj J, Lob H. Psychiatric and psychologic effects of ethosuximide treatment of epileptics. Encéphale. 1968;57(5):407–38.
108. Pakalnis A, Drake ME, John K, Kellum JB. Forced normalization. Acute psychosis after seizure control in seven patients. Arch Neurol. 1987;44(3):289–92.
109. McConnell H, Snyder PJ, Duffy JD, Weilburg J, Valeriano J, Brillman J, et al. Neuropsychiatric side effects related to treatment with felbamate. J Neuropsychiatry Clin Neurosci. 1996;8(3):341–6.
110. Mula M, Trimble MR. The importance of being seizure free: topiramate and psychopathology in epilepsy. Epilepsy Behav. 2003;4(4):430–4.
111. Sander JW, Hart YM, Trimble MR, Shorvon SD. Vigabatrin and psychosis. J Neurol Neurosurg Psychiatry. 1991;54(5):435–9.
112. Kimura S. Zonisamide-induced behavior disorder in two children. Epilepsia. 1994;35(2):403–5.
113. Tsuji M, Hori S, Asai N, Hamanaka T, Ishikawa T, Hiyoshi T, et al. Two epileptics showing antiepileptic drug-induced psychoses. Jpn J Psychiatry Neurol. 1993;47(2):298–9.
114. Brandt C, Fueratsch N, Boehme V, Kramme C, Pieridou M, Villagran A, et al. Development of psychosis in patients with epilepsy treated with lamotrigine: report of six cases and review of the literature. Epilepsy Behav. 2007;11(1):133–9.
115. Sackellares JC, Krauss G, Sommerville KW, Deaton R. Occurrence of psychosis in patients with epilepsy randomized to tiagabine or placebo treatment. Epilepsia. 2002;43(4):394–8.
116. Schapel G, Chadwick D. Tiagabine and non-convulsive status epilepticus. Seizure. 1996;5(2):153–6.
117. Trimble MR. New antiepileptic drugs and psychopathology. Neuropsychobiology. 1998;38(3):149–51.
118. Schmitz B. Psychiatric syndromes related to antiepileptic drugs. Epilepsia. 1999;40 Suppl 10:S65–70.
119. Pal DK. Phenobarbital for childhood epilepsy: systematic review. Paediatr Perinat Drug Ther. 2006;7(1):31–42.
120. Pal DK, Das T, Chaudhury G, Johnson AL, Neville BG. Randomised controlled trial to assess acceptability of phenobarbital for childhood epilepsy in rural India. Lancet. 1998;351(9095):19–23.
121. Bhaumik S, Branford D, Duggirala C, Ismail IA. A naturalistic study of the use of vigabatrin, lamotrigine and gabapentin in adults with learning disabilities. Seizure. 1997;6(2):127–33.
122. White JR, Walczak TS, Leppik IE, Rarick J, Tran T, Beniak TE, et al. Discontinuation of levetiracetam because of behavioral side effects: a case-control study. Neurology. 2003;61(9):1218–21.

123. Lynch BA, Lambeng N, Nocka K, Kensel-Hammes P, Bajjalieh SM, Matagne A, et al. The synaptic vesicle protein SV2A is the binding site for the antiepileptic drug levetiracetam. Proc Natl Acad Sci U S A. 2004;101(26):9861–6.
124. Muralidharan A, Bhagwagar Z. Potential of levetiracetam in mood disorders: a preliminary review. CNS Drugs. 2006;20(12):969–79.
125. Zhang W, Connor KM, Davidson JRT. Levetiracetam in social phobia: a placebo controlled pilot study. J Psychopharmacol Oxf Engl. 2005;19(5):551–3.
126. Saricicek A, Maloney K, Muralidharan A, Ruf B, Blumberg HP, Sanacora G, et al. Levetiracetam in the management of bipolar depression: a randomized, double-blind, placebo-controlled trial. J Clin Psychiatry. 2011;72(6):744–50.
127. Stein MB, Ravindran LN, Simon NM, Liebowitz MR, Khan A, Brawman-Mintzer O, et al. Levetiracetam in generalized social anxiety disorder: a double-blind, randomized controlled trial. J Clin Psychiatry. 2010;71(5):627–31.
128. Mattes JA. Levetiracetam in patients with impulsive aggression: a double-blind, placebo-controlled trial. J Clin Psychiatry. 2008;69(2):310–5.
129. Mula M, Trimble MR, Yuen A, Liu RSN, Sander JWAS. Psychiatric adverse events during levetiracetam therapy. Neurology. 2003;61(5):704–6.
130. Helmstaedter C, Mihov Y, Toliat MR, Thiele H, Nuernberg P, Schoch S, et al. Genetic variation in dopaminergic activity is associated with the risk for psychiatric side effects of levetiracetam. Epilepsia. 2013;54(1):36–44.
131. Lhatoo SD, Sander JW. The epidemiology of epilepsy and learning disability. Epilepsia. 2001;42 Suppl 1:6–9; discussion 19–20.
132. Besag FMC. Behavioural effects of the newer antiepileptic drugs: an update. Expert Opin Drug Saf. 2004;3(1):1–8.
133. Mantegazza M, Curia G, Biagini G, Ragsdale DS, Avoli M. Voltage-gated sodium channels as therapeutic targets in epilepsy and other neurological disorders. Lancet Neurol. 2010;9(4):413–24.
134. Delbello MP, Findling RL, Kushner S, Wang D, Olson WH, Capece JA, et al. A pilot controlled trial of topiramate for mania in children and adolescents with bipolar disorder. J Am Acad Child Adolesc Psychiatry. 2005;44(6):539–47.
135. Roy Chengappa KN, Schwarzman LK, Hulihan JF, Xiang J, Rosenthal NR, Clinical Affairs Product Support Study-168 Investigators. Adjunctive topiramate therapy in patients receiving a mood stabilizer for bipolar I disorder: a randomized, placebo-controlled trial. J Clin Psychiatry. 2006;67(11):1698–706.
136. Lindley SE, Carlson EB, Hill K. A randomized, double-blind, placebo-controlled trial of augmentation topiramate for chronic combat-related posttraumatic stress disorder. J Clin Psychopharmacol. 2007;27(6):677–81.
137. Tucker P, Trautman RP, Wyatt DB, Thompson J, Wu S-C, Capece JA, et al. Efficacy and safety of topiramate monotherapy in civilian posttraumatic stress disorder: a randomized, double-blind, placebo-controlled study. J Clin Psychiatry. 2007;68(2):201–6.
138. Wagner KD, Kowatch RA, Emslie GJ, Findling RL, Wilens TE, McCague K, et al. A double-blind, randomized, placebo-controlled trial of oxcarbazepine in the treatment of bipolar disorder in children and adolescents. Am J Psychiatry. 2006;163(7):1179–86.
139. Vasudev A, Macritchie K, Watson S, Geddes JR, Young AH. Oxcarbazepine in the maintenance treatment of bipolar disorder. Cochrane Database Syst Rev. 2008;(1):CD005171.
140. Vasudev A, Macritchie K, Vasudev K, Watson S, Geddes J, Young AH. Oxcarbazepine for acute affective episodes in bipolar disorder. Cochrane Database Syst Rev. 2011;(12):CD004857.
141. Bourgeois BFD. Valproate. In: Shorvon S, Perucca E, Engel Jr J, editors. The treatment of epilepsy. 3rd ed. Chichester: Wiley-Blackwell; 2009. p. 685–98.
142. Kelly KM, Gross RA, Macdonald RL. Valproic acid selectively reduces the low-threshold (T) calcium current in rat nodose neurons. Neurosci Lett. 1990;116(1–2):233–8.
143. Machado-Vieira R, Ibrahim L, Zarate CA. Histone deacetylases and mood disorders: epigenetic programming in gene-environment interactions. CNS Neurosci Ther. 2011;17(6): 699–704.

144. Macritchie K, Geddes J, Scott J, Haslam DR, Silva de Lima M, Goodwin G. Valproate for acute mood episodes in bipolar disorder. In: The Cochrane Collaboration, editor. Cochrane Database Syst Rev [Internet]. Chichester: Wiley; 2003 [Cited 28 Jan 2015]. Available from: http://doi.wiley.com/10.1002/14651858.CD004052.
145. Smith LA, Cornelius VR, Azorin JM, Perugi G, Vieta E, Young AH, et al. Valproate for the treatment of acute bipolar depression: systematic review and meta-analysis. J Affect Disord. 2010;122(1–2):1–9.
146. Bowden CL, Swann AC, Calabrese JR, Rubenfaer LM, Wozniak PJ, Collins MA, et al. A randomized, placebo-controlled, multicenter study of divalproex sodium extended release in the treatment of acute mania. J Clin Psychiatry. 2006;67(10):1501–10.
147. Gyulai L, Bowden CL, McElroy SL, Calabrese JR, Petty F, Swann AC, et al. Maintenance efficacy of divalproex in the prevention of bipolar depression. Neuropsychopharmacol Off Publ Am Coll Neuropsychopharmacol. 2003;28(7):1374–82.
148. Bond DJ, Lam RW, Yatham LN. Divalproex sodium versus placebo in the treatment of acute bipolar depression: a systematic review and meta-analysis. J Affect Disord. 2010;124(3):228–34.
149. Lindenmayer JP, Kotsaftis A. Use of sodium valproate in violent and aggressive behaviors: a critical review. J Clin Psychiatry. 2000;61(2):123–8.
150. Post RM, Ketter TA, Uhde T, Ballenger JC. Thirty years of clinical experience with carbamazepine in the treatment of bipolar illness: principles and practice. CNS Drugs. 2007;21(1):47–71.
151. Weisler RH, Kalali AH, Ketter TA, SPD417 Study Group. A multicenter, randomized, double-blind, placebo-controlled trial of extended-release carbamazepine capsules as monotherapy for bipolar disorder patients with manic or mixed episodes. J Clin Psychiatry. 2004;65(4):478–84.
152. Weisler RH, Keck PE, Swann AC, Cutler AJ, Ketter TA, Kalali AH, et al. Extended-release carbamazepine capsules as monotherapy for acute mania in bipolar disorder: a multicenter, randomized, double-blind, placebo-controlled trial. J Clin Psychiatry. 2005;66(3):323–30.
153. Greil W, Ludwig-Mayerhofer W, Erazo N, Schöchlin C, Schmidt S, Engel RR, et al. Lithium versus carbamazepine in the maintenance treatment of bipolar disorders – a randomised study. J Affect Disord. 1997;43(2):151–61.
154. Hartong EGTM, Moleman P, Hoogduin CAL, Broekman TG, Nolen WA, LitCar Group. Prophylactic efficacy of lithium versus carbamazepine in treatment-naive bipolar patients. J Clin Psychiatry. 2003;64(2):144–51.
155. Greil W, Kleindienst N, Erazo N, Müller-Oerlinghausen B. Differential response to lithium and carbamazepine in the prophylaxis of bipolar disorder. J Clin Psychopharmacol. 1998;18(6):455–60.
156. Zhang Z-J, Tan Q-R, Tong Y, Li Q, Kang W-H, Zhen X-C, et al. The effectiveness of carbamazepine in unipolar depression: a double-blind, randomized, placebo-controlled study. J Affect Disord. 2008;109(1–2):91–7.
157. Leucht S, Kissling W, McGrath J, White P. Carbamazepine for schizophrenia. Cochrane Database Syst Rev. 2007;(3):CD001258.
158. Cunningham MO, Jones RS. The anticonvulsant, lamotrigine decreases spontaneous glutamate release but increases spontaneous GABA release in the rat entorhinal cortex in vitro. Neuropharmacology. 2000;39(11):2139–46.
159. Meldrum BS. Lamotrigine – a novel approach. Seizure. 1994;3(Suppl A):41–5.
160. Wang SJ, Sihra TS, Gean PW. Lamotrigine inhibition of glutamate release from isolated cerebrocortical nerve terminals (synaptosomes) by suppression of voltage-activated calcium channel activity. Neuroreport. 2001;12(10):2255–8.
161. Zona C, Tancredi V, Longone P, D'Arcangelo G, D'Antuono M, Manfredi M, et al. Neocortical potassium currents are enhanced by the antiepileptic drug lamotrigine. Epilepsia. 2002;43(7):685–90.
162. Kocki T, Wielosz M, Turski WA, Urbanska EM. Enhancement of brain kynurenic acid production by anticonvulsants--novel mechanism of antiepileptic activity? Eur J Pharmacol. 2006;541(3):147–51.

163. Reid JG, Gitlin MJ, Altshuler LL. Lamotrigine in psychiatric disorders. J Clin Psychiatry. 2013;74(7):675–84.
164. Goodwin GM, Bowden CL, Calabrese JR, Grunze H, Kasper S, White R, et al. A pooled analysis of 2 placebo-controlled 18-month trials of lamotrigine and lithium maintenance in bipolar I disorder. J Clin Psychiatry. 2004;65(3):432–41.
165. Geddes JR, Calabrese JR, Goodwin GM. Lamotrigine for treatment of bipolar depression: independent meta-analysis and meta-regression of individual patient data from five randomised trials. Br J Psychiatry. 2009;194(1):4–9.
166. Schindler F, Anghelescu IG. Lithium versus lamotrigine augmentation in treatment resistant unipolar depression: a randomized, open-label study. Int Clin Psychopharmacol. 2007;22(3):179–82.
167. Ettinger AB, Kustra RP, Hammer AE. Effect of lamotrigine on depressive symptoms in adult patients with epilepsy. Epilepsy Behav. 2007;10(1):148–54.
168. Goff DC, Keefe R, Citrome L, Davy K, Krystal JH, Large C, et al. Lamotrigine as add-on therapy in schizophrenia: results of 2 placebo-controlled trials. J Clin Psychopharmacol. 2007;27(6):582–9.
169. Kremer I, Vass A, Gorelik I, Bar G, Blanaru M, Javitt DC, et al. Placebo-controlled trial of lamotrigine added to conventional and atypical antipsychotics in schizophrenia. Biol Psychiatry. 2004;56(6):441–6.
170. Reich DB, Zanarini MC, Bieri KA. A preliminary study of lamotrigine in the treatment of affective instability in borderline personality disorder. Int Clin Psychopharmacol. 2009;24(5): 270–5.
171. Tritt K, Nickel C, Lahmann C, Leiberich PK, Rother WK, Loew TH, et al. Lamotrigine treatment of aggression in female borderline-patients: a randomized, double-blind, placebo-controlled study. J Psychopharmacol Oxf Engl. 2005;19(3):287–91.
172. Beran RG, Gibson RJ. Aggressive behaviour in intellectually challenged patients with epilepsy treated with lamotrigine. Epilepsia. 1998;39(3):280–2.
173. Mishory A, Yaroslavsky Y, Bersudsky Y, Belmaker RH. Phenytoin as an antimanic anticonvulsant: a controlled study. Am J Psychiatry. 2000;157(3):463–5.
174. Mishory A, Winokur M, Bersudsky Y. Prophylactic effect of phenytoin in bipolar disorder: a controlled study. Bipolar Disord. 2003;5(6):464–7.
175. Nemets B, Bersudsky Y, Belmaker RH. Controlled double-blind trial of phenytoin vs. fluoxetine in major depressive disorder. J Clin Psychiatry. 2005;66(5):586–90.
176. Stanford MS, Helfritz LE, Conklin SM, Villemarette-Pittman NR, Greve KW, Adams D, et al. A comparison of anticonvulsants in the treatment of impulsive aggression. Exp Clin Psychopharmacol. 2005;13(1):72–7.
177. Andrews G. The treatment of anxiety disorders: clinician guides and patient manuals. 2nd ed. Cambridge: Cambridge University Press; 2003.
178. Mula M, Trimble MR. Antiepileptic drug-induced cognitive adverse effects: potential mechanisms and contributing factors. CNS Drugs. 2009;23(2):121–37.
179. Pande AC, Davidson JR, Jefferson JW, Janney CA, Katzelnick DJ, Weisler RH, et al. Treatment of social phobia with gabapentin: a placebo-controlled study. J Clin Psychopharmacol. 1999;19(4):341–8.
180. Pande AC, Crockatt JG, Janney CA, Werth JL, Tsaroucha G. Gabapentin in bipolar disorder: a placebo-controlled trial of adjunctive therapy. Gabapentin Bipolar Disorder Study Group. Bipolar Disord. 2000;2(3 Pt 2):249–55.
181. Frye MA, Ketter TA, Kimbrell TA, Dunn RT, Speer AM, Osuch EA, et al. A placebo-controlled study of lamotrigine and gabapentin monotherapy in refractory mood disorders. J Clin Psychopharmacol. 2000;20(6):607–14.
182. Vieta E, Manuel Goikolea J, Martínez-Arán A, Comes M, Verger K, Masramon X, et al. A double-blind, randomized, placebo-controlled, prophylaxis study of adjunctive gabapentin for bipolar disorder. J Clin Psychiatry. 2006;67(3):473–7.
183. Wolf SM, Shinnar S, Kang H, Gil KB, Moshé SL. Gabapentin toxicity in children manifesting as behavioral changes. Epilepsia. 1995;36(12):1203–5.

184. Lee DO, Steingard RJ, Cesena M, Helmers SL, Riviello JJ, Mikati MA. Behavioral side effects of gabapentin in children. Epilepsia. 1996;37(1):87–90.
185. Montgomery S, Chatamra K, Pauer L, Whalen E, Baldinetti F. Efficacy and safety of pregabalin in elderly people with generalised anxiety disorder. Br J Psychiatry. 2008;193(5): 389–94.
186. Kasper S, Herman B, Nivoli G, Van Ameringen M, Petralia A, Mandel FS, et al. Efficacy of pregabalin and venlafaxine-XR in generalized anxiety disorder: results of a double-blind, placebo-controlled 8-week trial. Int Clin Psychopharmacol. 2009;24(2):87–96.
187. Feltner DE, Liu-Dumaw M, Schweizer E, Bielski R. Efficacy of pregabalin in generalized social anxiety disorder: results of a double-blind, placebo-controlled, fixed-dose study. Int Clin Psychopharmacol. 2011;26(4):213–20.
188. Greist JH, Liu-Dumaw M, Schweizer E, Feltner D. Efficacy of pregabalin in preventing relapse in patients with generalized social anxiety disorder: results of a double-blind, placebo-controlled 26-week study. Int Clin Psychopharmacol. 2011;26(5):243–51.
189. Rickels K, Pollack MH, Feltner DE, Lydiard RB, Zimbroff DL, Bielski RJ, et al. Pregabalin for treatment of generalized anxiety disorder: a 4-week, multicenter, double-blind, placebo-controlled trial of pregabalin and alprazolam. Arch Gen Psychiatry. 2005;62(9):1022–30.
190. Montgomery SA, Tobias K, Zornberg GL, Kasper S, Pande AC. Efficacy and safety of pregabalin in the treatment of generalized anxiety disorder: a 6-week, multicenter, randomized, double-blind, placebo-controlled comparison of pregabalin and venlafaxine. J Clin Psychiatry. 2006;67(5):771–82.
191. Stein DJ, Baldwin DS, Baldinetti F, Mandel F. Efficacy of pregabalin in depressive symptoms associated with generalized anxiety disorder: a pooled analysis of 6 studies. Eur Neuropsychopharmacol J Eur Coll Neuropsychopharmacol. 2008;18(6):422–30.
192. Montgomery SA, Herman BK, Schweizer E, Mandel FS. The efficacy of pregabalin and benzodiazepines in generalized anxiety disorder presenting with high levels of insomnia. Int Clin Psychopharmacol. 2009;24(4):214–22.
193. Feltner D, Wittchen H-U, Kavoussi R, Brock J, Baldinetti F, Pande AC. Long-term efficacy of pregabalin in generalized anxiety disorder. Int Clin Psychopharmacol. 2008;23(1):18–28.
194. Englisch S, Esser A, Enning F, Hohmann S, Schanz H, Zink M. Augmentation with pregabalin in schizophrenia. J Clin Psychopharmacol. 2010;30(4):437–40.
195. Showraki M. Pregabalin in the treatment of depression. J Psychopharmacol Oxf Engl. 2007;21(8):883–4.
196. Zaccara G, Gangemi P, Perucca P, Specchio L. The adverse event profile of pregabalin: a systematic review and meta-analysis of randomized controlled trials. Epilepsia. 2011;52(4): 826–36.
197. Yuen AWC, Singh R, Bell GS, Bhattacharjee A, Neligan A, Heaney DC, et al. The long-term retention of pregabalin in a large cohort of patients with epilepsy at a tertiary referral centre. Epilepsy Res. 2009;87(2–3):120–3.

Chapter 19
The Role of Stimulation Techniques

Steven C. Schachter

Abstract Neuropsychiatric symptoms are common, under-recognized, and undertreated in patients with epilepsy (PWE), and have a profound impact on quality of life. Effective, safe, and well-tolerated treatments are urgently needed for patients whose neuropsychiatric symptoms do not respond to pharmacological or behavioral therapies. Some of the brain stimulation modalities that are effective for seizure control in patients with drug-resistant epilepsy may also be effective for neuropsychiatric symptoms of comorbid psychiatric disorders. This chapter first provides an overview of comorbid psychiatric disorders that have shown symptomatic improvement in brain stimulation studies. Next, the effects of different stimulation techniques on symptoms of these psychiatric disorders in PWE as well as in patients without epilepsy are reviewed. Limitations of our current understanding are then outlined with suggested directions for future research. The role of stimulation techniques in the care of PWE is only beginning to be understood and their potential application to the amelioration of neuropsychiatric symptoms in PWE should be actively pursued.

Keywords Neurostimulation • Epilepsy • Depression • Suicidality • Anxiety • Psychosis • Closed-loop

Introduction

For the nearly one in three patients with epilepsy (PWE) who continue to have seizures in spite of taking one or more properly selected and dosed antiepileptic drugs (AEDs) (drug-resistant epilepsy; DRE), physicians may turn to brain stimulation

S.C. Schachter, MD
Departments of Neurology, Consortia for Improving Medicine with Innovation and Technology, Beth Israel Deaconess Medical Center, Massachusetts General Hospital, Harvard Medical School, 125 Nashua Street, Boston, MA 02114, USA
e-mail: sschacht@bidmc.harvard.edu

M. Mula (ed.), *Neuropsychiatric Symptoms of Epilepsy*, Neuropsychiatric Symptoms of Neurological Disease, DOI 10.1007/978-3-319-22159-5_19

techniques. While it may seem paradoxical that stimulating the brain directly or via a peripheral pathway could have an antiepileptic effect [1], the therapeutic benefit of brain stimulation for epilepsy has been firmly established in clinical studies and practice, with many new techniques under evaluation.

During clinical trials of brain stimulation modalities for the treatment of epilepsy, improvement in symptoms of comorbid psychiatric disorders may be incidentally observed, similar to what has occurred in trials of AEDs. These observations have often led to trials of stimulation techniques specifically for those neuropsychiatric symptoms, whether in PWE or in patients with only psychiatric disorders.

A benefit for brain stimulation on both seizures and behavior is not surprising given their many inter-connections, as well as the pervasiveness of psychiatric comorbidities in PWE, which are presumed, at least in part, to arise from shared underlying pathophysiologic mechanisms. There are several possible explanations for an effect of brain stimulation on neuropsychiatric symptoms in PWE. First, the symptoms may improve (or paradoxically worsen) as an indirect effect of improved seizure frequency or severity resulting from stimulation. Second, there may be a direct effect of stimulation on mechanisms relevant to neuropsychiatric symptoms but not to epilepsy. Third, brain stimulation may have a direct effect on cellular or network mechanisms that are relevant to both seizures and neuropsychiatric symptoms.

Neuropsychiatric symptoms are common, under-recognized, and undertreated in PWE. It has been estimated that one of every three PWE will experience mood and/or anxiety symptoms during their life [2]. The causes are multifactorial and include a family history of psychiatric disorders; a personal psychiatric history antedating the onset of epilepsy; neurochemical (serotonin, norepinephrine, glutamate, and gamma-aminobutyric acid), neuroinflammatory, neuroendocrine, and brain structural changes related to epilepsy; psychosocial issues associated with living with epilepsy; and side effects of AEDs [3].

Enhanced clinical recognition and more effective therapies are urgently needed for the neuropsychiatric symptoms of comorbid psychiatric disorders in PWE. This chapter first provides an overview of depression, suicidality, anxiety disorders, and psychosis, which are comorbid with epilepsy and which have been reported to show symptomatic improvement in brain stimulation studies. Next, the specific clinical effects of different stimulation techniques on these psychiatric disorders in PWE as well as in patients without epilepsy will be reviewed. Finally, limitations of our current understanding will be outlined with suggestions for further research.

Specific details about the stimulation techniques such as effects in animal models, surgical implantation (where applicable), safety and tolerability, practical aspects of implementation in the clinic, costs/reimbursement, impact on seizure control, and use in children, as well as personality disorders in epilepsy, use of electroconvulsive therapy, and the differential diagnosis of neuropsychiatric symptoms are beyond the scope of this chapter.

Comorbid Psychiatric Disorders and Related Symptoms as Potential Therapeutic Targets for Brain Stimulation

Depression

Depression is a risk factor for the development of epilepsy and vice versa [4, 5]. Depression occurs more often in PWE than in the general population, affecting 10–20 % of patients with well-controlled epilepsy and up to 60 % of patients with DRE [6, 7]. Risk factors for depression include frequent seizures, symptomatic focal epilepsy, younger age, psychosocial difficulties with learned helplessness, and polypharmacy [8]. Among patients with temporal lobe epilepsy, mesial temporal sclerosis is especially predictive of depression compared to other pathologies.

Depression is often under-recognized and undertreated in PWE. The majority of neurologists may not screen for depression in PWE [9]. Nearly one-third of patients with a lifetime history of major depressive disorder may never receive treatment [10] and for many others, treatment is significantly delayed [11].

Depressive symptoms may occur between seizures (inter-ictal) or before, during or after a seizure [12]. A common inter-ictal presentation is the so-called inter-ictal dysphoric disorder (IDD) [13] or "dysthymic-like disorder of epilepsy" [14]. Symptoms are typically independent of seizures, occur intermittently with abrupt onset and offset, and include irritability, depressed or euphoric moods, anergia, insomnia, atypical pains, anxiety, and fears.

A dysphoric mood, sometimes accompanied by aggressive behavior, may precede a seizure by hours or days [15] and be terminated by the seizure. Ictal depression, typically anhedonia, guilt, or suicidal ideation (SI), may manifest as the only ictal symptom, or be followed by a complex partial seizure. Post-ictal depressive symptoms may be severe, including SI, and occur in up to 43 % of patients with partial seizures, often persisting for hours to several days [12].

Severe depressive symptoms may become manifest as seizure control or EEG abnormalities improve through epilepsy treatment [16, 17]. Landolt [18] originally described the development of severe mood changes or psychosis in the setting of normalization of the EEG, leading to the term "forced normalization." Tellenbach subsequently observed patients in whom neuropsychiatric symptoms emerged in association with improved seizure control, which he termed "alternative psychosis" [19]. Clinical observations since then have linked this phenomenon to virtually any form of epilepsy treatment, including drugs, stimulation devices, and resective surgery. Psychosis is the most common clinical presentation.

Suicidality

The lifetime prevalence of SI in PWE is approximately 12 %, nearly double that of the general population; up to 30 % of PWE attempt suicide, compared to 1.1–7 %

of controls; and PWE are approximately three times more likely than the general population to commit suicide [20]. Risk factors include comorbid psychiatric diagnoses, including ictal and post-ictal depression, psychosis, anxiety, personality disorders, and bipolar disorder, as well as psychosocial stressors, poor physical health, young age in men, early age of seizure onset (especially adolescence), temporal lobe epilepsy (TLE), cognitive impairment, brain lesions, inadequate follow-up or treatment of seizures, access to firearms or other methods of self-harm, and inter-ictal behavioral disorders such as viscosity [21–23].

While the validity of the U.S. Food and Drug Administration (FDA) alert [24] regarding suicidality and AED use has been challenged [3], it nonetheless raised awareness for the potential occurrence of suicidality in PWE and stimulated the development of screening instruments that are practical for use in clinical settings.

Anxiety

Anxiety disorders are subdivided into generalized anxiety disorder (GAD), panic disorder (PD), obsessive–compulsive disorder (OCD), phobias, and post-traumatic stress disorder (PTSD). The prevalence of anxiety disorders is up to 66 % of PWE compared to 29 % in the general population [2]. As with depression, the association between anxiety and epilepsy is bidirectional [5] and symptoms may occur between seizures as well as before, during, or after seizures.

Pre-ictal anxiety may precede seizures by hours to days. Ictal anxiety, usually fear, is more common with medial than lateral foci in TLE. Post-ictal anxiety typically persists for 24 h, and a personal psychiatric history is a risk factor [12]. Inter-ictal anxiety does not correlate with seizure frequency [25, 26], and as with depressive symptoms, anxiety may occur as seizures remit. In addition, symptoms of anxiety may occur as a side effect of AEDs or develop in association with withdrawal of GABAergic AEDs.

As many as one in five PWE have inter-ictal PD [27], compared to 1–3.5 % of the general population. Patients with ictal fear are particularly susceptible [28]. The prevalence of OCD in patients with TLE has been estimated at between 10 and 22 % [29–31] compared to a 2–3 % lifetime prevalence of OCD in the general population [32]. OCD may also occur in association with seizures localized to the anterior cingulate [33] or frontorolandic regions [34], as well as with primary generalized seizures [35]. Common obsessions include intrusive and persistent thoughts, particularly related to symmetry or exactness, contamination, and aggressiveness; and typical compulsions leading to excessive repetitive behaviors or mental acts to reduce distress include ordering, washing, and checking [31, 36]. Comorbid anxiety and depression are common with OCD [37].

PTSD is a disabling and often chronic condition associated with witnessing or sustaining a psychically traumatic event. There are few epidemiological or cohort studies investigating the prevalence of PTSD among PWE or determining whether PTSD may be a risk factor for epilepsy and vice versa [38]. Nonetheless, the prevalence of PTSD in epilepsy populations, particularly women, appears to be elevated [39]; and the rates are substantially higher in patients with both epilepsy and psychogenic non-epileptic seizures [40]. One study found evidence for the development of PTSD following epileptic seizures, with the severity of the symptoms related to difficulty in identifying internal feelings and emotions [41]. The lifetime prevalence of PTSD in community cohorts is up to 8 % [32, 42]. Symptoms of PTSD occur with re-experiencing the traumatic event, avoidance, and hypervigilence, and include hyperarousal, intrusive thoughts, flashbacks, emotional numbness, and sleep disturbances, including nightmares.

Psychosis

Psychosis occurs in 0.6–7 % of community-based PWE and 19–27 % of hospitalized PWE [43]. Psychosis may occur before or after epilepsy onset, consistent with a bidirectional relationship [5]. Epilepsy-related risk factors include TLE, particularly left TLE due to mesial temporal sclerosis [44, 45].

Psychosis may occur inter-ictally, which is the most common presentation, or emerge with forced normalization, for example, after epilepsy surgery [46]. Psychotic symptoms may also be present during or after seizures, especially the first 72 h of the post-ictal period [12], typically in patients with bilateral independent ictal foci [47] and following a cluster of seizures or status epilepticus. Symptoms may last up to several weeks and include visual or auditory hallucinations, paranoia, delusions, confusion, affective changes, amnesia, and violence. Violent behavior may be purposeful and directed in response to hallucinations or delusions towards those nearby [48, 49]. Post-ictal violent behavior may also result when a person is restrained after a seizure, called "resistive violence" [50], and typically seen in those with CNS pathology, mental retardation, and comorbid psychiatric illness.

Neuropsychiatric Effects of Brain Stimulation

This section describes the effects of brain stimulation on the neuropsychiatric symptoms discussed in the previous section as well as on similar symptoms in patients with psychiatric disorders but without epilepsy, where applicable.

Vagus Nerve Stimulation

Vagus nerve stimulation (VNS) with the VNS Therapy system (Cyberonics, Inc.) is a non-pharmacological, surgically implanted, device-based therapy approved in 1997 by the FDA as an adjunctive therapy in reducing the frequency of seizures in adults and adolescents over 12 years of age with partial onset seizures not controlled by medication or who experience intolerable side effects. In 2005, the FDA approved VNS as an adjunctive long-term treatment of chronic or recurrent depression for patients 18 years of age or older who are experiencing a major depressive episode and have not had an adequate response to four or more adequate antidepressant treatments. VNS Therapy is also approved in numerous countries worldwide for use in DRE, and in the United States, Europe, Canada, Mexico, Brazil, Australia, and New Zealand for treatment-resistant depression (TRD) [51].

The clinical effects of VNS are dependent on vagus nerve anatomy and synaptic connections. Once afferent vagus nerve fibers enter the brainstem, they synapse at medullary nuclei including the nucleus of the tractus solitarius (NTS) [52, 53]. Fibers ascending from the NTS project primarily to the pontine parabrachial nucleus (PBN) and to brainstem nuclei that modulate the noradrenergic (via the pontine locus coeruleus) and serotonergic systems (via the medullary and pontine raphe nuclei) [54]. Afferent vagal information also travels from the PBN via multi-synaptic pathways [55, 56] to other sites related to epilepsy and depression such as the amygdala, insula, and prefrontal cortex. In addition to these potential neurotransmitter-based mechanisms as the basis for effects in epilepsy and depression, VNS-induced neurogenesis may also play a role, at least for depression [51].

A unique feature of VNS Therapy for epilepsy compared to other stimulation techniques is on-demand stimulation, in which the patient or a companion can activate VNS using a hand-held magnet. In some patients, this may attenuate or end seizures [57, 58].

Patients with Epilepsy

Some, but not all, studies suggest that improvement in mood and depressive symptoms may occur with VNS Therapy in patients with DRE [59–61]. Three studies demonstrated mood improvements for up to 6 months [59, 60, 62], including two in which AEDs remained constant [59, 60]. The magnitudes of seizure reduction and mood improvement were unrelated, and in one study, there was no correlation between stimulation "dose" and mood improvement [60]. In another study, improvements in tenseness, negative arousal, and dysphoria—but not of depressive symptoms—were observed following 6 months of treatment in 28 patients with stable AED regimens and low baseline depression scores [61].

Recommendations for the treatment of mood disorders in PWE issued by the Canadian Network for Mood and Anxiety Treatments include VNS as a potential therapy [63]. Caution is warranted, however, inasmuch as a small percentage of patients with DRE whose seizures are significantly improved with VNS may develop mood disorders, presumably due to forced normalization [64, 65], which may be improved by decreasing the pulse intensity [66].

Patients Without Epilepsy

VNS Therapy for TRD initially evolved from studies of patients with DRE in which subjects with concomitant major depression experienced an improvement in their depressive symptoms with sustained VNS Therapy. Four clinical trials (with extension phases) have since evaluated the efficacy of VNS Therapy in TRD [67–74]. Extensive details of these studies are available elsewhere [75]. Each trial found that depressive symptoms in a substantial proportion of patients responded to VNS. Interestingly, symptoms in some subjects required 6–12 months of stimulation for a clinical response to occur. Three open-label studies showed that the benefit of VNS persisted over the long term [69, 73, 76]. A meta-analysis of 6 trials reported that 71 and 67 % of those who responded at 24 weeks to VNS plus treatment as usual had a sustained response at 48 and 96 weeks, respectively, compared to 56 and 48 % of responders receiving only treatment as usual [77].

Trigeminal Nerve Stimulation

Transcutaneous trigeminal nerve stimulation (TNS) is a relatively new technique that uses stimulation of another cranial nerve to affect brain function. The Monarch eTNS System received CE certification in Europe in 2012 for the adjunctive treatment of epilepsy and major depressive disorder for adults and children 9 years and older, and was given a Class 2 medical device license in Canada in 2013 for treatment of DRE, major depressive disorder, and treatment-resistant depression.

The trigeminal nerve transmits sensory information from the face via the trigeminal ganglion to the trigeminal nuclei in the brainstem. Similar to the central projections of the vagus nerve, the trigeminal nuclei then send projections to the thalamus, the locus coeruleus, and the NTS. The shared central projections of the trigeminal and vagus nerves and the anticonvulsant effects of TNS in a standard animal model of epilepsy [78] comprised the basis for proceeding to clinical studies of TNS in PWE.

Patients with Epilepsy

The first pilot study showed that TNS of the infraorbital and supraorbital branches was well tolerated [79] and was followed by a double-blind, randomized, multicenter trial of bilateral transcutaneous stimulation of the ophthalmic and supratrochlear nerves with the Monarch™ eTNS™ System in patients with DRE [80]. Although there were no statistically significant differences between the treatment groups for change in seizure frequency, proportion of participants who experienced at least a 50 % reduction in seizure frequency, and time to the fourth seizure, there were statistically significant improvements in mood associated with active stimulation as measured by the Beck Depression Inventory. One-year safety and efficacy results were recently published, but an evaluation of mood was not included [81].

Patients Without Epilepsy

Currently, limited data exist with regard to the use of TNS in TRD. Two studies evaluated open-label TNS in 11 patients with TRD [82, 83]. Treatment consisted of nightly (approximately 8 h/night) bilateral transcutaneous electrical stimulation of the forehead (V1 trigeminal branch) for 8 weeks (approximately 55 treatment sessions). A statistically significant reduction in depressive symptoms (both rater- and patient-rated) was reported. Of the 11 TRD patients enrolled, 6 had ≥50 % reduction in depressive symptoms and 4 achieved symptom remission. Shiozawa et al. subsequently conducted a randomized, sham-controlled trial of TNS in 40 patients with major depressive disorder using a 10-day intervention protocol [84]. The investigators found a significant benefit of TNS compared to sham stimulation. These data are promising, but larger, prospective, double-blind studies of TNS for TRD are needed.

Transcranial Magnetic Stimulation

Transcranial magnetic stimulation (TMS) is a noninvasive technique that utilizes brief pulses of electrical current sent to a coiled wire placed over the scalp to deliver rapidly changing magnetic fields that pass through the scalp and skull to modulate plasticity and excitability of cortex within the stimulated field. The specific cortical effects depend on pulse intensity and frequency as well as the targeted area of cortex. The pulse intensity is usually titrated by first determining the patient's motor-evoked potential threshold [85]. TMS is approved for depression in the United States, Canada, Brazil, Australia, and Israel, and it is also widely used in Europe [86]. Most clinical applications of TMS to the treatment of neuropsychiatric symptoms involve trains of stimulation pulses, called repetitive TMS (rTMS). Low stimulation frequencies (≤1 Hz) are generally inhibitory while faster frequencies (≥5 Hz) are usually excitatory.

Patients with Epilepsy

Though a number of studies have evaluated rTMS as a treatment for epilepsy, methodological weaknesses limit the strength of the available data to "possible efficacy," according to European evidence-based guidelines [86]. Unfortunately, given the demonstrated benefits of TMS for depression and other psychiatric disorders, effects on neuropsychiatric symptoms in PWE have not been systematically assessed.

Patients Without Epilepsy

Many studies and meta-analyses have evaluated the use of TMS for depression. Evidence-based guidelines published by European experts found Level A evidence (definite efficacy) for an antidepressant effect of high-frequency rTMS administered to the left DLPFC and Level B (probable efficacy) evidence for an antidepressant effect of low-frequency rTMS to the right DLPFC [86]. By contrast, another appraisal concluded that four health technology assessments of TMS for depression provided insufficient evidence "to draw conclusions regarding the use of TMS for treating patients with depression," largely due to "methodological limitations of the primary research studies" [87]. The American Psychiatric Association includes rTMS in their list of possible initial therapies for depression [88].

Besides depression, TMS has also been evaluated for anxiety disorders. Neuroimaging studies suggest that the medial and dorsolateral prefrontal cortexes are hypo-activated in patients with PTSD. Consequently, studies have evaluated the effect of rTMS targeting the DLPFC for symptoms of PTSD. Pooled results of meta-analyses [89] found statistically significant improvements associated with TMS compared to sham TMS, especially when applied to the right DLPFC, but larger samples with more focused inclusion criteria and further testing of stimulation parameters are needed [87, 90]. Low-frequency TMS may produce significant improvement for symptoms of OCD, but the effects are transient [91]. Two case reports provide suggestive benefit of rTMS for social anxiety disorder, and low-frequency rTMS over the right medial prefrontal cortex combined with high-frequency rTMS over the left medial prefrontal cortex has been proposed for further study [92]. There are few studies evaluating TMS for PD and GAD [93].

Transcranial Direct Current Stimulation

Transcranial direct current stimulation (tDCS) is another noninvasive technique in which a weak electrical current (usually 0.5–2 mA) generated by a battery-powered stimulator is administered via one of two electrodes (anode, cathode) placed on the scalp (the other is positioned elsewhere) and which thereby modulates resting membrane potentials of cortical neurons [94]. Cathodal stimulation is postulated to be inhibitory and anodal stimulation excitatory [95], and the effects of both forms of stimulation may last well beyond the period of stimulation [96], depending on charge density, duration of stimulation, and the distance to the targeted area of cortex. tDCS is not specifically approved for epilepsy or psychiatric disorders, but is widely available for clinical investigations.

Patients with Epilepsy

Only a couple studies of tDCS in PWE have been published and neither evaluated neuropsychiatric effects [97, 98].

Patients Without Epilepsy

Several systematic reviews and meta-analyses of randomized, controlled trials of tDCS for major depression concluded that active treatment was either no different than sham [99], or was associated with a statistically significant improvement in depressive symptoms [100, 101]. Therefore, further definitive trials are needed.

Two studies in patients with schizophrenia suggest that tDCS may have long-lasting effects in reducing auditory verbal hallucinations and other symptoms as measured by the Positive and Negative Syndrome Scale [95].

Deep Brain Stimulation

Deep brain stimulation (DBS) is delivered through one or more electrodes placed into one or more specific brain targets that are connected to an implanted battery-powered pulse generator in the upper chest. Though high-frequency DBS has both excitatory and inhibitory effects on neurons [102, 103], and DBS may disrupt neuronal transmission [104], the mechanism by which DBS reduces seizure occurrence is unclear. DBS of the thalamus is approved for the treatment of drug-resistant partial and secondarily generalized seizures in the European Union, Canada, Taiwan, Australia, New Zealand, and Israel, though not the United States at this time [105].

Patients with Epilepsy

DBS targeting a variety of intracranial sites has been studied in patients with DRE, including the anterior nucleus of the thalamus, centromedian nucleus of the thalamus, basal ganglia (caudate nucleus and subthalamic nucleus), cerebellum, corpus callosum, hippocampus, locus coeruleus, substantia nigra pars reticulata, and caudal zona incerta [105–107]. The primary outcome measure for studies of these stimulation sites has been seizure frequency. The impact of DBS on neuropsychiatric symptoms has either not been monitored or not evaluated with standard safety and tolerability assessments. Further, most of the DBS studies in epilepsy are underpowered, not blinded, or not designed to observe statistically significant effects on behavior. The exception is the SANTE trial, which randomized 110 patients [108]. While anterior thalamic DBS in this study was not associated with changes in neuropsychological function, there was a higher rate of self-reported depression in patients randomized to active treatment compared to controls (14.8 % vs. 1.8 %; $p=0.02$). Seven of the eight patients in the stimulation group who reported depressive symptoms had a prior history of depression, and three were on medications for depression at the study baseline.

Patients Without Epilepsy

A small number of open-label studies of DBS targeting the subcallosal cingulate white matter have shown suggestive benefit for TRD. Other DBS targets for treatment of TRD have been infrequently studied, including the ventral internal capsule/ventral striatum, the nucleus accumbens, and medial forebrain bundle, the latter showing the most rapid antidepressant effect [109]. With regard to OCD, it has been hypothesized that DBS targeted to the nucleus accumbens, ventral internal capsule/ventral striatum, or anterior limb of the internal capsule could regulate OCD-associated dysfunction of the nucleus accumbens and inhibit overactivity of the cortical-striatal-pallidal-thalamic network [36]. Consistent with this hypothesis, a meta-analysis of five double-blind, randomized, sham-controlled studies showed a statistically significant improvement of OCD-related symptoms with active treatment [36]. A DBS system received an FDA Humanitarian Device Exemption from the FDA for patients with chronic, severe, treatment-resistant OCD [110].

Subthalamic nucleus (STN) DBS is a well-established treatment for Parkinson's disease. A recent review noted new-onset or worsened preexisting behavioral disorders in association with STN DBS, including depression, apathy, and impulse disorders (especially with rapid increase in stimulation intensity), whereas a significant improvement of anxiety scores has also been observed [111].

Responsive Neurostimulation

Responsive neurostimulation (RNS) is a new, closed-loop technique for direct cortical stimulation. The RNS System (NeuroPace) delivers electrical stimulation to one or two cortical seizure foci in response to physician-configurable, algorithmic detection of paroxysmal abnormal electrocorticographic activity such as spike and slow waves or changes in frequency or amplitude. The RNS System was approved by the FDA in 2013 as an adjunctive therapy in reducing the frequency of seizures in individuals aged 18 years or older with partial onset seizures who have undergone diagnostic testing that localized seizure onsets to no more than 2 epileptogenic foci and that are refractory to ≥2 antiepileptic medications, and who currently have frequent and disabling seizures (motor partial seizures, complex partial seizures, and/or secondarily generalized seizures) [112]. The system consists of a neurostimulator implanted in the cranium that connects to one or two recording and stimulating depth and/or cortical strip leads placed at the seizure foci [112].

The RNS System was shown to have a statistically significant effect on seizure frequency compared to no stimulation in patients with DRE (all patients had the systems implanted). In addition, for both the double-blind and the open-label periods, patient-reported improvements in quality of life were observed, and no worsening of neuropsychological function or mood, as measured by validated mood inventories, was noted [113–115]. Encouragingly, there were statistically significant improvements in depressive symptoms among patients with mesial TLE after 1 year as well as 2 years of open-label treatment. To date, there have been no published studies of effects of RNS on neuropsychiatric symptoms in patients without epilepsy.

Limitations of Current Research and Future Directions

The existing evidence base suggests that stimulation techniques may have a role in the treatment of neuropsychiatric symptoms in PWE who have comorbid psychiatric disorders. However, with the exception of VNS for the treatment of depressive symptoms in PWE, the potential benefit and safety of stimulation techniques for neuropsychiatric symptoms in PWE is largely unknown. Therefore, further systematic, controlled, and blinded studies are needed. It would be of particular interest to determine whether a single stimulation technique could successfully treat both seizures and neuropsychiatric symptoms in the same patient. Fortunately, the technologies underlying stimulation systems are rapidly improving [75, 87, 116], giving hope that further research will demonstrate the effectiveness of open- and closed-loop stimulation modalities in the treatment of inter-ictal, pre-ictal, ictal, and post-ictal neuropsychiatric symptoms.

As noted by Sun and Morrell, there are numerous challenges for designing and implementing closed-loop stimulation systems, including (1) determining the appropriate physiological markers and the site to detect them using physiological sensors that add minimal risk; (2) developing algorithms that detect the markers in real-time and require low computational power; and (3) modulating the stimulation in response to the detection so that the markers are affected in the clinically desired manner [112]. With regard to the occurrence of neuropsychiatric symptoms, the appropriate physiological markers are yet to be defined, but progress in closed-loop systems for epilepsy offer possibilities. For example, the AspireSR system (Cyberonics, Inc.) is a closed-loop VNS system in which algorithmic-based detection of ictal heart rate changes triggers VNS [117]. It is conceivable, therefore, that heart rate changes which characteristically accompany neuropsychiatric symptoms such as anxiety could trigger a stimulation modality. Likewise, if characteristic changes in scalp or cortical EEG were shown to be associated with the occurrence of particular neuropsychiatric symptoms, then open- or closed-loop stimulation could become a consideration. With regard to implanted systems, the ideal scenario would be to stimulate a single site that effectively treats both seizures and neuropsychiatric symptoms in the same patient, such as the nucleus accumbens in a PWE who has OCD.

Neuropsychiatric symptoms are common, under-recognized, and undertreated in PWE, and have a profound impact on quality of life. Effective, safe, and well-tolerated treatments are urgently needed for patients whose neuropsychiatric symptoms do not respond to pharmacological or behavioral therapies. In this context, the role of stimulation techniques is only beginning to be understood and their potential application to the amelioration of neuropsychiatric symptoms in PWE should be actively pursued.

References

1. Cascino GD. When drugs and surgery don't work. Epilepsia. 2008;49 Suppl 9:79–84.
2. Tellez-Zenteno JF, Patten SB, Jette N, Williams J, Wiebe S. Psychiatric comorbidity in epilepsy: a population-based analysis. Epilepsia. 2007;48(12):2336–44.

3. Korczyn AD, Schachter SC, Brodie MJ, Dalal SS, Engel Jr J, Guekht A, et al. Epilepsy, cognition, and neuropsychiatry (epilepsy, brain and mind, part 2). Epilepsy Behav. 2013;28:283–302.
4. Kanner AM. Depression in epilepsy: a complex relation with unexpected consequences. Curr Opin Neurol. 2008;21(2):190–4.
5. Hesdorffer DC, Ishihara L, Mynepalli L, Webb DJ, Weil J, Hauser WA. Epilepsy, suicidality, and psychiatric disorders: a bidirectional association. Ann Neurol. 2012;72(2):184–91.
6. Mendez MF, Cummings JL, Benson DF. Depression in epilepsy. Significance and phenomenology. Arch Neurol. 1986;43:766–70.
7. O'Donoghue MF, Goodridge DM, Redhead K, Sander JW, Duncan JS. Assessing the psychosocial consequences of epilepsy: a community-based study. Br J Gen Pract. 1999;49: 211–4.
8. Kimiskidis VK, Triantafyllou NI, Kararizou E, Gatzonis SS, Fountoulakis KN, Siatouni A, et al. Depression and anxiety in epilepsy: the association with demographic and seizure-related variables. Ann Gen Psychiatr. 2007;6:28.
9. Gilliam FG, Santos J, Vahle V, Carter J, Brown K, Hecimovic H. Depression in epilepsy: ignoring clinical expression of neuronal network dysfunction? Epilepsia. 2004;45 Suppl 2: 28–33.
10. Wiegartz P, Seidenberg M, Woodard A, Gidal B, Hermann B. Co-morbid psychiatric disorder in chronic epilepsy: recognition and etiology of depression. Neurology. 1999;53(5 Suppl 2): S3–8.
11. Kanner AM, Palac S. Depression in epilepsy: a common but often unrecognized comorbid malady. Epilepsy Behav. 2000;1(1):37–51.
12. Kanner AM, Soto A, Gross-Kanner H. Prevalence and clinical characteristics of postictal psychiatric symptoms in partial epilepsy. Neurology. 2004;62(5):708–13.
13. Blumer D, Montouris G, Davies K. The interictal dysphoric disorder: recognition, pathogenesis, and treatment of the major psychiatric disorder of epilepsy. Epilepsy Behav. 2004;5(6): 826–40.
14. Kanner AM, Kozak AM, Frey M. The use of sertraline in patients with epilepsy: is it safe? Epilepsy Behav. 2000;1(2):100–5.
15. Blanchet P, Frommer GP. Mood change preceding epileptic seizures. J Nerv Ment Dis. 1986;174(8):471–6.
16. Macrodimitris S, Sherman EM, Forde S, Tellez-Zenteno JF, Metcalfe A, Hernandez-Ronquillo L, et al. Psychiatric outcomes of epilepsy surgery: a systematic review. Epilepsia. 2011;52(5):880–90.
17. Blumer D, Wakhlu S, Davies K, Hermann B. Psychiatric outcome of temporal lobectomy for epilepsy: incidence and treatment of psychiatric complications. Epilepsia. 1998;39(5): 478–86.
18. Landoldt H. Some clinical electroencephalographical correlations in epileptic psychosis (twilight states). Electroencephalogr Clin Neurophysiol. 1853;5:121.
19. Tellenbach H. Epilepsy as a convulsive disorder and as a psychosis, on alternative psychoses of paranoid nature in "forced normalization" (Landolt) of the electroencephalogram of epileptics. Nervenarzt. 1965;36:190–202.
20. Bell GS, Gaitatzis A, Bell CL, Johnson AL, Sander JW. Suicide in people with epilepsy: how great is the risk? Epilepsia. 2009;50:1933–42.
21. Jones JE, Hermann BP, Barry JJ, Gilliam FG, Kanner AM, Meador KJ. Rates and risk factors for suicide, suicidal ideation, and suicide attempts in chronic epilepsy. Epilepsy Behav. 2003; 4 Suppl 3:S31–8.
22. Nilsson L, Ahlbom A, Farahmand BY, Asberg M, Tomson T. Risk factors for suicide in epilepsy: a case control study. Epilepsia. 2002;43(6):644–51.
23. Kalinin VV, Polyanskiy DA. Gender differences in risk factors of suicidal behavior in epilepsy. Epilepsy Behav. 2005;6(3):424–9.
24. U.S. Food and Drug Administration. Information for healthcare professionals: suicidality and antiepileptic drugs. Available at: http://www.fda.gov/Drugs/DrugSafety/PostmarketDrugSafetyInformationforPatientsandProviders/ucm100192.htm. Accessed 18 Jan 2015.

25. Mattsson P, Tibblin B, Kihlgren M, Kumlien E. A prospective study of anxiety with respect to seizure outcome after epilepsy surgery. Seizure. 2005;14(1):40–5.
26. Goldstein MA, Harden CL. Epilepsy and anxiety. Epilepsy Behav. 2000;1(4):228–34.
27. Pariente PD, Lepine JP, Lellouch J. Lifetime history of panic attacks and epilepsy: an association from a general population survey. J Clin Psychiatry. 1991;52(2):88–9.
28. Mintzer S, Lopez F. Comorbidity of ictal fear and panic disorder. Epilepsy Behav. 2002;3(4):330–7.
29. de Oliveira GN, Kummer A, Salgado JV, Portela EJ, Sousa-Pereira SR, David AS, et al. Psychiatric disorders in temporal lobe epilepsy: an overview from a tertiary service in Brazil. Seizure. 2010;19(8):479–84.
30. Monaco F, Cavanna A, Magli E, Barbagli D, Collimedaglia L, Cantello R, et al. Obsessionality, obsessive-compulsive disorder, and temporal lobe epilepsy. Epilepsy Behav. 2005;7(3):491–6.
31. Ertekin BA, Kulaksizoglu IB, Ertekin E, Gurses C, Bebek N, Gokyiqit A, et al. A comparative study of obsessive-compulsive disorder and other psychiatric comorbidities in patients with temporal lobe epilepsy and idiopathic generalized epilepsy. Epilepsy Behav. 2009;14(4):634–9.
32. Kessler RC, Berglund P, Demler O, Jin R, Merikangas KR, Walters EE. Lifetime prevalence and age-of-onset distributions of DSM-IV disorders in the National Comorbidity Survey Replication. Arch Gen Psychiatry. 2005;62:593–602.
33. Levin B, Duchowny M. Childhood obsessive-compulsive disorder and cingulate epilepsy. Biol Psychiatry. 1991;30(10):1049–55.
34. Guarnieri R, Araujo D, Carlotti Jr CG, Assirati Jr JA, Hallak JE, Velasco TR, et al. Suppression of obsessive-compulsive symptoms after epilepsy surgery. Epilepsy Behav. 2005;7(2):316–9.
35. Koopowitz LF, Berk M. Response of obsessive compulsive disorder to carbamazepine in two patients with comorbid epilepsy. Ann Clin Psychiatry. 1997;9(3):171–3.
36. Kisely S, Hall K, Siskind D, Frater J, Olson S, Crompton D. Deep brain stimulation for obsessive-compulsive disorder: a systematic review and meta-analysis. Psychol Med. 2014;44: 3533–42.
37. Hamed SA, Elserogy YM, Abd-Elhafeez HA. Psychopathological and peripheral levels of neurobiological correlates of obsessive-compulsive symptoms in patients with epilepsy: a hospital-based study. Epilepsy Behav. 2013;27(2):409–15.
38. Martin RC, Faught E, Richman J, Funkhouser E, Kim Y, Clements K, et al. Psychiatric and neurologic risk factors for incident cases of new-onset epilepsy in older adults: data from U.S. Medicare beneficiaries. Epilepsia. 2014;55(7):1120–7.
39. Dikel TN, Fennell EB, Gilmore RL. Posttraumatic stress disorder, dissociation, and sexual abuse history in epileptic and nonepileptic seizure patients. Epilepsy Behav. 2003;4:644–50.
40. Fiszman A, Alves-Leon SV, Nunes RG, D'Andea I, Figueira I. Traumatic events and posttraumatic stress disorder in patients with psychogenic nonepileptic seizures: a critical review. Epilepsy Behav. 2004;5:818–25.
41. Chung MC, Allen RD. Alexithymia and posttraumatic stress disorder following epileptic seizure. Psychiatry Q. 2013;84(3):271–85.
42. Kessler RC, Sonnega A, Bromet E, Hughes M, Nelson CB. Posttraumatic stress disorder in the National Comorbidity Survey. Arch Gen Psychiatry. 1995;52:1048–60.
43. Torta R, Keller R. Behavioral, psychotic, and anxiety disorders in epilepsy: etiology, clinical features, and therapeutic implications. Epilepsia. 1999;40 Suppl 10:S2–20.
44. Filho GM, Rosa VP, Lin K, Caboclo LO, Sakamoto AC, Yacubian EM. Psychiatric comorbidity in epilepsy: a study comparing patients with mesial temporal sclerosis and juvenile myoclonic epilepsy. Epilepsy Behav. 2008;13(1):196–201.
45. de Araujo Filho GM, da Silva JM, Mazetto L, Marchetti RL, Yacubian EM. Psychoses of epilepsy: a study comparing the clinical features of patients with focal versus generalized epilepsies. Epilepsy Behav. 2011;20(4):655–8.
46. Kanner AM. Psychosis of epilepsy: a neurologist's perspective. Epilepsy Behav. 2000; 1:219–27.

47. Kanner AM, Ostrovskaya A. Long-term significance of postictal psychotic episodes. I. Are they predictive of bilateral ictal foci? Epilepsy Behav. 2008;12:150–3.
48. Kanemoto K, Kawasaki J, Mori E. Violence and epilepsy: a close relation between violence and postictal psychosis. Epilepsia. 1999;40(1):107–9.
49. Kanemoto K, Tadokoro Y, Oshima T. Violence and postictal psychosis: a comparison of postictal psychosis, interictal psychosis, and postictal confusion. Epilepsy Behav. 2010; 19(2):162–6.
50. Alper KR, Barry JJ, Balabanov AJ. Treatment of psychosis, aggression, and irritability in patients with epilepsy. Epilepsy Behav. 2002;3(5S):13–8.
51. Shah A, Carreno FR, Frazer A. Therapeutic modalities for treatment resistant depression: focus on vagal nerve stimulation and ketamine. Clin Psychopharmacol Neurosci. 2014; 12(2):83–93.
52. Rhoton AL, O'Leary JL, Ferguson JP. The trigeminal, facial, vagal, and glossopharyngeal nerves in the monkey. Afferent connections. Arch Neurol. 1966;14(5):530–40.
53. Kalia M, Sullivan JM. Brainstem projections of sensory and motor components of the vagus nerve in the rat. J Comp Neurol. 1982;211(3):248–65.
54. Saper CB. Diffuse cortical projection systems: anatomical organization and role in cortical function. In: Plum F, editor. Handbook of physiology, section 1, vol. V. Washington, DC: American Physiological Society; 1987. p. 169–210.
55. Agostoni E, Chinnock JE, Daly MB, Murray JG. Functional and histological studies of the vagus nerve and its branches to the heart, lungs and abdominal viscera in the cat. J Physiol. 1957;135(1):182–205.
56. Henry TR. Therapeutic mechanisms of vagus nerve stimulation. Neurology. 2002;59 Suppl 4:S3–14.
57. Boon P, Vonck K, Van Walleghem P, D'Havé M, Goossens L, Vandekerckhove T, et al. Programmed and magnet-induced vagus nerve stimulation for refractory epilepsy. J Clin Neurophysiol. 2001;18(5):402–7.
58. Tatum WO, Helmers SL. Vagus nerve stimulation and magnet use: optimizing benefits. Epilepsy Behav. 2009;15(3):299–302.
59. Elger G, Hoppe C, Falkai P, Rush AJ, Elger CE. Vagus nerve stimulation is associated with mood improvements in epilepsy patients. Epilepsy Res. 2000;42(2–3):203–10.
60. Harden CL, Pulver MC, Ravdin LD, Nikolov B, Halper JP, Labar DR. A pilot study of mood in epilepsy patients treated with vagus nerve stimulation. Epilepsy Behav. 2000;1(2):93–9.
61. Hoppe C, Helmstaedter C, Scherrmann J, Elger CE. Self-reported mood changes following 6 months of vagus nerve stimulation in epilepsy patients. Epilepsy Behav. 2001;2(4):335–42.
62. Klinkenberg S, Majoie HJ, van der Heijden MM, Rijkers K, Leenen L, Aldenkamp AP. Vagus nerve stimulation has a positive effect on mood in patients with refractory epilepsy. Clin Neurol Neurosurg. 2012;114(4):336–40.
63. Ramasubbu R, Taylor VH, Samaan Z, Sockalingham S, Li M, Patten S, et al. The Canadian Network for Mood and Anxiety Treatments (CANMAT) task force recommendations for the management of patients with mood disorders and select comorbid medical conditions. Ann Clin Psychiatry. 2012;24(1):91–109.
64. Blumer D, Davies K, Alexander A, Morgan S. Major psychiatric disorders subsequent to treating epilepsy by vagus nerve stimulation. Epilepsy Behav. 2001;2(5):466–72.
65. Prater JF. Recurrent depression with vagus nerve stimulation. Am J Psychiatry. 2001;158(5): 816–7.
66. Keller S, Lichtenberg P. Psychotic exacerbation in a patient with seizure disorder treated with vagus nerve stimulation. Isr Med Assoc J. 2008;10(7):550–1.
67. Rush AJ, George MS, Sackeim HA, Marangell LB, Husain MM, Giller C, et al. Vagus nerve stimulation (VNS) for treatment-resistant depressions: a multicenter study. Biol Psychiatry. 2000;47(4):276–86.
68. Marangell LB, Rush AJ, George MS, Sackeim HA, Johnson CR, Husain MM, et al. Vagus nerve stimulation (VNS) for major depressive episodes: one year outcomes. Biol Psychiatry. 2002;51(4):280–7.

69. Nahas Z, Marangell LB, Husain MM, Rush AJ, Sackeim HA, Lisanby SH, et al. Two-year outcome of vagus nerve stimulation (VNS) for treatment of major depressive episodes. J Clin Psychiatry. 2005;66(9):1097–104.
70. Rush AJ, Marangell LB, Sackeim HA, George MS, Brannan SK, Davis SM, et al. Vagus nerve stimulation for treatment-resistant depression: a randomized, controlled acute phase trial. Biol Psychiatry. 2005;58(5):347–54.
71. Rush AJ, Sackeim HA, Marangell LB, George MS, Brannan SK, Davis SM, et al. Effects of 12 months of vagus nerve stimulation in treatment-resistant depression: a naturalistic study. Biol Psychiatry. 2005;58(5):355–63.
72. Schlaepfer TE, Frick C, Zobel A, Maier W, Heuser I, Bajbouj M, et al. Vagus nerve stimulation for depression: efficacy and safety in a European study. Psychol Med. 2008;38(5):651–61.
73. Bajbouj M, Merkl A, Schlaepfer TE, Frick C, Zobel A, Maier W, et al. Two-year outcome of vagus nerve stimulation in treatment-resistant depression. J Clin Psychopharmacol. 2010;30(3):273–81.
74. Aaronson ST, Carpenter LL, Conway CR, Reimherr FW, Lisanby SH, Schwartz TL, et al. Vagus nerve stimulation therapy randomized to different amounts of electrical charge for treatment-resistant depression: acute and chronic effects. Brain Stimul. 2013;6(4):631–40.
75. Conway CR, Colijn MA, Schachter SC. Vagus nerve stimulation for epilepsy and depression. In: Reti IM, editor. Brain stimulation: methodologies and interventions. Hoboken: John Wiley & Sons, Inc; 2015. p. 305–35.
76. Mauro MPS, Patronelli F, Spinelli E, Cordero A, Covello D, Gorostiaga JA. Nerves of the heart: a comprehensive review with a clinical point of view. Neuroanatomy. 2009;8(1): 26–31.
77. Berry SM, Broglio K, Bunker M, Jayewardene A, Olin B, Rush AJ. A patient-level meta-analysis of studies evaluating vagus nerve stimulation therapy for treatment-resistant depression. Med Devices (Auckl). 2013;6:17–35.
78. Fanselow EE, Reid AP, Nicolelis MA. Reduction of pentylenetetrazol-induced seizure activity in awake rats by seizure-triggered trigeminal nerve stimulation. J Neurosci. 2000;20:8160–8.
79. DeGiorgio CM, Shewmon A, Murray D, Whitehurst T. Pilot study of trigeminal nerve stimulation (TNS) for epilepsy: a proof-of-concept trial. Epilepsia. 2006;47:1213–5.
80. DeGiorgio CM, Soss J, Cook IA, Markovic D, Gornbein J, Murray D, et al. Randomized controlled trial of trigeminal nerve stimulation for drug-resistant epilepsy. Neurology. 2013;80:786–91.
81. Soss J, Heck C, Murray D, Markovic D, Oviedo S, Corrale-Leyva G, et al. A prospective long-term study of external trigeminal nerve stimulation for drug-resistant epilepsy. Epilepsy Behav. 2015;42:44–7.
82. Schrader LM, Cook IA, Miller PR, Maremont ER, DeGiorgio CM. Trigeminal nerve stimulation in major depressive disorder: first proof of concept in an open pilot trial. Epilepsy Behav. 2011;22(3):475–8.
83. Cook IA, Schrader LM, DeGiorgio CM, Miller PR, Maremont ER, Leuchter AF. Trigeminal nerve stimulation in major depressive disorder: acute outcomes in an open pilot study. Epilepsy Behav. 2013;28(2):221–6.
84. Shiozawa P, da Silva ME, Netto GTM, Taiar I, Cordeiro Q. Effect of a 10-day trigeminal nerve stimulation (TNS) protocol for treating major depressive disorder: a phase II, sham-controlled, randomized clinical trial. Epilepsy Behav. 2015;44:23–6.
85. Sandrini M, Umilta C, Rusconi E. The use of transcranial magnetic stimulation in cognitive neuroscience: a new synthesis of methodological issues. Neurosci Biobehav Rev. 2011;35:516–36.
86. Lefaucheur JP, Andre-Obadia N, Antal A, Ayache SS, Baeken C, Benninger DH, et al. Evidence-based guidelines on the therapeutic use of repetitive transcranial magnetic stimulation (rTMS). Clin Neurophysiol. 2014;125:2150–206.
87. CADTH Rapid Response Reports. Transcranial magnetic stimulation for the treatment of adults with PTSD, GAD, or depression: a review of clinical effectiveness and guidelines. Ottawa: Canadian Agency for Drugs and Technologies in Health; 2014. p. 1–44.

88. American Psychiatric Association. Practice guideline for the treatment of patients with major depressive disorder. Available at: http://psychiatryonline.org/pb/assets/raw/sitewide/practice_guidelines/guidelines/mdd.pdf. Accessed 18 Jan 2015.
89. Karsen EF, Watts BV, Holtzheimer PE. Review of the effectiveness of transcranial magnetic stimulation for post-traumatic stress disorder. Brain Stimul. 2014;7(2):151–7.
90. Berlim MT, Van den Eynde F. Repetitive transcranial magnetic stimulation over the dorsolateral prefrontal cortex for treating posttraumatic stress disorder: an exploratory meta-analysis of randomized, double-blind and sham-controlled trials. Can J Psychiatry. 2014;59(9): 487–96.
91. Bais M, Figee M, Denys D. Neuromodulation in obsessive-compulsive disorder. Psychiatr Clin North Am. 2014;37(3):393–413.
92. Paes F, Baczynski T, Novaes F, Marinho T, Arias-Carrion O, Budde H, et al. Repetitive transcranial magnetic stimulation (rTMS) to treat social anxiety disorder: case reports and a review of the literature. Clin Pract Epidemiol Ment Health. 2013;9:180–8.
93. Cristancho MA, Cristancho P, O'Reardon JP. Other therapeutic psychiatric uses of superficial brain stimulation. Handb Clin Neurol. 2013;116:415–22.
94. Stagg CJ, Nitsche MA. Physiological basis of transcranial direct current stimulation. Neuroscientist. 2011;17:37–53.
95. David CN, Rapoport JL, Gogtay N. Treatments in context: transcranial direct current brain stimulation as a potential treatment in pediatric psychosis. Expert Rev Neurother. 2013;13(4):447–58.
96. Bennabi D, Pedron S, Haffen E, Monnin J, Peterschmitt Y, Van Waes V. Transcranial direct current stimulation for memory enhancement: from clinical research to animal models. Front Syst Neurosci. 2014;8:159.
97. Assenza G, Campana C, Formica D, Schena E, Taffoni F, Di Pino G, et al. Efficacy of cathodal transcranial direct current stimulation in drug-resistant epilepsy: a proof of principle. Conf Proc IEEE Eng Med Biol Soc. 2014;2014:530–3.
98. Auvichayapat N, Rotenberg A, Gersner R, Ngodklang S, Tiamkao S, Tassaneeyakul W, et al. Transcranial direct current stimulation for treatment of refractory childhood focal epilepsy. Brain Stimul. 2013;6(4):696–700.
99. Berlim MT, Van den Eynde F, Daskalakis ZJ. Clinical utility of transcranial direct current stimulation (tDCS) for treating major depression: a systematic review and meta-analysis of randomized, double-blind and sham-controlled trials. J Psychiatr Res. 2013;47: 1–7.
100. Kalu UG, Sexton CE, Loo CK, Ebmeier KP. Transcranial direct current stimulation in the treatment of major depression: a meta-analysis. Psychol Med. 2012;42:1791–800.
101. Shiozawa P, Fregni F, Bensenor IM, Lotufo PA, Berlim MT, Daskalakis JZ, et al. Transcranial direct current stimulation for major depression: an updated systematic review and meta-analysis. Int J Neuropsychopharmacol. 2014;17:1443–52.
102. McIntyre CC, Savasta M, Kerkerian-Le Goff L, Vitek JL. Uncovering the mechanism(s) of action of deep brain stimulation: activation, inhibition, or both. Clin Neurophysiol. 2004;115:1239–48.
103. Iremonger KJ, Anderson TR, Hu B, Kiss ZH. Cellular mechanisms preventing sustained activation of cortex during subcortical high-frequency stimulation. J Neurophysiol. 2006;96:613–21.
104. Chiken S, Nambu A. Disrupting neuronal transmission: mechanism of DBS? Front Syst Neurosci. 2014;8:33.
105. Fisher RS, Velasco AL. Electrical brain stimulation for epilepsy. Nat Rev Neurol. 2014;10: 261–70.
106. Cox JH, Seri S, Cavanna AE. Clinical utility of implantable neurostimulation devices as adjunctive treatment of uncontrolled seizures. Neuropsychiatr Dis Treat. 2014;10: 2191–200.
107. Heck C, King-Stephens D, Massey A, Nair D, Jobst B, Barkley G, et al. Responsive neurostimulation: the hope and the challenges. Epilepsy Curr. 2014;14:270–1.

108. Fisher R, Salanova V, Witt T, Worth R, Henry T, Gross R, et al. Electrical stimulation of the anterior nucleus of thalamus for treatment of refractory epilepsy. Epilepsia. 2010;51(5):899–908.
109. Delaloye S, Holtzheimer PE. Deep brain stimulation in the treatment of depression. Dialoques Clin Neurosci. 2014;16(1):83–91.
110. Medtronic. About deep brain stimulation for psychiatric disorders. Available at: https://professional.medtronic.com/pt/neuro/dbs-pd/edu/about/index.htm#tabs-1. Accessed 18 Jan 18 2015.
111. Castrioto A, Lhommee E, Moro E, Krack P. Mood and behavioural effects of subthalamic stimulation in Parkinson's disease. Lancet Neurol. 2014;13(3):287–305.
112. Sun FT, Morrell MJ. Closed-loop neurostimulation: the clinical experience. Neurotherapeutics. 2014;11:553–63.
113. Morrell MJ, RNS System in Epilepsy Study Group. Responsive cortical stimulation for the treatment of medically intractable partial epilepsy. Neurology. 2011;77(13):1295–304.
114. Heck C, King-Stephens D, Massey A, Nair D, Jobst B, Barkley G, et al. Two-year seizure reduction in adults with medically intractable partial onset epilepsy treated with responsive neurostimulation: final results of the RNS System Pivotal trial. Epilepsia. 2014;55(3):432–41.
115. Meador KJ, Kapur R, Loring DW, Kanner AM, Morrell MJ, the RNS System Pivotal Trial Investigators. Quality of life and mood in patients with medically intractable epilepsy treated with targeted responsive neurostimulation. Epilepsy Behav. 2015;45:242–7.
116. Kavirajan HC, Lueck K, Chuang, K. Alternating current cranial electrotherapy stimulation (CES) for depression. Cochrane Database Syst Rev. 2014;(7):CD010521.
117. Cyberonics, Inc. Available at: http://ir.cyberonics.com/releasedetail.cfm?ReleaseID=826981. Accessed 18 Jan 2015.